Diagnosis and Clinical Management of Prostate Cancer

Diagnosis and Clinical Management of Prostate Cancer

Editor: Olivier Douglas

AMERICAN
MEDICAL PUBLISHERS
www.americanmedicalpublishers.com

AMERICAN
MEDICAL PUBLISHERS
www.americanmedicalpublishers.com

Cataloging-in-Publication Data

Diagnosis and clinical management of prostate cancer / edited by Olivier Douglas.
p. cm.
Includes bibliographical references and index.
ISBN 978-1-63927-791-9
1. Prostate--Cancer. 2. Prostate--Cancer--Diagnosis. 3. Prostate--Cancer--Treatment. I. Douglas, Olivier.
RC280.P7 D53 2023
616.994 63--dc23

American Medical Publishers,
41 Flatbush Avenue,
1st Floor, New York,
NY 11217, USA

ISBN 978-1-63927-791-9 (Hardback)

Contents

Preface

I am honored to present to you this unique book which encompasses the most up-to-date data in the field. I was extremely pleased to get this opportunity of editing the work of experts from across the globe. I have also written papers in this field and researched the various aspects revolving around the progress of the discipline. I have tried to unify my knowledge along with that of stalwarts from every corner of the world, to produce a text which not only benefits the readers but also facilitates the growth of the field.

Prostate cancer affects the prostate gland found in male reproductive system. The gland surrounds the urethra and is located below the bladder. Prostate cancer may not cause any symptoms at first, but a few symptoms can be seen in the later stages, such as pain in the back or pelvis, trouble or pain while urinating, and blood in the urine. There are several factors that enhance the risk of prostate cancer, such as family history, race and older age. Other risk factors include a diet rich in red meat and processed meat. Biopsy, used for the diagnosis of prostate cancer can also be used to determine the presence of metastasis. In many circumstances, watchful waiting or active surveillance is used to manage the situation. Several other treatment options include radiation therapy, surgery, chemotherapy or hormone therapy. Various drugs utilized for the treatment of advanced castration-sensitive and castration-resistant prostate cancer include apalutamide, cabazitaxel, abiraterone and enzalutamide. From diagnosis to clinical management, case studies related to all contemporary topics of relevance to prostate cancer have been included in this book. Those with an interest in this disease would find it helpful.

Finally, I would like to thank all the contributing authors for their valuable time and contributions. This book would not have been possible without their efforts. I would also like to thank my friends and family for their constant support.

Editor

1

Incorporating Prognostic Biomarkers into Risk Assessment Models and TNM Staging for Prostate Cancer

Ragheed Saoud [1], Nassib Abou Heidar [2], Alessia Cimadamore [3] and Gladell P. Paner [1,4,*]

1 Department of Surgery (Section of Urology), University of Chicago, Chicago, IL 60637, USA; Ragheed.Saoud@uchospitals.edu
2 Department of Surgery (Division of Urology), American University of Beirut Medical Center, Beirut 11-0236, Lebanon; na192@aub.edu.lb
3 Section of Pathological Anatomy, Polytechnic University of the Marche Region, School of Medicine, 60126 Ancona, Italy; alessiacimadamore@gmail.com
4 Department of Pathology, University of Chicago, Chicago, IL 60637, USA
* Correspondence: Gladell.Paner@uchospitals.edu

Abstract: In current practice, prostate cancer staging alone is not sufficient to adequately assess the patient's prognosis and plan the management strategies. Multiple clinicopathological parameters and risk tools for prostate cancer have been developed over the past decades to better characterize the disease and provide an enhanced assessment of prognosis. Herein, we review novel prognostic biomarkers and their integration into risk assessment models for prostate cancer focusing on their capability to help avoid unnecessary imaging studies, biopsies and diagnosis of low risk prostate cancers, to help in the decision-making process between active surveillance and treatment intervention, and to predict recurrence after radical prostatectomy. There is an imperative need of reliable biomarkers to stratify prostate cancer patients that may benefit from different management approaches. The integration of biomarkers panel with risk assessment models appears to improve prostate cancer diagnosis and management. However, integration of novel genomic biomarkers in future prognostic models requires further validation in their clinical efficacy, standardization, and cost-effectiveness in routine application.

Keywords: prostate cancer; biomarkers; staging; risk assessment models; predictive scores; prognosis; molecular classifier

---

1. Introduction

Extent of urological cancers is now assessed universally by the tumor-node-metastasis (TNM) system which is considered the "gold standard" for staging and benchmark for prognostication [1]. Currently, the goals of modifications in TNM staging classifications are being tailored towards a more "personalized" model rather than being based solely on anatomical factors. The 8th edition of the American Joint Committee on Cancer (8th AJCC) staging system provides major evidence-based changes by incorporating clinical and pathological variables in prostate cancer to make staging more relevant for precision medicine [2,3]. The AJCC aims at building on the anatomic basis of disease while incorporating additional clinical and pathological variables including biomarkers and risk assessment models that have been rigorously studied to predict prognosis [2].

When dealing with prostate cancer, the clinical T stage might not be optimally correlated with the biological behavior of the tumor, as demonstrated previously to be an inadequate predictor of recurrence after radical prostatectomy (RP). Moreover, it is well known that clinical staging of prostate cancer is variable due to differences in imaging modalities and subjectivity of rectal examination [2,4]. Therefore, clinical stage may vary significantly from pathological stage on RP specimens.

In current practice, prostate cancer anatomical staging alone may not be sufficient to adequately assess patient prognosis as well as to plan for management strategies. Over the past decades, multiple clinicopathological parameters and risk assessment tools for prostate cancer have been developed to better discriminate the risk and provide an adequate assessment of outcome. These clinical parameters are mainly the D'Amico derived systems that include National Comprehensive Cancer Network (NCCN), American Urologic Association (AUA), and European Association of Urology (EAU) risk stratification groups; these mainly use anatomical TNM staging, Gleason grade, as well as Prostate Specific Antigen (PSA) levels. Risk stratification models proved to be well correlated with cancer specific mortality [5–9].

2. Discussion

2.1. *8th AJCC Changes for Prostate Cancer Staging*

Adoption of clinical and pathological data is a step forward towards more individualized and personalized medicine in order to better stratify patients in terms of prognosis. For the aforementioned reasons, AJCC had already incorporated non-anatomic factors such as serum PSA and Gleason score into "prognostic stage groups" [3]. The most recent 8th AJCC version abandoned the pathological T2 subcategorization of pT2a, pT2b, and pT2c due to the lack of prognostic significance between the subcategories [9–11]. More importantly, the 8th AJCC endorsed statistical models to predict survival in prostate cancer. However, the only approved prognostic models by the AJCC are for metastatic castration-resistant prostate cancer that include clinical (non-anatomic) parameters such as PSA, hemoglobin and performance status [12,13]. The AJCC did not accept prognostic models in their stringent inclusion criteria for localized prostate cancer, which included endpoints of overall survival and generalizability of the models [14].

2.2. *Molecular Biomarkers and Gene Alterations in Prostate Cancer*

The traditional PSA as well as imaging and Gleason scores provide certain prostate cancer risk stratification; however, these alone may not accurately predict the patient's prognosis [15]. This has led to the search for additional biomarkers and prostate cancer genetic alterations that when present, can help in decision making and accurately predict prognosis. Multiple somatic single gene mutations in prostate cancer have been explored. Though it is present in about 50% of prostate cancer, *TMPRSS2-ERG* fusion has not been consistently associated with clinical outcomes [16], while the loss of *PTEN* tumor suppressor gene was found to be of clinical prognostic value [17]. Emerging data has also linked several germline DNA mutations to prostate cancer, namely *BRCA1, BRCA2, MSH, ATM, PALB2, CHEK2,* and *MUTYH* [18]. Individuals who may have family history of prostate cancer and positive for *BRCA2* mutation have higher rates of progression/grade reclassification while on active surveillance (AS), and lower metastasis free and overall survival after primary treatment [19–23]. Guidelines now recommend testing germline mutations in men diagnosed with prostate cancer and any of the following: a positive family history, high risk, regional, or metastatic prostate cancer regardless of family history, Ashkenazi Jewish ancestry, and intraductal carcinoma histology [6]. Currently, there is insufficient data to incorporate genetic mutations into prognostic algorithms or predictive models as their value in the setting of localized prostate cancer is not yet clear. However, patients with germline mutations may be counselled to follow-up closely if opting for AS [22].

Biomarkers in prostate cancer provide diagnostic, prognostic or predictive information [21]. Several diagnostic biomarkers have been explored to better detect patients with clinically significant prostate cancer while decreasing the need for prostate biopsies [24]. On the other hand, prognostic biomarkers can help stratify patients in terms of disease aggressiveness and ultimately cancer prognosis.

So far, no single molecular biomarker in prostate cancer has translated into clinical use and the current trend is to explore multiple gene panels or classifiers, some of which are already commercially available.

Not all available biomarkers however have been thoroughly evaluated and validated. Currently, three mRNA-based classifiers (Prolaris, Oncotype Dx, and Decipher) are useful to evaluate tissue from biopsy or RP specimens. One protein-based biomarker (Promark) based on the expression of 8 prostate cancer specific proteins in biopsy tissue, can predict the aggressiveness of prostate cancer by providing a score from 1–100 [22].

According to the American Society of Clinical Oncology (ASCO), validated prostate cancer biomarkers should be used only in particular clinical settings, when assay result along with routine clinical factors may affect management [22]. Each of the aforementioned biomarkers can independently improve the prognostic accuracy of clinical multivariable models for identifying men with biologically significant prostate cancer [25–28]. However, there is no high-quality comparative data to determine which of the markers is the most accurate prognosticator. Longer term data is needed to determine whether their utility will impact patient quality of life and prostate cancer specific outcomes [22,29,30]. They may be useful when combined with known risk stratification systems in prostate cancer. Examples include patients who are diagnosed with low risk prostate cancer according to the D'Amico classification, but either have high volume Grade Group (GG) 1, low volume GG 2, or those who have higher risk features (e.g., Germline/somatic mutations, high PSA density) associated with GG 1 disease [21]. Though such patients may not be ideal candidates for AS, prognostic information provided by biomarkers may assist the treating physician and the patient in choosing AS vs. primary treatment [24].

2.3. Novel Biomarkers Integrated into Risk Assessment Models for Prostate Cancer Screening and Prognostication

2.3.1. Prolaris

Prolaris is a test that can be performed on either biopsy or RP tissue. It is a sum of 31 cell cycle progression (CCP) genes and 15 reference genes [31]. It may help guide decision making in patients opting for AS versus surgery/radiation. It provides a score from 1–10; the higher the score, the higher the risk of disease progression. This score should not be utilized alone to alter decision making but rather combined with the patient's age, PSA, clinical stage, percent positive cores, Gleason score, and AUA risk category to predict 10-year prostate cancer-specific mortality risk [31,32]. In a study of 585 men with clinically localized prostate cancer, Prolaris score was shown to be an independent predictor of prostate cancer death [32]. Per NCCN guidelines, the Prolaris biopsy score is recommended for patients with very low- and low-risk disease on biopsy and a life expectancy of 10 years [6]. However, it is also useful in men with high risk features after RP. Prolaris, combined with PSA, Gleason score, and other clinicopathologic factors including known T categories (extraprostatic extension [pT3a], seminal vesicle invasion [pT3b]), and lymph node invasion (N1) can predict 10-year risk of biochemical recurrence (BCR) after surgery (Table 1) [33,34].

Table 1. Available biomarkers and risk assessment tools to guide prostate cancer treatment and decision making.

Test	Type of Tissue	Genes/Biomarkers Encoded	Tool in Risk Assessment	Utility	Result
Prolaris	Biopsy	31 CCP + 15 reference genes	Combined with age, PSA, clinical stage, % positive cores, Gleason score, AUA risk category	Decision making: Active surveillance vs. Treatment	Higher score implies higher risk of cancer progression/independent predictor of prostate cancer death.
	Radical Prostatectomy		Combined with PSA, Gleason score, pathologic features of surgical specimen.	Prognostication/Need for adjuvant therapy	Predicts 10-year risk of BCR after radical prostatectomy
4-K Score	Blood	4 biomarkers: free PSA, total PSA, intact PSA, and human glandular kallikrein 2 (hk2)	Combined with ERSPC RPCRC risk calculator	Screening	Predicts presence of clinically significant prostate cancer
PCA3	Urine after DRE	Prostate Cancer Antigen 3	Combined with PSA, DRE, and risk calculator	Screening	Predicts presence of clinically significant prostate cancer: (a) On initial biopsy (b) Avoids unnecessary re-biopsy in patients with an initial negative biopsy.
Select MDx	Urine after DRE	HOXC6 and DLX1 genes	Combined with MRI, PSA, DRE, prostate volume, age, family history	Screening	Predicts presence of clinically significant prostate cancer: (a) Avoids detection of low risk prostate cancer (b) Avoids unnecessary re-biopsy
Stockholm-3 Model (S3M)		232 genetic polymorphisms + protein biomarkers (fPSA, iPSA)	Combined with age, DRE	Screening + patient selection: which patients deserve MRI +/− Biopsy.	Predicts presence of clinically significant prostate cancer (a) Avoids detection of low risk prostate cancer (b) Avoids unnecessary MRI +/- Biopsy
Oncotype Dx	Prostate biopsy	17 gene assay	Combined with CAPRA score	Decision making: Active surveillance vs. Treatment	Predicts high risk (stage & grade) disease upon eventual radical prostatectomy

2.3.2. 4K-score and European Randomized Study of Screening for Prostate Cancer Rotterdam Prostate Cancer Risk Calculator (ERSPC RPCRC)

Numerous risk calculators (RC) are available for prostate cancer, but only six are externally validated in multiple study populations [35]. Among those, ERSPC RPCRC is the most commonly used RC as it has shown superiority in predicting men at risk for clinically significant prostate cancer [36]. However, when ERSPC RPCRC is combined with 4K score, together they are able to predict clinically significant prostate cancer more accurately than either alone and decreasing the need of unnecessary biopsies [35,37] (Figure 1).

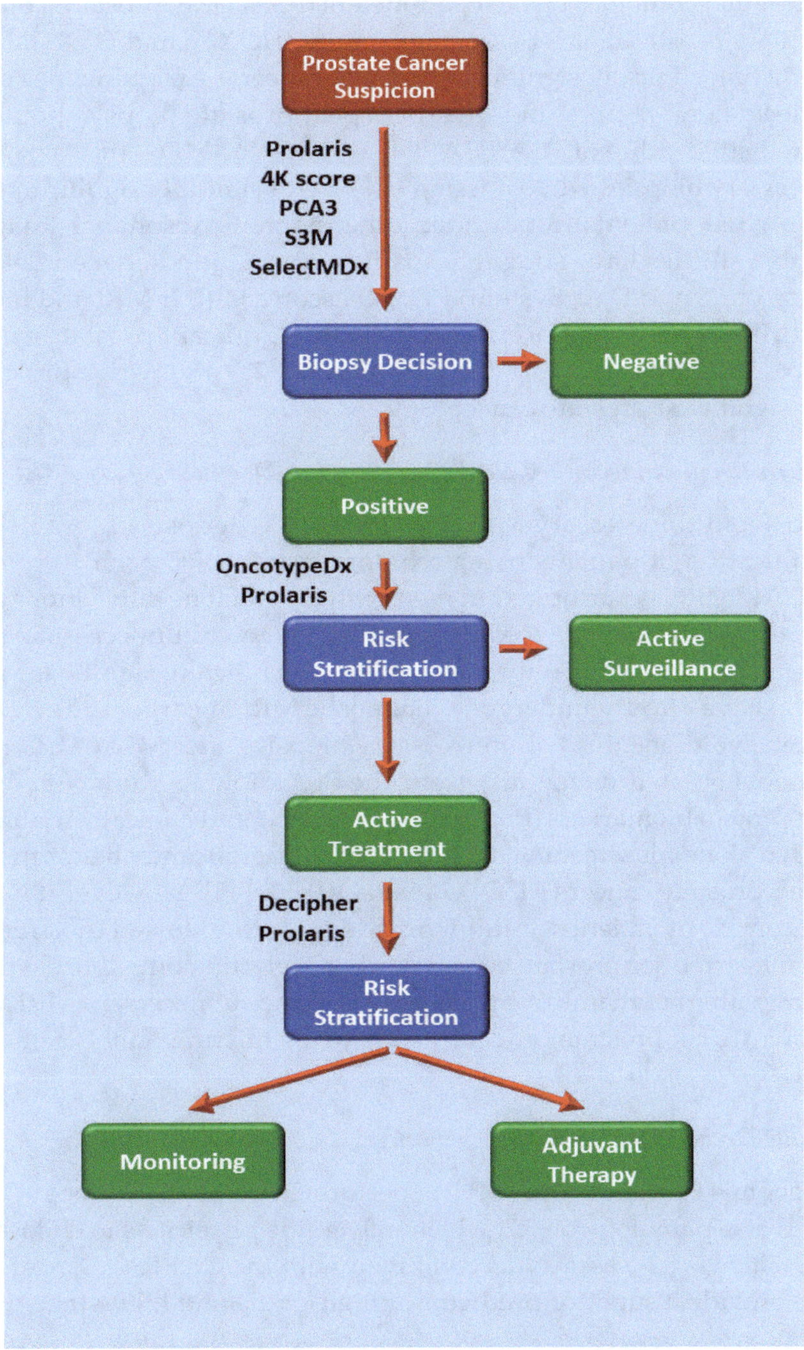

Figure 1. Algorithm describing the utility of prostate cancer biomarkers and risk assessment tools in clinical practice.

2.3.3. PCA3

Prostate cancer antigen 3 (*PCA3*) is a gene that codes for a mRNA that is overexpressed in prostate cancer tissue. It is detectable in urine after digital rectal examination (DRE) and can be used alone to predict the presence of clinically significant prostate cancer. However, when combined with a RC, *PCA3* enhances diagnostic accuracy particularly in men undergoing initial or repeat biopsy [38]. *PCA3* based nomograms could predict initial biopsy results and avoid unnecessary biopsy in 55% of patients while missing only 2% of patients with clinically significant prostate cancer [39].

2.3.4. SelectMDx

SelectMDx is a test that combines clinical parameters (PSA, DRE, prostate volume, age and family history) with two urinary prostate cancer associated genes (*HOXC6* and *DLX1*). Due to its suggested high accuracy in predicting clinically significant prostate cancer, EAU guidelines state that SelectMDx may be utilized to decide on whether an initial or repeat prostate biopsy should be performed [7]. Due to the strong predictive value of PSA/PSA density in SelectMDx, this risk assessment tool can prevent 42% of unnecessary biopsies while missing only 2% of clinically significant prostate cancer [38]. It can also exclude low risk patients from undergoing magnetic resonance imaging (MRI) prior to biopsy, as retrospective studies have shown a positive association between SelectMDx scores and (Prostate Imaging Reporting and Data System) PIRADS scores [40]. If MRI and biopsy are performed only when the SelectMDx score reflects a risk of clinically significant prostate cancer >10%, this will reduce 35% of unnecessary biopsies, avoid the detection of 52% of low risk prostate cancer and only miss 2% of clinically significant prostate cancer [36].

2.4. What Strategies Can Avoid Unnecessary MRI, Biopsies, and Diagnosis of Low Risk Prostate Cancer?

The best way to avoid unnecessary MRI, biopsies and diagnosis of low risk prostate cancer is to perform risk stratification of patients using a biomarker or a RC prior to pursuing unnecessary workup. When ERSPC RPCRC is performed in men with an initial negative biopsy but high suspicion of harboring cancer, the RC is able to avoid 51% of MRI's, 69% of unnecessary repeat biopsies and 25% of low risk prostate cancer, while only missing 10% of clinically significant prostate cancer [41]. Moreover, in men who have already undergone diagnostic MRI, incorporating age and PIRADS score into the ERSPC RC can avoid one third of unnecessary biopsies after MRI (AUC = 0.84) (Table 1) [42].

S3M is a risk model created using data from the Stockholm-3 study. It combines 232 genetic polymorphisms with protein biomarkers (PSA, fPSA, iPSA etc.) and clinical variables (age, DRE, family history etc.) When used alone for screening, S3M performed significantly better than PSA for detection of clinically significant prostate cancer (AUC 0.74 versus 0.56) [43]. However it has proven especially advantageous in the context of patient selection to undergo MRI followed by targeted prostate biopsy. In a cohort of 532 men referred for prostate cancer workup, selecting only those with a risk of clinically significant prostate cancer higher than 10% by S3M could reduce unnecessary MRI and biopsies by 38%, decrease diagnosis of low risk prostate cancer by 42% while missing only 8% of clinically significant prostate cancer [43].

2.5. Biomarkers to Guide Decision for Active Surveillance

Oncotype Dx Genomic Prostate Score (GPS) is performed on prostate biopsy sample that provides a risk prediction of adverse pathology on RP, which may guide physicians to choose active surveillance or pursue treatment. This 17-gene assay was combined with the CAPRA (Cancer of the Prostate Risk Assessment) score to provide a superior predictor of high-grade and high-stage disease at the time of prostatectomy [29].

Similarly, Prolaris is a 46-gene panel that can be performed on RP or biopsy specimens and helps in decision making between active surveillance and treatment [44]. Cooperberg et al. validated that the incorporation of Prolaris with CAPRA score has superior prognostic risk stratification for patients with localized prostate cancer [33].

2.6. Biomarkers to Predict Recurrence after Radical Prostatectomy

Biochemical recurrence and metastasis after RP are important measurable outcomes that have an implication on prognosis. Classical adverse pathologic features such as extraprostatic extension (pT3a), seminal vesicle involvement (pT3b), and positive surgical margins have been used to stratify patients into high risk of biochemical recurrence. Treating these patients with adjuvant radiation has been implicated with improved biochemical-free survival [45–47] and overall survival [48]. However, many practices offer watchful waiting for adverse pathologic features due to the indolent disease process and to decrease the risk of unwarranted radiation toxicities, especially that many trials have shown that early salvage radiation is equivalent to adjuvant radiation therapy [49].

Therefore, an accurate risk assessment model is needed, and not solely based on pathologic parameters, to better manage patients after RP. Genomic testing, such as the Decipher RP test, have been found to better stratify post-RP patients and identify the patients who need adjuvant radiation therapy and those who can afford to go for watchful waiting [50,51].

Many clinical nomograms and risk scores have been developed to predict biochemical recurrence after RP, such as the Stephenson nomogram and CAPRA-S [52–54]. These risk calculators rely only on clinical and pathologic information; however, if genomic information could be added to individualize stratification, this would yield more accurate information about prognosis of the disease. Indeed, Spratt et al., [55] has found that Decipher testing independently adds prognostic benefit over routine clinicopathologic variables to predict metastasis. Moreover, Spratt et al. has developed an internally validated integrated clinical-genomic risk group stratification for localized prostate cancer that outperforms traditional NCCN risk classification [56]. In addition, prospective trials confer that genomic testing post RP confers both decreased patient-related anxiety and improved decision making [57,58]. Subsequently, a defined role of genomic testing after RP has been included in the most recent NCCN guidelines [6]. However, the routine use of these genomic biomarkers and their integration in TNM/risk assessment models is still modest because of the lack of extensive cost-effectiveness studies and long-term prospective data on clinical utility.

2.7. Future Potential Perspectives

Since its first edition in 1968 [59], the TNM staging system has experienced regular updates and integrations, although preserving the same predominantly-anatomic based structure. With the application of new genomic technologies, the assessment of risk of cancer progression and development of metastatic diseases has improved. A modified staging system has been proposed recently by Yang et al. In addition to the traditional TNM, the authors proposed to integrate the results of the liquid biopsy designed as "B" (representing blood), as "B0" for absence and "B1" for presence of detectable circulating tumor DNA (ctDNA) [60]. So far, there are no available data on integration of ctDNA and/or circulating tumor cells with TNM or risk assessment models in prostate cancer. Moreover, the potential theranostic utility of circulating tumor cells (CTC) in the context of localized prostate cancer is still debatable and the sensitivity and specificity of technical approaches used for isolation and characterization of CTC need to be improved and standardized [61].

3. Conclusions

With the vast advancements in the field of personalized medicine, there is a crucial need for reliable prostate cancer prognostic biomarkers to identify patients that may benefit from different management strategies. Integration of biomarkers into risk assessment models appears to enhance prostate cancer stratification for both diagnosis and management. However, to be integrated in future prognostic and predictive models, genomic biomarkers need greater standardization to improve generalizability, validation of their clinical efficacy, and cost-effectiveness in routine application.

Author Contributions: Conception and design: all authors; Drafting the manuscript and final editing: all authors; Review of the literature: R.S., N.A.H.; Critical revision of the manuscript: A.C., G.P.P. All authors have read and agreed to the published version of the manuscript.

References

1. Varma, M.; Cochlin, D.; Delahunt, B.; Kynaston, H.; Rees, J.; Rous, B.; Narahari, K. TNM clinical staging of prostate cancer: Issues and solutions. *BJU Int.* **2019**, *123*, 382–384. [CrossRef] [PubMed]
2. Paner, G.P.; Stadler, W.M.; Hansel, D.E.; Montironi, R.; Lin, D.W.; Amin, M.B. Updates in the Eighth Edition of the Tumor-Node-Metastasis Staging Classification for Urologic Cancers. *Eur. Urol.* **2018**, *73*, 560–569. [CrossRef] [PubMed]
3. Amin, M.B.; Greene, F.L.; Edge, S.B.; Compton, C.C.; Gershenwald, J.E.; Brookland, R.K.; Meyer, L.; Gress, D.M.; Byrd, D.R.; Winchester, D.P. The Eighth Edition AJCC Cancer Staging Manual: Continuing to build a bridge from a population-based to a more "personalized" approach to cancer staging. *CA A Cancer J. Clin.* **2017**, *67*, 93–99. [CrossRef] [PubMed]
4. de Rooij, M.; Hamoen, E.H.J.; Witjes, J.A.; Barentsz, J.O.; Rovers, M.M. Accuracy of Magnetic Resonance Imaging for Local Staging of Prostate Cancer: A Diagnostic Meta-analysis. *Eur. Urol.* **2016**, *70*, 233–245. [CrossRef]
5. Olleik, G.; Kassouf, W.; Aprikian, A.; Hu, J.; Vanhuyse, M.; Cury, F.; Peacock, S.; Bonnevier, E.; Palenius, E.; Dragomir, A. Evaluation of New Tests and Interventions for Prostate Cancer Management: A Systematic Review. *J. Natl. Compr. Cancer Netw. JNCCN* **2018**, *16*, 1340–1351. [CrossRef]
6. Mohler, J.L.; Antonarakis, E.S.; Armstrong, A.J.; D'Amico, A.V.; Davis, B.J.; Dorff, T.; Eastham, J.A.; Enke, C.A.; Farrington, T.A.; Higano, C.S.; et al. Prostate Cancer, Version 2.2019, NCCN Clinical Practice Guidelines in Oncology. *J. Natl. Compr. Cancer Netw. JNCCN* **2019**, *17*, 479–505. [CrossRef]
7. Mottet, N.; Bellmunt, J.; Bolla, M.; Briers, E.; Cumberbatch, M.G.; De Santis, M.; Fossati, N.; Gross, T.; Henry, A.M.; Joniau, S.; et al. EAU-ESTRO-SIOG Guidelines on Prostate Cancer. Part 1: Screening, Diagnosis, and Local Treatment with Curative Intent. *Eur. Urol.* **2017**, *71*, 618–629. [CrossRef]
8. Sanda, M.G.; Cadeddu, J.A.; Kirkby, E.; Chen, R.C.; Crispino, T.; Fontanarosa, J.; Freedland, S.J.; Greene, K.; Klotz, L.H.; Makarov, D.V.; et al. Clinically Localized Prostate Cancer: AUA/ASTRO/SUO Guideline. Part I: Risk Stratification, Shared Decision Making, and Care Options. *J. Urol.* **2018**, *199*, 683–690. [CrossRef]
9. Kordan, Y.; Chang, S.S.; Salem, S.; Cookson, M.S.; Clark, P.E.; Davis, R.; Herrell, S.D.; Baumgartner, R.; Phillips, S.; Smith, J.A.; et al. Pathological Stage T2 Subgroups to Predict Biochemical Recurrence After Prostatectomy. *J. Urol.* **2009**, *182*, 2291–2295. [CrossRef]
10. Chun, F.K.H.; Graefen, M.; Zacharias, M.; Haese, A.; Steuber, T.; Schlomm, T.; Walz, J.; Karakiewicz, P.I.; Huland, H. Anatomic radical retropubic prostatectomy—long-term recurrence-free survival rates for localized prostate cancer. *World J. Urol.* **2006**, *24*, 273–280. [CrossRef]
11. Epstein, J.I. Prognostic Significance of Tumor Volume in Radical Prostatectomy and Needle Biopsy Specimens. *J. Urol.* **2011**, *186*, 790–797. [CrossRef] [PubMed]
12. Halabi, S.; Lin, C.Y.; Kelly, W.K.; Fizazi, K.; Moul, J.W.; Kaplan, E.B.; Morris, M.J.; Small, E.J. Updated prognostic model for predicting overall survival in first-line chemotherapy for patients with metastatic castration-resistant prostate cancer. *J. Clin. Oncol.* **2014**, *32*, 671–677. [CrossRef] [PubMed]
13. Halabi, S.; Lin, C.-Y.; Small, E.J.; Armstrong, A.J.; Kaplan, E.B.; Petrylak, D.; Sternberg, C.N.; Shen, L.; Oudard, S.; de Bono, J.; et al. Prognostic Model Predicting Metastatic Castration-Resistant Prostate Cancer Survival in Men Treated With Second-Line Chemotherapy. *JNCI: J. Natl. Cancer Inst.* **2013**, *105*, 1729–1737. [CrossRef] [PubMed]
14. Buyyounouski, M.K.; Choyke, P.L.; McKenney, J.K.; Sartor, O.; Sandler, H.M.; Amin, M.B.; Kattan, M.W.; Lin, D.W. Prostate cancer—Major changes in the American Joint Committee on Cancer eighth edition cancer staging manual. *CA A Cancer J. Clin.* **2017**, *67*, 245–253. [CrossRef]
15. Wang, S.Y.; Cowan, J.E.; Cary, K.C.; Chan, J.M.; Carroll, P.R.; Cooperberg, M.R. Limited ability of existing nomograms to predict outcomes in men undergoing active surveillance for prostate cancer. *BJU Int.* **2014**, *114*, E18–E24. [CrossRef]

16. Beltran, H.; Rubin, M.A. New strategies in prostate cancer: Translating genomics into the clinic. *Clin. Cancer Res. Off. J. Am. Assoc. Cancer Res.* **2013**, *19*, 517–523. [CrossRef]
17. Jamaspishvili, T.; Berman, D.M.; Ross, A.E.; Scher, H.I.; De Marzo, A.M.; Squire, J.A.; Lotan, T.L. Clinical implications of PTEN loss in prostate cancer. *Nat. Rev. Urol.* **2018**, *15*, 222–234. [CrossRef]
18. Giri, V.N.; Obeid, E.; Gross, L.; Bealin, L.; Hyatt, C.; Hegarty, S.E.; Montgomery, S.; Forman, A.; Bingler, R.; Kelly, W.K.; et al. Inherited Mutations in Men Undergoing Multigene Panel Testing for Prostate Cancer: Emerging Implications for Personalized Prostate Cancer Genetic Evaluation. *JCO Precis. Oncol.* **2017**, 1–17. [CrossRef]
19. Castro, E.; Goh, C.; Olmos, D.; Saunders, E.; Leongamornlert, D.; Tymrakiewicz, M.; Mahmud, N.; Dadaev, T.; Govindasami, K.; Guy, M.; et al. Germline BRCA mutations are associated with higher risk of nodal involvement, distant metastasis, and poor survival outcomes in prostate cancer. *J. Clin. Oncol. Off. J. Am. Soc. Clin. Oncol.* **2013**, *31*, 1748–1757. [CrossRef]
20. Castro, E.; Goh, C.; Leongamornlert, D.; Saunders, E.; Tymrakiewicz, M.; Dadaev, T.; Govindasami, K.; Guy, M.; Ellis, S.; Frost, D.; et al. Effect of BRCA Mutations on Metastatic Relapse and Cause-specific Survival After Radical Treatment for Localised Prostate Cancer. *Eur. Urol.* **2015**, *68*, 186–193. [CrossRef]
21. Castro, E.; Romero-Laorden, N.; Del Pozo, A.; Lozano, R.; Medina, A.; Puente, J.; Piulats, J.M.; Lorente, D.; Saez, M.I.; Morales-Barrera, R.; et al. PROREPAIR-B: A Prospective Cohort Study of the Impact of Germline DNA Repair Mutations on the Outcomes of Patients With Metastatic Castration-Resistant Prostate Cancer. *J. Clin. Oncol. Off. J. Am. Soc. Clin. Oncol.* **2019**, *37*, 490–503. [CrossRef] [PubMed]
22. Eggener, S.E.; Rumble, R.B.; Armstrong, A.J.; Morgan, T.M.; Crispino, T.; Cornford, P.; van der Kwast, T.; Grignon, D.J.; Rai, A.J.; Agarwal, N.; et al. Molecular Biomarkers in Localized Prostate Cancer: ASCO Guideline. *J. Clin. Oncol. Off. J. Am. Soc. Clin. Oncol.* **2020**, *38*, 1474–1494. [CrossRef]
23. Carter, H.B.; Helfand, B.; Mamawala, M.; Wu, Y.; Landis, P.; Yu, H.; Wiley, K.; Na, R.; Shi, Z.; Petkewicz, J.; et al. Germline Mutations in ATM and BRCA1/2 Are Associated with Grade Reclassification in Men on Active Surveillance for Prostate Cancer. *Eur. Urol.* **2019**, *75*, 743–749. [CrossRef]
24. Becerra, M.F.; Atluri, V.S.; Bhattu, A.S.; Punnen, S. Serum and urine biomarkers for detecting clinically significant prostate cancer. *Urol. Oncol.* **2020**. [CrossRef]
25. Van Den Eeden, S.K.; Lu, R.; Zhang, N.; Quesenberry, C.P., Jr.; Shan, J.; Han, J.S.; Tsiatis, A.C.; Leimpeter, A.D.; Lawrence, H.J.; Febbo, P.G.; et al. A Biopsy-based 17-gene Genomic Prostate Score as a Predictor of Metastases and Prostate Cancer Death in Surgically Treated Men with Clinically Localized Disease. *Eur. Urol.* **2018**, *73*, 129–138. [CrossRef]
26. Cullen, J.; Rosner, I.L.; Brand, T.C.; Zhang, N.; Tsiatis, A.C.; Moncur, J.; Ali, A.; Chen, Y.; Knezevic, D.; Maddala, T.; et al. A Biopsy-based 17-gene Genomic Prostate Score Predicts Recurrence After Radical Prostatectomy and Adverse Surgical Pathology in a Racially Diverse Population of Men with Clinically Low- and Intermediate-risk Prostate Cancer. *Eur. Urol.* **2015**, *68*, 123–131. [CrossRef]
27. Klein, E.A.; Cooperberg, M.R.; Magi-Galluzzi, C.; Simko, J.P.; Falzarano, S.M.; Maddala, T.; Chan, J.M.; Li, J.; Cowan, J.E.; Tsiatis, A.C.; et al. A 17-gene assay to predict prostate cancer aggressiveness in the context of Gleason grade heterogeneity, tumor multifocality, and biopsy undersampling. *Eur. Urol.* **2014**, *66*, 550–560. [CrossRef] [PubMed]
28. Cuzick, J.; Berney, D.M.; Fisher, G.; Mesher, D.; Møller, H.; Reid, J.E.; Perry, M.; Park, J.; Younus, A.; Gutin, A.; et al. Prognostic value of a cell cycle progression signature for prostate cancer death in a conservatively managed needle biopsy cohort. *Br. J. Cancer* **2012**, *106*, 1095–1099. [CrossRef]
29. Shore, N.D.; Kella, N.; Moran, B.; Boczko, J.; Bianco, F.J.; Crawford, E.D.; Davis, T.; Roundy, K.M.; Rushton, K.; Grier, C.; et al. Impact of the Cell Cycle Progression Test on Physician and Patient Treatment Selection for Localized Prostate Cancer. *J. Urol.* **2016**, *195*, 612–618. [CrossRef]
30. Hu, J.C.; Tosoian, J.J.; Qi, J.; Kaye, D.; Johnson, A.; Linsell, S.; Montie, J.E.; Ghani, K.R.; Miller, D.C.; Wojno, K.; et al. Clinical Utility of Gene Expression Classifiers in Men With Newly Diagnosed Prostate Cancer. *JCOPrecis. Oncol.* **2018**, 1–15. [CrossRef]
31. Alford, A.V.; Brito, J.M.; Yadav, K.K.; Yadav, S.S.; Tewari, A.K.; Renzulli, J. The Use of Biomarkers in Prostate Cancer Screening and Treatment. *Rev. Urol.* **2017**, *19*, 221–234. [CrossRef] [PubMed]
32. Cuzick, J.; Stone, S.; Fisher, G.; Yang, Z.H.; North, B.V.; Berney, D.M.; Beltran, L.; Greenberg, D.; Møller, H.; Reid, J.E.; et al. Validation of an RNA cell cycle progression score for predicting death from prostate cancer in a conservatively managed needle biopsy cohort. *Br. J. Cancer* **2015**, *113*, 382–389. [CrossRef]

33. Cooperberg, M.R.; Simko, J.P.; Cowan, J.E.; Reid, J.E.; Djalilvand, A.; Bhatnagar, S.; Gutin, A.; Lanchbury, J.S.; Swanson, G.P.; Stone, S.; et al. Validation of a cell-cycle progression gene panel to improve risk stratification in a contemporary prostatectomy cohort. *J. Clin. Oncol. Off. J. Am. Soc. Clin. Oncol.* **2013**, *31*, 1428–1434. [CrossRef] [PubMed]
34. Erho, N.; Crisan, A.; Vergara, I.A.; Mitra, A.P.; Ghadessi, M.; Buerki, C.; Bergstralh, E.J.; Kollmeyer, T.; Fink, S.; Haddad, Z.; et al. Discovery and validation of a prostate cancer genomic classifier that predicts early metastasis following radical prostatectomy. *PLoS ONE* **2013**, *8*, e66855. [CrossRef]
35. Roobol, M.J.; Verbeek, J.F.M.; van der Kwast, T.; Kümmerlin, I.P.; Kweldam, C.F.; van Leenders, G. Improving the Rotterdam European Randomized Study of Screening for Prostate Cancer Risk Calculator for Initial Prostate Biopsy by Incorporating the 2014 International Society of Urological Pathology Gleason Grading and Cribriform growth. *Eur. Urol.* **2017**, *72*, 45–51. [CrossRef]
36. Osses, D.F.; Roobol, M.J.; Schoots, I.G. Prediction Medicine: Biomarkers, Risk Calculators and Magnetic Resonance Imaging as Risk Stratification Tools in Prostate Cancer Diagnosis. *Int. J. Mol. Sci.* **2019**, 1637. [CrossRef]
37. Verbeek, J.F.M.; Bangma, C.H.; Kweldam, C.F.; van der Kwast, T.H.; Kümmerlin, I.P.; van Leenders, G.; Roobol, M.J. Reducing unnecessary biopsies while detecting clinically significant prostate cancer including cribriform growth with the ERSPC Rotterdam risk calculator and 4Kscore. *Urol. Oncol.* **2019**, *37*, 138–144. [CrossRef]
38. Van Neste, L.; Hendriks, R.J.; Dijkstra, S.; Trooskens, G.; Cornel, E.B.; Jannink, S.A.; de Jong, H.; Hessels, D.; Smit, F.P.; Melchers, W.J.; et al. Detection of High-grade Prostate Cancer Using a Urinary Molecular Biomarker-Based Risk Score. *Eur. Urol.* **2016**, *70*, 740–748. [CrossRef]
39. Hansen, J.; Auprich, M.; Ahyai, S.A.; de la Taille, A.; van Poppel, H.; Marberger, M.; Stenzl, A.; Mulders, P.F.; Huland, H.; Fisch, M.; et al. Initial prostate biopsy: Development and internal validation of a biopsy-specific nomogram based on the prostate cancer antigen 3 assay. *Eur. Urol.* **2013**, *63*, 201–209. [CrossRef]
40. Hendriks, R.J.; van der Leest, M.M.G.; Dijkstra, S.; Barentsz, J.O.; Van Criekinge, W.; Hulsbergen-van de Kaa, C.A.; Schalken, J.A.; Mulders, P.F.A.; van Oort, I.M. A urinary biomarker-based risk score correlates with multiparametric MRI for prostate cancer detection. *Prostate* **2017**, *77*, 1401–1407. [CrossRef]
41. Alberts, A.R.; Schoots, I.G.; Bokhorst, L.P.; van Leenders, G.J.; Bangma, C.H.; Roobol, M.J. Risk-based Patient Selection for Magnetic Resonance Imaging-targeted Prostate Biopsy after Negative Transrectal Ultrasound-guided Random Biopsy Avoids Unnecessary Magnetic Resonance Imaging Scans. *Eur. Urol.* **2016**, *69*, 1129–1134. [CrossRef] [PubMed]
42. Alberts, A.R.; Roobol, M.J.; Verbeek, J.F.M.; Schoots, I.G.; Chiu, P.K.; Osses, D.F.; Tijsterman, J.D.; Beerlage, H.P.; Mannaerts, C.K.; Schimmöller, L.; et al. Prediction of High-grade Prostate Cancer Following Multiparametric Magnetic Resonance Imaging: Improving the Rotterdam European Randomized Study of Screening for Prostate Cancer Risk Calculators. *Eur. Urol.* **2019**, *75*, 310–318. [CrossRef]
43. Nordström, T.; Grönberg, H.; Adolfsson, J.; Egevad, L.; Aly, M.; Eklund, M. Balancing Overdiagnosis and Early Detection of Prostate Cancer using the Stockholm-3 Model. *Eur. Urol. Focus* **2018**, *4*, 385–387. [CrossRef] [PubMed]
44. Cucchiara, V.; Cooperberg, M.R.; Dall'Era, M.; Lin, D.W.; Montorsi, F.; Schalken, J.A.; Evans, C.P. Genomic Markers in Prostate Cancer Decision Making. *Eur. Urol.* **2018**, *73*, 572–582. [CrossRef]
45. Thompson, I.M., Jr.; Tangen, C.M.; Paradelo, J.; Lucia, M.S.; Miller, G.; Troyer, D.; Messing, E.; Forman, J.; Chin, J.; Swanson, G.; et al. Adjuvant radiotherapy for pathologically advanced prostate cancer: A randomized clinical trial. *JAMA* **2006**, *296*, 2329–2335. [CrossRef] [PubMed]
46. Wiegel, T.; Bottke, D.; Steiner, U.; Siegmann, A.; Golz, R.; Störkel, S.; Willich, N.; Semjonow, A.; Souchon, R.; Stöckle, M.; et al. Phase III postoperative adjuvant radiotherapy after radical prostatectomy compared with radical prostatectomy alone in pT3 prostate cancer with postoperative undetectable prostate-specific antigen: ARO 96-02/AUO AP 09/95. *J. Clin. Oncol. Off. J. Am. Soc. Clin. Oncol.* **2009**, *27*, 2924–2930. [CrossRef]
47. Ritter, M.A. Commentary on "Postoperative radiotherapy after radical prostatectomy for high-risk prostate cancer: Long-term results of a randomised controlled trial (EORTC trial 22911)." Bolla M, van Poppel H, Tombal B, Vekemans K, Da Pozzo L, de Reijke TM, Verbaeys A, Bosset JF, van Velthoven R, Colombel M, van de Beek C, Verhagen P, van den Bergh A, Sternberg C, Gasser T, van Tienhoven G, Scalliet P, Haustermans K,

Collette L.; European Organisation for Research and Treatment of Cancer, Radiation Oncology and Genito-Urinary Groups. Department of Radiation Oncology, Centre Hospitalier Universitaire A Michallon, Grenoble, France.: Lancet 2012;380(9858):2018-27. doi: 10.1016/S0140-6736(12)61253-7. [Epub 2012 Oct 19]. *Urol. Oncol.* **2014**, *32*, 372–373. [CrossRef]

48. Thompson, I.M.; Tangen, C.M.; Paradelo, J.; Lucia, M.S.; Miller, G.; Troyer, D.; Messing, E.; Forman, J.; Chin, J.; Swanson, G.; et al. Adjuvant radiotherapy for pathological T3N0M0 prostate cancer significantly reduces risk of metastases and improves survival: Long-term followup of a randomized clinical trial. *J. Urol.* **2009**, *181*, 956–962. [CrossRef]
49. Fossati, N.; Karnes, R.J.; Boorjian, S.A.; Moschini, M.; Morlacco, A.; Bossi, A.; Seisen, T.; Cozzarini, C.; Fiorino, C.; Noris Chiorda, B.; et al. Long-term Impact of Adjuvant Versus Early Salvage Radiation Therapy in pT3N0 Prostate Cancer Patients Treated with Radical Prostatectomy: Results from a Multi-institutional Series. *Eur. Urol.* **2017**, *71*, 886–893. [CrossRef]
50. Den, R.B.; Yousefi, K.; Trabulsi, E.J.; Abdollah, F.; Choeurng, V.; Feng, F.Y.; Dicker, A.P.; Lallas, C.D.; Gomella, L.G.; Davicioni, E.; et al. Genomic classifier identifies men with adverse pathology after radical prostatectomy who benefit from adjuvant radiation therapy. *J. Clin. Oncol. Off. J. Am. Soc. Clin. Oncol.* **2015**, *33*, 944–951. [CrossRef]
51. Dalela, D.; Santiago-Jiménez, M.; Yousefi, K.; Karnes, R.J.; Ross, A.E.; Den, R.B.; Freedland, S.J.; Schaeffer, E.M.; Dicker, A.P.; Menon, M.; et al. Genomic Classifier Augments the Role of Pathological Features in Identifying Optimal Candidates for Adjuvant Radiation Therapy in Patients With Prostate Cancer: Development and Internal Validation of a Multivariable Prognostic Model. *J. Clin. Oncol. Off. J. Am. Soc. Clin. Oncol.* **2017**, *35*, 1982–1990. [CrossRef] [PubMed]
52. Kattan, M.W.; Eastham, J.A.; Stapleton, A.M.; Wheeler, T.M.; Scardino, P.T. A preoperative nomogram for disease recurrence following radical prostatectomy for prostate cancer. *J. Natl. Cancer Inst.* **1998**, *90*, 766–771. [CrossRef] [PubMed]
53. Stephenson, A.J.; Scardino, P.T.; Eastham, J.A.; Bianco, F.J., Jr.; Dotan, Z.A.; DiBlasio, C.J.; Reuther, A.; Klein, E.A.; Kattan, M.W. Postoperative nomogram predicting the 10-year probability of prostate cancer recurrence after radical prostatectomy. *J. Clin. Oncol. Off. J. Am. Soc. Clin. Oncol.* **2005**, *23*, 7005–7012. [CrossRef]
54. Cooperberg, M.R.; Hilton, J.F.; Carroll, P.R. The CAPRA-S score: A straightforward tool for improved prediction of outcomes after radical prostatectomy. *Cancer* **2011**, *117*, 5039–5046. [CrossRef]
55. Spratt, D.E.; Yousefi, K.; Deheshi, S.; Ross, A.E.; Den, R.B.; Schaeffer, E.M.; Trock, B.J.; Zhang, J.; Glass, A.G.; Dicker, A.P.; et al. Individual Patient-Level Meta-Analysis of the Performance of the Decipher Genomic Classifier in High-Risk Men After Prostatectomy to Predict Development of Metastatic Disease. *J. Clin. Oncol. Off. J. Am. Soc. Clin. Oncol.* **2017**, *35*, 1991–1998. [CrossRef]
56. Spratt, D.E.; Zhang, J.; Santiago-Jiménez, M.; Dess, R.T.; Davis, J.W.; Den, R.B.; Dicker, A.P.; Kane, C.J.; Pollack, A.; Stoyanova, R.; et al. Development and Validation of a Novel Integrated Clinical-Genomic Risk Group Classification for Localized Prostate Cancer. *J. Clin. Oncol. Off. J. Am. Soc. Clin. Oncol.* **2018**, *36*, 581–590. [CrossRef]
57. Gore, J.L.; du Plessis, M.; Santiago-Jiménez, M.; Yousefi, K.; Thompson, D.J.S.; Karsh, L.; Lane, B.R.; Franks, M.; Chen, D.Y.T.; Bandyk, M.; et al. Decipher test impacts decision making among patients considering adjuvant and salvage treatment after radical prostatectomy: Interim results from the Multicenter Prospective PRO-IMPACT study. *Cancer* **2017**, *123*, 2850–2859. [CrossRef] [PubMed]
58. Marascio, J.; Spratt, D.E.; Zhang, J.; Trabulsi, E.J.; Le, T.; Sedzorme, W.S.; Beeler, W.H.; Davicioni, E.; Dabbas, B.; Lin, D.W.; et al. Prospective study to define the clinical utility and benefit of Decipher testing in men following prostatectomy. *Prostate Cancer Prostatic Dis.* **2020**, *23*, 295–302. [CrossRef]
59. Harmer, M.; Denoix, P.; Hamperl, H. Das TNM-System zur Klassifikation von Tumorkrankheiten. *Klin. Wochenschr.* **1968**, *46*, 1181–1185. [CrossRef]
60. Yang, M.; Forbes, M.E.; Bitting, R.L.; O'Neill, S.S.; Chou, P.C.; Topaloglu, U.; Miller, L.D.; Hawkins, G.A.; Grant, S.C.; DeYoung, B.R.; et al. Incorporating blood-based liquid biopsy information into cancer staging: Time for a TNMB system? *Ann. Oncol. Off. J. Eur. Soc. Med Oncol.* **2018**, *29*, 311–323. [CrossRef]
61. Broncy, L.; Paterlini-Bréchot, P. Clinical Impact of Circulating Tumor Cells in Patients with Localized Prostate Cancer. *Cells* **2019**, 676. [CrossRef] [PubMed]

2

Advances in Prognostic Methylation Biomarkers for Prostate Cancer

Dilys Lam [1], Susan Clark [1,2], Clare Stirzaker [1,2,†] and Ruth Pidsley [1,2,*,†]

1 Epigenetics Research Laboratory, Genomics and Epigenetics Division, Garvan Institute of Medical Research, Sydney, New South Wales 2010, Australia; d.lam@garvan.org.au (D.L.); s.clark@garvan.org.au (S.C.); c.stirzaker@garvan.org.au (C.S.)
2 St. Vincent's Clinical School, University of New South Wales, Sydney, New South Wales 2010, Australia
* Correspondence: r.pidsley@garvan.org.au
† These authors have contributed equally.

Simple Summary: Prostate cancer is a major cause of cancer-related death in men worldwide. There is an urgent clinical need for improved prognostic biomarkers to better predict the likely outcome and course of the disease and thus inform the clinical management of these patients. Currently, clinically recognised prognostic markers lack sensitivity and specificity in distinguishing aggressive from indolent disease, particularly in patients with localised, intermediate grade prostate cancer. Thus, there is major interest in identifying new molecular biomarkers to complement existing standard clinicopathological markers. DNA methylation is a frequent alteration in the cancer genome and offers potential as a reliable and robust biomarker. In this review, we provide a comprehensive overview of the current state of DNA methylation biomarker studies in prostate cancer prognosis. We highlight advances in this field that have enabled the discovery of novel prognostic genes and discuss the potential of methylation biomarkers for noninvasive liquid-biopsy testing.

Abstract: There is a major clinical need for accurate biomarkers for prostate cancer prognosis, to better inform treatment strategies and disease monitoring. Current clinically recognised prognostic factors, including prostate-specific antigen (PSA) levels, lack sensitivity and specificity in distinguishing aggressive from indolent disease, particularly in patients with localised intermediate grade prostate cancer. There has therefore been a major focus on identifying molecular biomarkers that can add prognostic value to existing markers, including investigation of DNA methylation, which has a known role in tumorigenesis. In this review, we will provide a comprehensive overview of the current state of DNA methylation biomarker studies in prostate cancer prognosis, and highlight the advances that have been made in this field. We cover the numerous studies into well-established candidate genes, and explore the technological transition that has enabled hypothesis-free genome-wide studies and the subsequent discovery of novel prognostic genes.

Keywords: DNA methylation; epigenetics; biomarkers; circulating DNA; cfDNA; prostate cancer; early detection; prognosis

---

1. Introduction

Prostate cancer (PCa) is the most commonly diagnosed noncutaneous cancer in men and one of the leading causes of cancer death in males. Globally, 1,276,106 new cases were diagnosed in 2018 alone [1,2], and this number is projected to rise by approximately 80%, to more than two million new cases a year, by 2040 [3–5]. Currently, PCa diagnosis is achieved through assessment of blood prostate-specific antigen (PSA) levels, digital rectal examination (clinical T-stage) and histological examination of needle biopsies (Gleason Score (GS)/ISUP Grade) [6]. PSA-based screening was introduced in the late 1980s, and has significantly increased the early detection of localized disease [7–9]. Diagnosis at this early organ-confined stage of disease is crucial as it is potentially curable by radical prostatectomy (RP), a procedure to surgically remove the whole prostate gland. While this is curative for most prostate cancers, approximately 30% of patients treated by RP experience biochemical recurrence (BCR) [10], and 17–22% of these relapsed patients progress to metastatic-lethal PCa [11–13]. There is therefore a need to identify the men at high risk of metastatic progression, so that additional interventions can be offered earlier (e.g., adjuvant therapies such as chemotherapy and radiotherapy) [14].

On the other hand, many men diagnosed with PCa have an indolent form of the disease, which is characterised by slow progression with no eventual clinical manifestation [15,16]. For these men, RP represents an overtreatment given the risk of unnecessary side effects and compromised quality of life [17,18]. Thus, strategies such as 'watchful waiting' and 'active surveillance' have emerged for men diagnosed with low grade disease, in which regular monitoring is used to detect tumour progression, with the aim of delaying RP until it is clinically necessary [19]. However, 13–45% of low-risk men on active surveillance exhibit a PSA rise and progress to surgery or other treatments [20–22], indicating that they may have been inappropriately assigned to monitoring, and should have been treated earlier.

PCa has a heterogeneous clinical course which makes it challenging to decide the most appropriate treatment or monitoring strategy for individual patients [23]. There is a major unmet clinical need for specific prognostic biomarkers that can accurately differentiate indolent from aggressive tumours that are likely to metastasise and lead to lethal disease [24]. The ability to identify the risk of progression at initial diagnosis would inform decisions about personalized treatment and/or monitoring strategies, as well as the use of adjuvant therapy, for improved clinical management and enhanced outcomes for PCa patients (Figure 1).

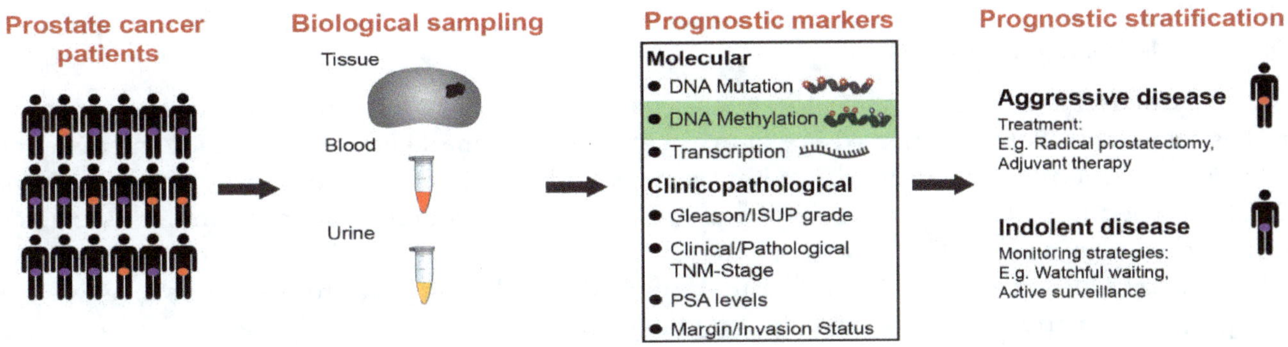

Figure 1. Schematic showing the pathway for the application of biomarkers for improved prognostic stratification in prostate cancer patients. Prostate cancer is a heterogeneous disease and identifying those patients at diagnosis that have aggressive vs. indolent disease is critical in informing the clinical management of these patients. Biological sampling includes tissue biopsies, and blood and urine samples. These are assayed using molecular biomarkers, including DNA mutations, DNA methylation and transcription, and clinicopathological markers, such as GS/ISUP grade and tumour staging. The ultimate goal is to improve the prognostic stratification of patients to inform the optimal treatment strategies for prostate cancer patients. TNM: tumour/nodes/metastasis staging; PSA: prostate-specific antigen.

1.1. Current Clinicopathological Prognostic Markers

The existing scoring systems and nomograms that are used to identify patients at high risk of progression are based solely on routine clinical and pathological variables at the time of diagnosis or surgery, including preoperative (pre-op) PSA levels, GS/ISUP grade scoring, tumour staging (clinical or pathological T-stage) and margin status (Figure 1) [11,25–30]. These tools, whilst useful in the diagnostic assessment of the tumour, lack sensitivity and specificity in classifying the risk of an individual patient's disease [6,31–33]. One problem with the current prognostic approach is that a number of scoring systems exist, with no single accepted standard system being used in clinical practice [29,34]. Furthermore, these prognostic variables are based on histological assessment, which may not capture the underlying biology of a tumour and its potential to progress to an aggressive, lethal cancer. Advances in molecular profiling techniques mean that we can now access another layer of biological information in tumours, including early molecular changes that may precede histologically visible alterations [23,35]. Much research is now being dedicated to investigating whether molecular information can better inform clinical decisions about individualised treatment and/or monitoring strategies, as well as providing new biological insights to guide the development of new therapies [35].

1.2. Molecular Biomarkers for Prognosis

There is increasing evidence for the value of prognostic molecular biomarkers to complement existing standard clinicopathological markers. Molecular prognostication of PCa has been investigated in various contexts, including at the level of genetic, epigenetic and gene expression alterations [36,37], from both tumour tissue [37,38] and liquid biopsies [39,40] (Figure 1). To date, the major success stories of prognostic molecular biomarkers are the commercialised tissue-based tests centred on panels of gene expression signatures. These tests include Prolaris (Myriad Genetics, Salt Lake City, UT, USA), Oncotype DX Prostate (Genomic Health, Redwood City, CA, USA) and Decipher (GenomeDX Biosciences, Vancouver, BC, Canada) [37]. The Prolaris test determines risk of progression (BCR, cancer-specific death) by measuring a proliferation signature of 31 cell cycle progression transcripts [41], whilst Oncotype DX predicts adverse pathology (high grade/stage disease) or poor outcome (BCR) based on 12 genes [42]. Decipher is based on 22 markers which have been trained to predict early metastasis and aggressive PCa [43]. Whilst these tests demonstrate the potential for molecular biomarkers, they have yet to be integrated into the standard clinical routine following the initial diagnosis [37].

1.3. DNA Methylation Biomarkers

DNA methylation is one of the earliest, most stable and frequent alterations in the cancer genome and has been extensively investigated as a source of molecular biomarkers [36,44–46]. DNA methylation is an epigenetic modification, in which a methyl group is added to the cytosine base of a cytosine-guanine (CpG) dinucleotide. It is associated with gene regulation and function, with promoter-associated clusters of marks, termed CpG islands, often linked to gene silencing [47,48]. In the context of PCa, aberrant DNA methylation is a key feature observed during early tumorigenesis, as well as in its progression and metastatic development [49–51], and occurs at a much higher frequency and more consistently than genetic mutations [52]. Additionally, DNA methylation has been shown to outperform gene expression in detecting cancer from prostate biopsies [53]. The feasibility of using DNA methylation as a biomarker is further supported by the fact that DNA is more stable than RNA [54] and its methylation patterns are retained following long-term storage of clinical material, including as formalin-fixed paraffin-embedded tissue (FFPET). DNA methylation assays can also be easily integrated into routine clinical practice as many diagnostic labs already have the infrastructure in place, due to their similarity with DNA-sequence-based biomarker approaches [55]. There is currently one validated epigenetic test commercially available, ConfirmMDx (MDxHealth, Irvine, CA, USA), designed for diagnostic rather than prognostic purposes, that uses the methylation profile of three genes (*APC, RASSF1, GSTP1*) to detect cancer in histologically negative biopsies [56]. PCa-derived aberrant DNA methylation patterns have also been detected in liquid biopsies such as blood and urine samples, paving the way for the development of noninvasive molecular tests [57–60].

2. Current State of Prognostic Methylated Biomarkers

A plethora of studies have been conducted over the last two decades investigating DNA methylation-based biomarkers to aid PCa prognosis. The majority of these studies have interrogated primary prostate tumours extracted from RP tissue, whilst others have used prostate tissue from core or needle biopsies, transurethral resection of the prostate (TURP) specimens, as well as tumour-adjacent and benign nonneoplastic prostate specimens. The studies reviewed in this section have been primarily performed on RP tissue, and studies that have used other types of prostate specimens will be noted accordingly. Initial studies in this field, limited by the laboratory techniques available, took the traditional a priori approach of examining genes that had been implicated in biological pathways of PCa. These studies used targeted methylation profiling techniques including methylation-specific PCR (MSP) [61], quantitative methylation-specific PCR (qMSP) [62], pyrosequencing [63,64] and mass spectrometry (MassARRAY EpiTYPER, Agena Bioscience, San Diego, California, USA) [65] to assess the methylation profile of a specific gene of interest (Figure 2). Figure 2 lists other targeted approaches that have also been used to assess methylation in cancer, including ddPCR [66], COBRA [67], high resolution melt curve [68] and headloop MSP [69–71]. With recent advances in the technological capabilities to interrogate the methylome more broadly, the field has transitioned into conducting hypothesis-free genome-wide screens for novel prognostic methylation biomarkers. The candidate and genome-wide studies reviewed below use a range of outcome measures to assess the prognostic value of methylated genes, including low vs. high grade cancers, localised vs. advanced disease, and clinical outcomes such as BCR, metastatic relapse and PCa-specific death (PCa death). Importantly, the clinical outcome most often studied is BCR, defined by an increase in serum PSA levels post-RP. However, there is increasing evidence that BCR is not a sufficient indicator of progression to aggressive lethal disease, with metastatic relapse instead being the clinically relevant endpoint for predicting survival [72,73]. This requires long-term follow-up (≥15 years) for metastatic relapse and PCa death to manifest [16], which many study populations lack, thus reducing their ability to fully evaluate and assess molecular biomarkers of PCa prognosis.

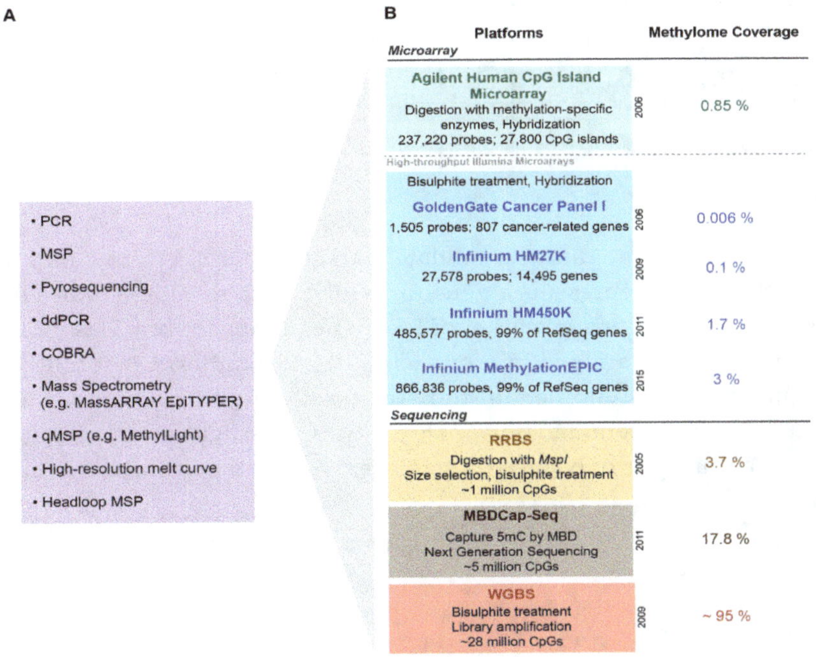

Figure 2. Methylation profiling approaches for biomarker discovery and validation. (**A**) Candidate gene approaches: Targeted candidate gene approaches used in a priori studies and for the validation of novel candidate markers. (**B**) Genome wide approaches: Microarray and sequencing-based genome-wide approaches used for the discovery of novel biomarkers—comparison of the methodology, number of CpGs (cytosine-guanine dinucleotides) and/or genes targeted and coverage of the methylome across the different platforms. RefSeq: Reference Sequences; PCR: polymerase chain reaction; MSP: methylation-specific PCR; ddPCR: droplet digital PCR; COBRA: combined bisulphite restriction analysis; qMSP: quantitative methylation-specific PCR; HM: human methylation; RRBS: reduced representation bisulphite sequencing; MBDCap-Seq: methyl-CpG binding domain capture sequencing; WGBS: whole genome bisulphite sequencing.

2.1. Candidate (A Priori) Markers

To date, DNA methylation of over 60 candidate genes has been investigated. To summarise the top candidate markers with the greatest prognostic evidence, this review focuses on genes that have been investigated in at least three studies and used well-defined prognostic outcomes. The studies reporting on these genes are detailed in Table 1. The majority of these studies were performed on RP-derived tissue, when other types of tissue were used (for example, needle biopsies of prostate tissue or urine) this is specified below or within Table 1. Figure 3 visualises the 20 genes examined in these studies and specifies which of these were found to have potential prognostic value in univariate (U) and/or multivariate (M) statistical models (adjusted for clinicopathological variables) of prognosis. Below we discuss the genes that have been most extensively studied and validated across independent studies: *GSTP1*, *APC*, *RARB*, *PITX2*, *CCND2* and *PTGS2*.

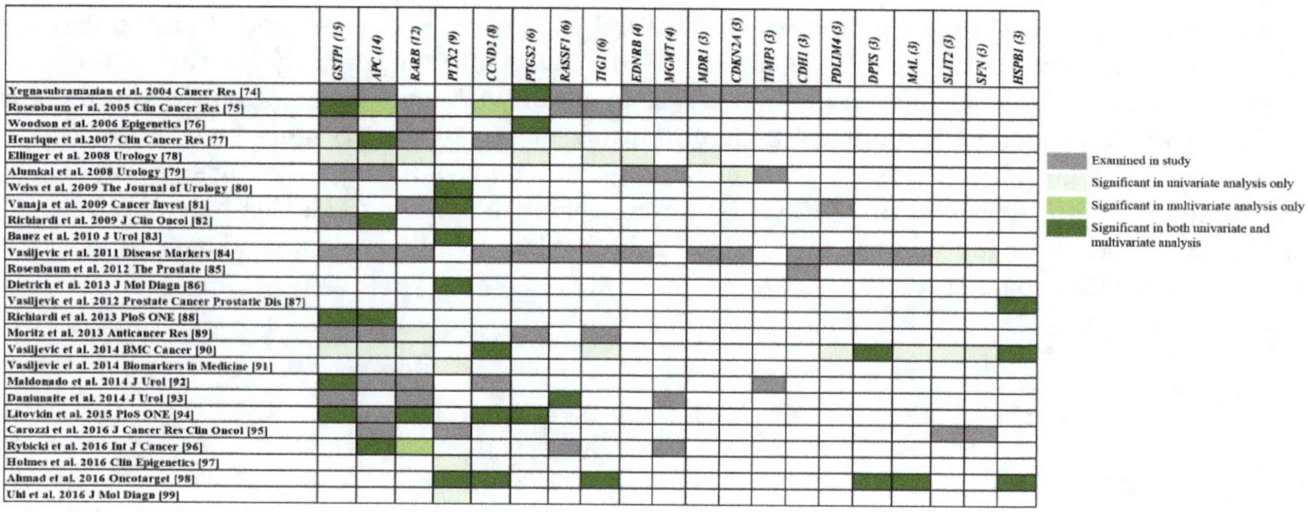

Figure 3. Genes studied in ≥ 3 prognostic candidate marker studies. Each row represents a candidate gene study, and each column represents a gene for which three or more studies have investigated its methylation profile as a prognostic marker of PCa. The number in brackets indicates the number of studies the gene has been examined in. For each of the 26 studies, genes that were investigated have been highlighted: grey = examined in study but no significant associations were found; faded green = significant associations found in univariate analysis only; light green = significant associations observed in multivariate analysis only; green = significant associations reported in both univariate and multivariate analysis.

Table 1. Candidate (a priori) prognostic methylated tissue-based biomarker studies.

Study [Ref] [a]	Primary Outcomes Examined	Total COHORT SIZE	Additional COHORT DETAILS	Follow-Up (Years)	Method	Genes Examined	Genes Validated [b,c,d,e]	Results [g]
Yegnasubramanian et al. [74]	BCR	$n = 36$	n = ns BCR	Range: 8–13	qMSP	*GSTP1, APC, RASSF1, PTGS2, MDR1, HIC1, EDNRB, ESR1, CDKN2a, CDKN2b, p14/QRF, MGMT, hMLH1, TIMP3, DAPK1, CDH1*	U: *PTGS2* M: *PTGS2* [+ GS + pathological T-stage]	U: HR 2.82 (1.07–7.44), $p = 0.04$ M: HR 4.26 (1.36–13.36), $p = 0.01$
Rosenbaum et al. [75]	Primary: Progression Secondary: Metastatic relapse and/or PCa death	$n = 74$	$n = 37$ no progression, $n = 37$ progression ($n = 14$ BCR, $n = 16$ metastatic relapse, $n = 7$ PCa death) [all GS 7 (3 + 4)]	Min: 7, Median: 9	qMSP	*APC, CCND2, GSTP1, TIG1, RASSF1, RARB*	Progression: U: *GSTP1* M: [+ age > 60] (1) *GSTP1* + *APC*; (2) *GSTP1* + *APC* and/or *CCND2* Metastatic relapse and/or PCa death: U: None M: None	Progression: U: HR 0.34 (0.13–0.88), $p = 0.03$ M: (1) *GSTP1* [HR 0.23 (0.09–0.64), $p = 0.004$], *APC* [HR 3.0 (1.42–6.32), $p = 0.0004$; (2) *GSTP1* [HR 0.29 (0.11–0.77), $p = 0.01$], *APC* or *CCND2* methylated: [HR 1.84 (0.92–3.72), $p = 0.09$], *APC* + *CCND2* [HR 4.33 (1.52–12.33), $p = 0.01$] Metastatic relapse and/or PCa death: U: non-sig; M: non-sig
Woodson et al. [76]	BCR	$n = 60$	$n = 49$ no BCR, $n = 11$ BCR	Mean (SD): No BCR-6.5 (3.2) BCR-4.7 (2.8)	qMSP	*GSTP1, RARB, CD44, PTGS2*	U: (1) *CD44*; (2) *PTGS2* M: *CD44* + *PTGS2* [+ GS]	U: (1) OR 6.83 (1.67–27.99), $p = 0.008$; (2) OR 4.38 (1.13–17.40), $p = 0.04$ M: *CD44* + *PTGS2* [OR 8.87 (1.85–42.56), $p = 0.006$]
Henrique et al. [77]	Primary: PCa death Secondary: BCR	$n = 83$	$n = 15$ PCa death, $n = 37$ BCR [Sextant biopsy cores]	Median (range): 3.7 (0.5–5)	qMSP	*APC, CCND2, GSTP1, RARB, RASSF1*	PCa death: U: *APC* M: *APC* [+ Clinical T-stage] BCR: U: (1) *APC*; (2) *GSTP1*; (3) *RASSF1* M: *APC* [+ Clinical T-stage]	PCa death: U: Log-rank $p = 0.010$ M: OR 3.51 (1.23–9.96), $p = 0.018$ BCR: U: Log-rank (1) $p = 0.002$; (2) $p = 0.047$; (3) $p = 0.019$ M: OR 2.58 (1.29–5.16), $p = 0.008$
Ellinger et al. [78]	BCR	$n = 41$	$n = 28$ no BCR, $n = 13$ BCR	Mean; median (range): 2.3; 1.7 (0.5–6)	qMSP	*Annexin2, APC, EDNRB, GSTP1, PTGS2, MDR1, RARB, Reprimo, TIG1*	U: (1) *APC* + *Reprimo*, (2) > 5 genes hypermethylated together M: None	U: Log-rank (1) $p = 0.0078$; (2) $p = 0.0074$ M: non-sig
Alumkal et al. [79]	BCR	$n = 151$	$n = 104$ no BCR, $n = 47$ BCR	At least 5 years	Nested MSP	*GSTP1, MGMT, ASC, CDKN2A, EDNRB, CDH13, CD44, TIMP3, RUNX3, APC, WIF1–*	U: *CDKN2A* M: *CDH13* and/or *ASC* [+ *GS* + extra capsular penetration + seminal vesicle involvement +margin status]	U: OR 0.43 (0.19–0.98), $p = 0.05$ M: *CDH13* [OR 5.51 (1.34–22.67), $p = 0.02$], *CDH13* and/or *ASC* [OR 5.64 (1.47–21.7), $p = 0.01$, sensitivity = 72.3%, specificity = 48%]

Table 1. *Cont.*

Study [Ref] [a]	Primary Outcomes Examined	Total COHORT SIZE	Additional COHORT DETAILS	Follow-Up (Years)	Method	Genes Examined	Genes Validated [b,c,d,e]	Results [g]
Weiss et al. [80]	BCR	$n = 605$	$n = 540$ no BCR, $n = 65$ BCR	Median: 5.5	qMSP	*ABHD9, Chr3-EST, GPR7, HIST2H 2B F, CCND2, PITX2*	U: (1) *ABHD9*; (2) *Chr3-EST*; (3) *GPR7*; (4) *HIST2H 2B F*; (5) *PITX2* (also in GS7 only and GS8 only patients) M: *PITX2* [+ GS + pathological T-stage]	U: (1) HR 1.9 (1.1–3.1), $p = 0.02$; (2) HR 2.1 (12–3.5), $p = 0.007$; (3) HR 2.3 (1.4–3.9), $p = 0.002$; (4) HR 1.9 (1.1–3.1), $p = 0.018$; (5) HR 3.4 (1.9–6.0), $p < 0.001$, GS7 log-rank $p = 0.007$, GS8 log-rank $p = 0.023$ M: HR 2.5 (1.1–5.8), $p = 0.032$
Vanaja et al. [81]	Recurrence within 5 years	$n = 64$	$n = 32$ no recurrence, $n = 32$ recurrence ($n = 10$ BCR, $n = 10$ local, $n = 12$ metastatic relapse)	Range: 0–5	MassARRAY EpiTYPER	*FLNC, EFS, ECRG4, RARB, PITX2, GSTP1, PDLIM4, KCNMA1*	U: (1) *FLNC* (6 CpG units), (2) *GSTP1* (3 CpG units), (3) *PITX2* (1 CpG unit), (4) *EFS* (1 CpG unit) (5) Methylation score: top 11 CpG units from *FLNC, EFS, PITX2, PDLIM4, KCNMA1* (also subgroups of patients with local recurrence, metastatic relapse and BCR) M: Methylation score [+p re-op PSA + GPSM prognostic score using weighted sum of GS, PSA, seminal vesicle involvement and marginal status]	U: (1) Sensitivity = 71.43–78.57%/Specificity = 62.52–75.12%; (2) 63.33–76.92%/72.73–81.82%; (3) 66.67%/64.29%; (4) 62.50%/60.02%; (5) 71.12%/71.90%; local recurrence only: 80.32%/81.2%; metastatic relapse only: 72.72%/75.14%; BCR: 60.26%/59.42% M: Sensitivity = 80%, Specificity = 81.2%, AUC 0.852
Richiardi et al. [82]	PCa death	1980s cohort: $n = 216$ 1990s cohort: $n = 243$	1980s cohort: $n = 95$ no PCa death, $n = 121$ PCa death 1990s cohort: $n = 167$ no PCa death $n = 76$ PCa death	Median (range): 1980s cohort—3.1 (0–14) 1990s cohort—6.3 (0–14)	MSP	*APC, RUNX3, GSTP1*	1980s cohort: U: *APC* M: *APC* [+ source of tumour tissue + GS + follow-up duration] 1990s cohort: U: (1) *APC*, (2) *RUNX3* M: [+ source of tumour tissue + GS + follow-up duration] (1) *APC*; (2) *APC* (GS < 8 only); (3) *RUNX3*; (4) *RUNX3* (GS < 8 only)	(p-values not specified in this study) 1980s cohort: U: HR 1.46 M: HR 1.42 (0.98–2.07) 1990s cohort: U: (1) HR 1.99; (2) HR 1.74 M: (1) HR 1.57 (0.95–2.62); (2) HR 2.09 (1.02–4.28); (3) HR 1.56 (0.95–2.56); (4) HR 2.40 (1.18–4.91)
Banez et al. [83]	BCR	$n = 476$	$n = 370$ no BCR, $n = 106$ BCR	ns	qMSP	*PITX2*	U: *PITX2* (also in GS7 patients only) M: *PITX2* [+ GS + pathological T-stage + margin status] (also in GS7 patients only)	U: HR 2.99 (1.99–4.48), $p < 0.001$; GS7 only: HR 2.0 (1.2–3.3), $p = 0.005$; M: HR 2.39 (1.45–3.94), $p < 0.001$, C-index = 0.77; GS7 only: HR 1.87 (1.1–3.1), $p = 0.02$

Table 1. *Cont.*

Study [Ref] [a]	Primary Outcomes Examined	Total COHORT SIZE	Additional COHORT DETAILS	Follow-Up (Years)	Method	Genes Examined	Genes Validated [b,c,d,e]	Results [g]
Vasiljevis et al. [84]	Low vs. High GS	$n = 48$	$n = 9$ GS6, $n = 23$ GS7, $n = 7$ GS8, $n = 9$ GS9–10	NA	Pyro sequencing	*RARB, GSTP1, HIN1, APC, BCL2, CCND2, CDH13, EGFR5, NKX2–5, RASSF1, DPYS, MDR1, PTGS2, EDNRB, MAL, PDLIM4, HLAa, TIG1, ESR1, SLIT2, CDKN2A, MCAM, SFN, THRB, CDH1, TWIST1*	U: *SFN, SLIT2, SERPINB5* (pairwise measures) M: Not conducted	U: *SFN* + *SERPINB5*: correctly classified 81% of high GS; *SFN* + *SLIT2*: 62%; *SERPINB5* + *SLIT2*: 62% M: NA
Rosenbaum et al. [85]	Primary: Progression Secondary: Metastatic relapse and/or PCa death	$n = 95$	$n = 47$ no progression, $n = 48$ progression ($n = 22$ BCR only, $n = 17$ metastatic relapse, $n = 9$ PCa death) [all GS 7 (3 + 4)]	All: At least 8 years No progression (Median (range))—10 (8–14) Progression (Median)—8	qMSP	*RBM6, MT1G, CDH1, AIM1, KIF1A, PAK3*	Progression: U: *AIM1* M: *AIM1* [+ age at diagnosis + lymph node status] Metastatic relapse and/or PCa death: U: None M: None	Progression: U: HR 0.4 (0.18–0.89), $p = 0.02$ M: HR = 0.45 (0.2–1.0), $p = 0.05$ Metastatic relapse and/or PCa death: U: non-sig M: non-sig
Vasiljevic et al. [86]	PCa death	$n = 349$	$n = 258$ no PCa death, $n = 91$ PCa death	Median (max): 9.5 (20)	Pyro sequencing	*HSPB1*	U: *HSPB1* (in all samples and in subgroup of GS < 7) M: *HSPB1* [+ GS + extent of disease (proportion of TURP) + PSA + *HSPB1* × GS interaction term]	U: HR 1.77 (per 50% increase) (1.13–2.79), $p = 0.02$; GS < 7: $p = 0.028$ M: *HSPB1* [HR 1.18 (per 10% increase) (0.98–1.41), $p = 0.075$], *HSPB1* × *GS* [0.98 (0.97–0.99), $p = 0.014$]; model with *HSPB1* vs. clinical variables only: $\Delta\chi^2 = 6.673$, df = 2, $p = 0.036$
Dietrich et al. [87]	BCR	Training cohort: $n = 157$ Testing cohort: $n = 523$	Training cohort: n = ns BCR Testing cohort: $n = 414$ no BCR, $n = 109$ BCR (same cohort as Banez et al. [83])	ns	qMSP	*PITX2*	Training cohort: U: *PITX2* M: Not conducted Testing cohort: U: *PITX2*, (2) *PITX2* (subgroup of ≥ 75% tumour content), (3) *PITX2* (subgroup of GS7 and ≥ 75% tumour content) M: (1) *PITX2* [+ GS + pathological T-stage + PSA + surgical margins]; (2) *PITX2* [+ tumour cell content + pathological T-stage]	Training cohort: U: 3.479 (1.2599˘C.614), *p*-value not given M: NA Testing cohort: U: HR 2.614 (1.79–53.807), $p < 0.001$; (2) log-rank $p < 0.001$; (3) log-rank $p = 0.003$ M: (1) HR 1.814 (1.232–2.673), $p = 0.003$; (2) HR 1.889 (1.259–2.832), $p = 0.002$

Table 1. *Cont.*

Study [Ref] [a]	Primary Outcomes Examined	Total COHORT SIZE	Additional COHORT DETAILS	Follow-Up (Years)	Method	Genes Examined	Genes Validated [b,c,d,e]	Results [g]
Richiardi et al. [88]	PCa death	$n = 157$	$n = 114$ no PCa death, $n = 43$ PCa death [Non-neoplastic tissue adjacent to prostate tumour] [nested in the 2 cohorts of Richiardi et al. [82]]	Median (range): 6.8 (0.03–24.1)	qMSP	*APC, GSTP1*	U: (1) *APC*, (2) *GSTP1* M: *APC* + *GSTP1* [+ age at diagnosis + year of diagnosis + source of tumour tissue + methylation in prostate tumour tissue + GS] (also in restricted analyses of first 5 years of follow-up)	U: (1) HR 2.38 (1.23–4.61), *p*-value not given; (2) HR 2.92 (1.49–5.74), *p*-value not given M: *APC* + *GSTP1* [HR 2.40 (1.15–5.01), $p = 0.032$]; first 5 yrs follow-up: HR 3.29 (1.27–8.52), $p = 0.019$
Moritz et al. [89]	BCR	$n = 84$	$n = 31$ no BCR, $n = 53$ BCR [GS 5–7]	Mean; median (range): 4; 1.8 (0–10.9)	qMSP	*APC, GSTP1, PTGS2, RARB, TIG1*	U: *RARB* M: None	U: HR 2.686 (1.147–6.291), $p = 0.023$ M: non-sig
Vasiljevic et al. [90]	PCa death	$n = 367$	$n = 268$ no PCa death, $n = 99$ PCa death [TURP tissues of men who chose not to be treated for at least 6 months following diagnosis—TAPG cohort]	Median (range): 9.5 (0.7–19.6)	Pyro sequencing	*GSTP1, APC, RARB, CCND2, SLIT2, SFN, SERPINB5, MAL, DPYS, TIG1, HIN1, PDLIM4* and *HSPB1*	U: (1) *GSTP1*; (2) *APC*; (3) *RARB*; (4) *CCND2*; (5) *SLIT2*; (6) *SFN*; (7) *MAL*; (8) *DPYS*; (9) *TIG1*; (10) *HIN1*; (11) *PDLIM4*; and (12) *HSPB1* M: *DPYS* + *HSPB1* + *CCND2* [+ GS, PSA + HSPB1 × GS interaction term]	U: All genes had an HR (per 10% increment) between 1.09 and 1.28, and *p* between 2.9×10^{-6} and 0.029. M: *DPYS* [HR 1.13 (1.03–1.25), $p = 0.012$], *HSPB1* [HR 2.39 (1.15–4.97), $p = 0.019$], *CCND2* [HR 0.86 (0.75–0.98), $p = 0.024$], *HSPB1* × *GS* [HR 0.89 (0.81–0.97), $p = 0.012$], C-index = 0.83 (vs. 0.74 for GS + PSA only)
Vasiljevic et al. [91]	PCa death	$n = 135$	$n = 90$ no PCa death, $n = 45$ PCa death [all GS ≤ 7] [subset of cohort from Vasiljevic et al. [90]]	No PCa death (Mean)—7.8 PCa death (Median (max))—15.3 (20)	Pyro sequencing	*PITX2, WNT5A, SPARC, EPB4L 1L 3* and *TPM4*	U: *PITX2* (FDR adjustment = 5%) M: not conducted	U: OR 1.56 (per 10% increment) (1.17–2.08), adjusted $p = 0.005$ M: NA
Maldonado et al. [92]	Progression	$n = 452$	$n = 193$ no progression, $n = 259$ progression	Range: 3–11	qMSP	*AIM1, APC, CCND2, GPX3, GSTP1, MCAM, RARB, SSBP2, TIMP3*	U: *GSTP1* M: *GSTP1* [+ age at surgery + pre-op PSA + positive surgical margins + surgery year + pathological T-stage + GS] (organ confined disease only)	U: Wilcoxon rank sum test $p = 0.01$ M: OR 1.73 (1.00–3.02), $p = 0.05$
Daniunaite et al. [93]	BCR	$n = 149$	n = ns BCR	No BCR (Median (range))—3.4 (0.2–5.5)	qMSP	*RARB, GSTP1, RASSF1, MGMT, DAPK1, p16* and *p14*	U: (1) *RASSF1*; (2) *DAPK*; (3) *RASSF1* +/or *DAPK1* M: *RASSF1* [+pT] (GS6 only)	U: (1) HR 2.27 (1.12–4.63), $p = 0.019$; (2) HR 2.55 (1.11–5.84), $p = 0.045$; (3) HR 2.20 (1.06–4.54), $p = 0.027$ M: HR 5.81 (1.08–31.22), $p = 0.042$

Table 1. *Cont.*

Study [Ref] [a]	Primary Outcomes Examined	Total COHORT SIZE	Additional COHORT DETAILS	Follow-Up (Years)	Method	Genes Examined	Genes Validated [b,c,d,e]	Results [g]
Litovkin et al. [94]	Clinical Failure	Training cohort: $n = 147$ Validation cohort: $n = 71$	Training cohort: $n = 117$ no CF $n = 30$ CF Validation cohort: $n = 58$ no CF $n = 13$ CF [High-risk PCa patients: Clinical stage ≥ T3a, GS 8–10 and/or PSA > 20 ng/mL]	Median (range): Training cohort—6.8 (0.1–12.8) Validation cohort—11.5 (1.4–18.8)	Multiplex qMSP	*APC*, *CCND2*, *GSTP1*, *PTGS2* and *RARB*	Training cohort: U: (1) *GSTP1* (trichotomized); *PTGS2* M: [+ pathological T-stage + GS + pre-op PSA] (1) *GSTP1* (trichotomized); (2) *PTGS2* Validation cohort: U: (1) *GSTP1* (trichotomized); (2) *CCND2*; (3) *RARB* M: [+ pathological T-stage + GS + pre-op PSA] (1) *GSTP1* (trichotomized); (2); (3) *RARB*	Training cohort: U: (1) HR 2.96 (1.38–6.36), $p = 0.005$; (2) HR 0.39 (0.18–0.81), $p = 0.013$ M: (1) HR 3.65 (1.65–8.07), $p = 0.001$, C-index = 0.72 (vs. 0.68 for stage + GS + PSA only); (2) HR 0.21 (0.09–0.50), $p < 0.001$ Validation cohort: U: (1) HR 3.34 (1.38–4.87), $p = 0.003$; (2) HR 0.21 (0.07–0.65), $p = 0.007$; (3) HR 3.45 (1.09–10.87), $p = 0.035$ M: (1)HR 4.27 (1.03–17.72), $p = 0.046$, C-index = 0.80 (vs. 0.75 for stage + GS + PSA only); (2) HR 0.19 (0.05–0.79), $p = 0.022$; (3) HR 3.81 (1.09–13.34), $p = 0.036$
Carozzi et al. [95]	PCa death (within 10 yrs of diagnosis)	$n = 129$	$n = 91$ alive > 10 yrs, $n = 38$ died ≤ 10 years [Needle biopsy specimens]	ns	Pyro sequencing	*APC*, *SFN*, *SERPINB5*, *SLIT2*, *PITX2*, *AR*	U: *SERPINB5* [f] M: None	U: 2nd quartile [OR 1.54 (0.56–4.23)], 3rd quartile [HR 2.42 (0.91–6.49); $p = 0.0474$ M: non-sig
Rybicki et al. [96]	BCR	$n = 353$	$n = 262$ no BCR, $n = 91$ BCR (White: $n = 152$ no BCR, $n = 54$ BCR African American: $n = 110$ no BCR, $n = 37$ BCR) [Benign prostate specimens—patients who eventually developed PCa]	Median (range): No BCR-6.3 (1–19) BCR-1.9 (0.2–14)	Nested MSP	*RARB*, *APC*, *CTNND2*, *RASSF1* and *MGMT*	U: APC (White patients) M: (1) *APC* (White patients) [+ age at diagnosis + tumour stage + GS + pre-op PSA, treatment type]; (2) *APC* (White patients) [+ no other gene methylated + low PSA at cohort entry + inflammation was present]; (3) *RARB* (African American patients) [+ another gene methylated + absence of inflammation]	U: HR 2.07 (1.15–3.74), $p = 0.02$ M: (1) HR 2.26 (1.23–4.16), $p = 0.01$; (2) HR 3.28 (1.33–8.11), $p = 0.01$; (3) HR = 3.80 (1.07–13.53), $p = 0.04$
Holmes et al. [97]	BCR	Cohort 1 (TCGA): $n = 498$ Cohort 2: $n = 300$	Cohort 1: $n =$ ns BCR Cohort 2: $n =$ ns BCR	Mean; median: Cohort 1—1.83; 1.3 Cohort 2—5.5; 5.2	Cohort 1—HM450K Microarray Cohort 2—qMSP	*PITX3*, *PITX2*	Cohort 1: U: (1) *PITX3*; (2) *PITX3* + *PITX2* M: Not conducted Cohort 2: U: (1) *PITX3*; (2) *PITX2*; (3) *PITX3* + *PITX2* M: Not conducted	Cohort 1 U: (1) HR 1.83 (1.07–3.11), $p = 0.027$; (2) HR 2.20 (1.25–3.87), $p = 0.006$; (3) LR = 12.70, log-rank $p = 0.002$ M: NA Cohort 2: U: (1) HR 2.56 (1.44–4.54), $p = 0.001$; (2) see Reference 99; (3) LR = 12.14, log-rank $p = 0.002$ M: NA

Table 1. *Cont.*

Study [Ref] [a]	Primary Outcomes Examined	Total COHORT SIZE	Additional COHORT DETAILS	Follow-Up (Years)	Method	Genes Examined	Genes Validated [b,c,d,e]	Results [g]
Ahmad et al. [98]	PCa death	$n = 385$	$n = 328$ no PCa death, $n = 57$ PCa death [low (0–2) to intermediate (3–5) risk CAPRA scores] [from TAPG cohort in Vasiljevic et al. [90]]	Median (IQR): 11.36 (6.20–14.72)	Pyro sequencing	*HSPB1, CCND2, TIG1, DPYS, PITX2, MAL*	Methylation score: HSPB1 + CCND2 + TIG1 + NPYS + PITX2 + MAL + CCND2 · HSPB1 interaction term. U: Methylation score M: Methylation score [+ CAPRA]	U: HR 2.72 (1.933.8), $p < 10^{-8}$ M: HR 2.02 (1.402.92), $p < 10^{-3}$, C-index of full model = 0.74 Sensitivity = 83%, Specificity = 44% (vs. CAPRA only: 68%/44%) At 10 yr follow-up: AUC = 0.74 (vs. CAPRA only: 0.62)
Uhl et al. [99]	Cohort 1: BCR Cohort 2: ISUP grade group (as surrogate for survival)	$n = 206$	Cohort 1: $n = 208$ no BCR, $n = 52$ BCR [same cohort as Cohort 2 in Holmes et al. [97]] Cohort 2: $n = 32$ [core needle biopsy specimens]	Cohort 1 (Mean; median (range))—5.5; 5.2 (0–12.1) Cohort 2—NA	qMSP	*PITX2*	Cohort 1: U: *PITX2* M: None Cohort 2: U: *PITX2* (median, mean and maximum levels) M: Not conducted	Cohort 1: U: HR 1.77 (1.01–3.10), $p = 0.046$ M: non-sig Cohort 2: U: median [$r = 0.456, p = 0.010$]; mean [$r = 0.478, p = 0.007$]; maximum [$r = 0.495; p = 0.005$] M: NA

Abbreviations: AUC = area under the curve; CF = clinical failure; df = degrees of freedom; GS = Gleason Score; HR = hazard ratio; IQR = interquartile range; LR = likelihood ratio; M = multivariate analysis; MSP = methylation-specific PCR; NA = not applicable; non-sig = nonsignificant; ns = not specified; OR = odds ratio; PCa = prostate cancer; PSA = prostate-specific antigen; qMSP = quantitative methylation-specific PCR; r = correlation coefficient; U = univariate analysis. Definitions: BCR: Biochemical recurrence—PSA elevations ≥ 0.2 ng/mL post-RP, except [77] >0.4 ng/mL and [89] >0.1 ng/mL; clinical failure: either of local recurrence or metastatic relapse; clinical T-stage: tumour staging based on results of digital rectal examination, PSA levels and GS. Local recurrence: cancer observed on prostatic bed, confirmed by histological analysis of biopsies; metastatic relapse: metastatic deposits (visceral, bony metastasis) confirmed by positive biopsies or cT/bone scans; pathological T-stage: tumour staging based on pathological examination of surgically removed prostate tissue; PCa death: prostate cancer-specific death; progression: either of BCR, metastatic relapse or PCa death; recurrence: either of BCR, local recurrence or metastatic relapse. [a] All studies are on prostate cancer tissues from radical prostatectomy, unless specified. [b] Univariate (U) or Multivariate (M) analyses. [c] Plus (+) sign indicates variables in the same multivariate model or methylation score together. [d] Square bracket ([[]) indicate the clinicopathological factors adjusted for in each multivariate model. [e] The use of bracketed numbers; e.g., (1), (2), indicates different genes, sets of genes or multivariate models validated in the respective study. [f] Genes validated may have been impacted by high number of missing cases. [g] Number in brackets following HR or OR indicate the 95% confidence interval.

2.1.1. GSTP1

The *glutathione S-transferase pi* gene (*GSTP1*) is the most well-studied DNA methylation biomarker of PCa, particularly in diagnosis [100]. It encodes glutathione *S*-transferase, a detoxifying enzyme and tumour suppressor involved in drug metabolism and protecting DNA from oxidative damage [101]. Hypermethylation (increased methylation) of *GSTP1* is observed frequently in PCa tissue but rarely in histologically negative prostate tissues [102]. We identified 15 candidate prognostic biomarker studies that have studied *GSTP1* methylation, with its prognostic value validated in 8 of these studies (Table 1). The earliest of these studies assessed *GSTP1* methylation using qMSP in a cohort of GS 7 (3 + 4) patients (n = 74), and reported that *GSTP1* hypermethylation was significantly associated with time to progression (any of BCR, metastatic relapse and/or PCa death) in univariate analysis, and as an independent predictor in multivariate analysis with other candidate genes [75]. Subsequent studies of RP tissue, using qMSP, have again found *GSTP1* to be an independent prognostic factor. Briefly, Maldonado et al. used a large cohort (n = 452) to show that *GSTP1* methylation was a significant independent prognostic factor of progression in a multivariate model adjusting for age at surgery, pre-op PSA, surgery year, surgical margins, pathological T-stage and GS; but only in samples from early, organ-confined disease (n = 183) [92]. Litovkin et. al. found trichotomised *GSTP1* methylation to be an independent prognostic predictor (when adjusted for GS, pathological T-stage and pre-op PSA levels) of clinical failure (see Table 1 for definition) in two cohorts (Training: n = 147, Validation: n = 71) of high-risk PCa patients [94]. In a study of non-neoplastic tissue adjacent to the prostate tumour from PCa patients with follow-up up to 24 years (n = 157), the presence of *GSTP1* methylation increased risk of PCa death by almost 3-fold, and remained an independent prognostic factor in multivariate models in combination with *APC* methylation, GS, age at diagnosis, year of diagnosis, source of tumour tissue and methylation in matched tumour tissue [88]. Another study assessing PCa death, using pyrosequencing of TURP tissue (n = 367), also found univariate associations with *GSTP1* methylation [90].

Two small studies with BCR as the clinical endpoint observed associations with *GSTP1* methylation: (1) in a univariate analysis, using sextant biopsy cores (n = 83) [77] and (2) as part of a multigene signature, using RP tissue (n = 41) [78]. Another small study (n = 64) investigating the broader outcome of recurrence (any of BCR, local recurrence or metastatic relapse) observed associations with *GSTP1* methylation at 3 CpG units in univariate analysis only [81]. Importantly, of the 15 studies assessing *GSTP1* methylation as a prognostic biomarker, 7 studies did not find any prognostic value in *GSTP1* methylation in the prediction of BCR [74,76,79,89,93], low vs. high GS cancers [84] or PCa death [77,82].

2.1.2. APC

APC is a tumour suppressor gene which encodes the adenomatous polyposis coli (APC) protein, with a known role in the cellular processes of tumourigenesis [103]. Hypermethylation of *APC* is observed in PCa tumours [104] and a number of studies have demonstrated its prognostic potential (Table 1). In two of these studies, *APC* hypermethylation was included in multivariate models alongside *GSTP1* methylation to predict progression in GS 7 patients [75] and PCa death (using DNA from non-neoplastic adjacent tissue) [88]. *APC* methylation has also been observed to be an individual methylation marker of BCR [77,96] and PCa death [77,82]. In the study by Henrique et al., methylation levels of 5 genes (*APC, CCND2, GSTP1, RARB, RASSF1*) were quantified by qMSP of DNA extracted from sextant biopsies (n = 83), of which *APC* was the only gene significantly associated with both BCR and PCa death in univariate and multivariate analyses with other clinicopathological factors. [77]. A separate study that used MSP to quantify *APC, RUNX3, GSTP1* reported that *APC* was the only independent prognostic gene in the prediction of PCa death across two cohorts of RP patients, one before PSA-testing was widespread (1980s cohort: n = 216) and one after the introduction of PSA-testing (1990s cohort: n = 243); adjusting for source of tumour tissue, GS and follow-up duration [82]. One study looking at BCR examined *APC* methylation using nested MSP in benign prostate specimens (needle biopsy or TURP) from patients who eventually developed PCa (n = 353) and found associations between *APC* and risk of BCR in White patients only (n = 206), adjusting for age, tumour stage, GS, PSA level and treatment type [96]. Two other studies of *APC* methylation levels reported only univariate associations with risk of BCR [78] and PCa death in TURP tissues [90]. It should be noted that, while these studies provide evidence for the potential prognostic value of *APC* methylation, a number of other studies did not observe such associations with predicting risk of BCR [74,79,89], low vs. high GS [84], clinical failure [94], progression [92] and PCa death within 10 years of diagnosis [95].

2.1.3. RARB

The *RARB* gene encodes the retinoic acid receptor beta protein, a nuclear transcriptional regulator important in cellular signalling in cell growth and differentiation processes, and often silenced and hypermethylated in PCa [105]. In total, 5 of the 12 studies examining *RARB* methylation have reported its potential prognostic utility, of which 2 studies have observed *RARB* methylation levels to be an independent prognostic variable in multivariate models including other clinicopathological factors [94,96]. Briefly, the qMSP study by Litovkin et al., examining prediction of clinical failure in high-risk patients, found dichotomised *RARB* methylation, significant in univariate and multivariate analyses (adjusted for GS, pathological T-stage and PSA) in a small validation cohort (n = 41), but not in the training cohort (n = 71) [94]. In their more recent study, methylation of the *RARB* promoter region significantly increased risk of BCR in African American patients (n = 147), but only when another gene was methylated (*APC, CTNND2, RASSF1* or *MGMT*) and no inflammation was present in the prostate specimen [96]. Other studies reported only univariate associations between methylation and prognosis with the clinical endpoints of PCa death [90] and BCR if hypermethylated alongside four or more candidate genes [78] or in RP patients with GS ≤ 7 [89]. Other studies assessing BCR [76,93], recurrence or progression [75,81,92] and PCa death [77] found no associations with *RARB* methylation.

2.1.4. PITX2

PITX2 encodes the paired-like homeodomain transcription factor 2, induced by the WNT pathway to activate growth regulating genes required for cell-type specific proliferation [106]. Aberrant *PITX2* methylation has been observed in multiple tumour types including breast [107] and PCa [80]. Of nine studies on *PITX2* methylation in Table 1, all but one study, which assessed methylation in benign prostate specimens [96], reported significant associations with risk of progression. The first study by Weiss and colleagues, observed *PITX2* methylation, quantified by qMSP, as the strongest and only independent predictor of BCR, providing additional prognostic information to existing clinicopathological factors of GS and pathological T-stage [80]. A subsequent study of n = 476 patients confirmed the association between *PITX2* hypermethylation, also quantified by qMSP, and increased BCR risk in a multivariate model with GS, pathological T-stage, surgical margin, age and PSA levels [83]. Another study, using samples from the same cohort as [83], plus a smaller training cohort (training cohort: n = 157, testing cohort: n = 523) observed that *PITX2* methylation added prognostic information to GS, pathological T-stage and surgical margins in the prediction of BCR in multivariate cox analysis. Vanaja et al. constructed a methylation score consisting of 11 CpG units across 5 genes (from the EpiTYPER MassARRAY platform, see Table 1) including sites in the *PITX2* promoter region to predict recurrence within 5 years, in a model combined with GS, pre-op PSA, seminal vesicle involvement and margin status, achieving an AUC of 0.852 (Sensitivity/Specificity = 80/81.2%) [81]. In a more recent study investigating PCa death as the clinical endpoint in a large cohort of patient-derived TURP tissue (n = 385), a prognostic model was built on 6 methylation biomarkers (see Table 1) including *PITX2*, and was able to improve on the sensitivity of the Cancer of the Prostate Risk

Assessment (CAPRA) score to predict aggressive PCa at 10 years follow-up with an AUC of 0.74 (Table 1) [98]. A smaller study of risk of PCa death in patients with GS ≤ 7 ($n = 135$, median follow-up of 15 years, TURP tissue specimens), also using pyrosequencing, reported a significant association with increased *PITX2* methylation levels [91]. Two additional studies from the same lab likewise reported univariate associations between *PITX2* methylation and BCR, with no multivariate analysis with clinicopathological factors conducted [97,99]. Additional analyses showed that combinations of both *PITX2* and *PITX3* methylation were associated with BCR [97] and that there was a strong correlation between *PITX2* methylation and ISUP grade group in core needle biopsy specimens [99].

2.1.5. CCND2 and PTGS2

CCND2 and *PTGS2* have been studied in eight and six studies respectively, with four studies reporting modest evidence of potential prognostic value for each gene. Hypermethylation of *CCND2* has been reported as an independent prognostic marker of clinical failure [94], and for prediction of progression [75] and PCa death [90,98] in combination with other markers. Three small studies (each $n \leq 60$) observed associations between higher *PTGS2* methylation and increased risk of BCR [74,76,78] with one study reporting a nine-fold increased risk when combined with *CD44* methylation [76], whilst a larger two-cohort study reported associations with clinical failure in the training cohort only [94].

2.1.6. Other Candidate Genes

Other candidate genes that have been investigated in at least three studies include *RASSF1, TIG1, EDNRB, MGMT, MDR1, CDKN2A, TIMP3, CDH1, PDLIM4, DPYS, MAL, SLIT2, SFN* and *HSPB1* (Table 1). Methylation of four of these genes (*MGMT, CDKN2A, TIMP3, CDH1*) was not found to have any prognostic utility, whilst *EDNRB, MDR1* and *PDLIM4* methylation was only reported to have significant univariate associations with disease risk in one study each (Figure 3). Surprisingly, *RASSF1*, frequently hypermethylated in PCa and part of the ConfirmMDX panel [56], has only been reported to have associations with risk of BCR in two small studies [77,93]. *TIG1* was not observed to be an independent prognostic factor alone, only in combination with other genes for prediction of PCa death in low-to-intermediate-risk patients [98]. Pairwise combinations of high *SLIT2, SFN* and *SERPINB5* methylation were able to classify high from low GS patients in random forest modelling of a small cohort ($n = 48$) [84]. *DPYS, MAL* and *HSPB1* emerge as potential prognostic biomarkers, with *HSPB1* in particular validating as an independent prognostic factor of PCa death in the three studies it has been investigated in [86,90,98]. *SERPINB5* and *AIM1*, the only markers found to have significant associations with progression [95] and overall survival [85] have only been investigated in two small independent studies each thus far, and require further validation in larger cohorts. And finally, new candidate genes from different biological pathways have been explored recently (e.g., *PD1−, PD-L1, CDO1, TFF3, ZNF660*) [108–112] and also require further validation.

In summary, the evidence for the prognostic value of the most extensively studied candidate genes (e.g., *GSTP1, APC, RARB, CCND2, PTGS2*) is conflicting, potentially due to differences in study designs including diversity in sample type, cohort size, clinical endpoints examined, methylation profiling methodologies, analytical approach and clinicopathological factors adjusted for in multivariate analyses. Thus far, *PITX2* methylation has shown the most robust evidence of providing additive prognostic information to traditional clinicopathological markers, in particular in the prediction of BCR progression.

2.2. *Genome-Wide Prognostic Biomarker Discovery Studies*

Technological advancements in microarray and next-generation sequencing technologies over the last decade have enabled hypothesis-free, genome-wide screening for new prognostic methylation biomarkers. Platforms that have been used for epigenome-wide screens include restriction enzyme-based, capture-based and microarray-based platforms, together with next-generation sequencing, summarised in Figure 2. In this section, we summarise genome-wide prognostic methylation biomarker discovery studies in primary PCa tumours, with all but one study performed on RP tissue (Table 2). Table 2 highlights the novel biomarkers that were further validated within the original or subsequent studies, and details the top 20 genes for studies that found a large number of significantly associated markers. We refer readers to the original studies for the full lists of methylation markers. We focus on those studies that used measures of disease risk to identify potential biomarkers (for example, comparing methylation of patients of different GS, or different survival outcomes), rather than studies that compared methylation differences between benign and tumour tissue to identify disease-specific biomarkers, with assessment of their prognostic value as only a secondary step [113–119].

Table 2. Candidate (a priori) prognostic methylated tissue-based biomarker studies.

Study [Ref] [a]	Approach (Discovery)	Cohort Size (Discovery)	Follow-Up (Discovery) [Years]	Approach (Validation)	Cohort Size (Validation)	Method (Validation)	Follow-Up (Validation) [Years]	Final Markers Identified (Validation) [c,d,e,f]	Key Results (Validation) [g]
Restriction-based methylation sequencing platforms [h]									
1. Methylation sensitive arbitrarily primed PCR and methylated CpG island amplification									
Cottrell et al. [120]	Low GS (2–6 with no grade 4 or 5 patterns) vs. High GS (8–10) Early BCR (< 2 yrs post-RP) vs. no early BCR (> 4 yrs)	n = 5 Low GS, n = 5 High GS, n = 5 no early BCR, n = 5 early BCR	Range: 2–4	Low GS vs. High GS Early BCR vs. no early BCR	Cohort 1: n = 304 (130 low GS, 96 high GS; 88 no BCR, 63 BCR) Cohort 2: n = 233 (28 low GS, 27 high GS; 134 no BCR, 59 BCR)	1. Custom methylation oligonucleotide microarray 2. MethyLight (qMSP) [b]	Range: 2–4	Low GS vs. High GS: Cohort 1—U: (1) *ABDH9*, (2) *Chr3-EST*, (3) *GPR7*, (4) *NOTCH*, (5) *KBTBD6*; M: not conducted Cohort 2—U: (1) *ABDH9*, (2) *Chr3-EST*; M: not conducted Early BCR vs. no early BCR: Cohort 1—U: (1) *ABDH9*, (2) *ABDH9* (intermediate GS 6, 7 patients only) (3) *Chr3-EST*, (4) *Chr3-EST* (intermediate GS), (5) *GPR7*, (6) *GPR7* (intermediate GS); M: not conducted Cohort 2—U: (1) *ABDH9*, (2) *ABDH9* (intermediate GS), (3) *Chr3-EST*, (4) *Chr3-EST* (intermediate GS); M: (1) *ABDH9* [+ GS + pathological T-stage + margin status], (2) *Chr3-EST* [+ GS + pathological T-stage + margin status]	Low GS vs. High GS: Cohort 1—U: AUC (all Wilcoxon's $p < 0.001$) (1) 0.71, (2) 0.70, (3) 0.72, (4) 0.71, (5) 0.71; M: NA Cohort 2—U: AUC (all Wilcoxon's $p < 0.001$) (1) 0.77, (2) 0.79; M: NA Early BCR vs. no early BCR: Cohort 1—U: AUC (Wilcoxon's) (1) 0.71 ($p = 0.002$), (2) 0.63 ($p = 0.072$), (3) 0.66 ($p = 0.05$), (4) 0.72 ($p = 0.002$), (5) 0.72 ($p = 0.0002$), (6) 0.70 ($p = 0.005$); M: NA Cohort 2—U: AUC (Wilcoxon's) (1) 0.65 ($p < 0.001$), (2) 0.66 ($p < 0.01$), (3) 0.67 ($p < 0.001$), (4) 0.67 ($p < 0.01$); M: Logistic regression (1) $p = 0.016$; (2) $p = 0.043$, AUC = 0.81 & 0.79 (vs. 0.75 of GS + stage + margin status only)
2. Enhanced Reduced Representation Bisulphite Sequencing									
Lin et al. [121]	Indolent (localised disease, no recurrence) vs. Advanced (aggressive CRPC) PCa	n = 7 indolent, n = 6 advanced	Indolent (range) 5–6 years	Indolent vs. aggressive PCa	n = 16 indolent, n = 8 advanced	MassARRAY EpiTYPER	Indolent 3–7 years	Panel of 13 CpG islands: *KCNC2, ZDHHC1, TBX1, CAPG, RARRES2, GRASP, SAC3D1, TPM4, GSTP1, NKX2–1, FAM107A, SLC13A3, FILIP1L* U: Panel M: Not conducted	U: AUC = 0.975 (Sensitivity = 95%; Specificity = 95%) M: NA
Capture-based methylation sequencing platforms									
MBD (methyl-CpG binding domain)-isolated genome sequencing (MiGS)									
Bhasin et al. [122]	Low GS (6) vs. High GS (8–10)	n = 6 Low GS, n = 9 High GS	NA	Low GS vs. High GS	n = 46 Low GS, n = 203 High GS (TCGA)	HM450K Microarray	NA	U: 101 DMRs including at *CD14, PCDHGA11, EYA1, CCDC8, HOXC4*; M: not conducted	U: LIMMA $p = 2.81 \times 10^{28}$–0.05 (range) M: NA

Table 2. *Cont.*

Study [Ref] [a]	Approach (Discovery)	Cohort Size (Discovery)	Follow-Up (Discovery) [Years]	Approach (Validation)	Cohort Size (Validation)	Method (Validation)	Follow-Up (Validation) [Years]	Final Markers Identified (Validation) [c,d,e,f]	Key Results (Validation) [g]
Microarray-based platforms									
1. Agilent Human CpG Island Microarray									
Kron et al. [123]	Low GS (6 (3 + 3)) vs. High GS (8 (4 + 4))	$n = 10$ Low GS, $n = 10$ High GS	NA	1. Low GS vs. High GS	$n = 20$ low GS vs. $n = 19$ high GS (MethyLight)	MethyLight	NA	U: *HOXD3* (detected in $n = 2$ GS6 vs. $n = 6$ GS8); M: not conducted	Sample size too low for statistical U: 17.3% difference in methylation M: NA
				2. Kron et al. [124] GS ≤ 6 vs. GS7 BCR	$n = 232$ ($n = 101$ GS ≤ 6, $n = 107$ GS 7, $n = 147$ no BCR, $n = 85$ BCR)	MethyLight	Mean (range): 4.4 (0.2–9.5)	GS ≤ 6 vs. GS7-U: *HOXD3*; M: not conducted BCR-U: *HOXD3*; M: *HOXD3* x pathological T-stage interaction term [+ GS + pathological T-stage + margin status]	GS ≤ 6 vs. GS7-U: 10.1% difference in av. PMR values, Mann-Whitney U test $p < 0.001$; M: NA BCR-U: Log-rank $p = 0.043$; M: HOXD3 x pT3a [HR 3.78 (1.09–13.17), $p = 0.037$], HOXD3 x pT3b/pT4 [HR 5.23 (1.31–20.96), $p = 0.019$]
				3. Liu et al. [125] GS≤6 vs. GS7 BCR	$n = 219$ ($n = 138$ GS ≤6, $n = 98$ GS 7, n = ns BCR) (reduced cohort from Kron et al. [124])	MethyLight	ns	GS ≤ 6 vs. GS7-U: (1) *APC*, (2) *TGFβ2*; M: not conducted BCR-U: (1) *APC*, (2) *HOXD3* + *TGFβ2* + *APC*; M: (1) *HOXD3* + *TGFβ2* + *APC* [+ pathological T-stage + GS (7 and ≥8 groups)], (2) *HOXD3* + *TGFβ2* + *APC* [+ pathological T-stage + GS (7 (3 + 4), 7 (4 + 3) and ≥ 8 groups)]	GS ≤ 6 vs. GS7-U: Mann-Whitney U test (1) $p = 0.018$, (2) $p = 0.028$; M: NA BCR-U: Log-rank (1) $p = 0.028$, (2) $p < 0.001$; M: (1) HR 2.01 (1.14–3.57), $p = 0.017$, (2) HR 2.068 (1.155–3.704), $p = 0.014$
				4. Jeyapala et al. [126] BCR	Cohort 1: $n = 435$, $n = 43$ BCR	Cohort 1: HM450K Microarray (TCGA)	Mean (range): Cohort 1: 1.9 (0–12.6)	Cohort 1—U: *GBX2*; M: not conducted	Cohort 1—U: Mann-Whitney Test cg09094860 [$p = 0.003$], cg00302494 [$p = 0.01$]; M: not conducted
					Cohort 2: $n = 254$ ($n = 202$, $n = 52$ BCR, $n = 58$ IDC/C-positive, $n = 196$ IDC/C-negative)	Cohort 2: MethyLight	Cohort 2: 5.7 (0.1–12.3)	Cohort 2—U: *GBX2* (and in IDC/C-negative patients only); M: (1) *GBX2* [+ GS + Pathological T-stage + pre-op PSA], 2) *GBX2* [+ pre-op PSA]	Cohort 2—U: Mann-Whitney Test $p = 0.0001$, IDC/C-negative patients: Log-rank $p = 0.002$; M: (1) HR 1.02 (1.006–1.034), $p = 0.004$, (2) C-index 0.78 (vs. 0.71 for PSA alone)

Table 2. *Cont.*

Study [Ref] [a]	Approach (Discovery)	Cohort Size (Discovery)	Follow-Up (Discovery) [Years]	Approach (Validation)	Cohort Size (Validation)	Method (Validation)	Follow-Up (Validation) [Years]	Final Markers Identified (Validation) [c,d,e,f]	Key Results (Validation) [g]
				5. Jeyapala et al. [127] BCR salvage RT/hormone therapy	Cohort 1: $n = 254$ ($n = 202$ no BCR, $n = 52$ BCR, $n = 205$ no salvage RT, $n = 42$ salvage RT, $n = 226$ no hormone therapy, $n = 21$ hormone therapy) Cohort 2: $n = 199$ ($n = 159$ no BCR, $n = 40$ BCR, $n = 180$ no salvage RT, $n = 19$ salvage RT, $n = 177$ no hormone therapy, $n = 22$ hormone therapy)	MethyLight	Median (range): Cohort 1: 6.7 (0.1–12.8); Cohort 2: 6.7 (0.2–18.6)	4-G model: *HOXD3*, *TGFβ2*, *CRIP3*, *APC* (candidate) Cohort 1 BCR-U: 4-G model; M: Integrative model = 4-G model [+ CAPRA-S] Salvage RT/hormone therapy: U: 4-G model; M: Integrative model Cohort 2 BCR-U: 4-G model; M: Integrative model Salvage RT/hormone therapy: U: 4-G model; M: Integrative model	Cohort 1 BCR-U: HR 2.72 (1.77–4.17), $p < 0.001$, Sensitivity = 90.9%, Specificity = 35.2%, AUC = 0.740; M: HR 1.49 (1.12–1.99), $p = 0.006$, Sensitivity = 92.9%, Specificity = 43.4%, AUC = 0.846 Salvage RT/hormone therapy: U: HR 2.20 (1.48–3.29), $p < 0.001$;M: HR 1.34 (1.03–1.75), $p = 0.027$ Cohort 2 BCR-U: HR 2.48 (1.59–3.86), $p < 0.001$, Sensitivity = 95.0%, Specificity = 27.5%, AUC = 0.670; M: HR 1.62 (1.17–2.24), $p = 0.004$, Sensitivity = 89.5%, Specificity = 37.3%, AUC = 0.726 (vs. 0.698 for CAPRA-S alone) Salvage RT/hormone therapy-U: HR 1.97 (1.21–3.21), $p < 0.001$, Sensitivity = 91.2%, Specificity = 27.4%, AUC = 0.636; M: HR 1.17 (0.79–1.72), $p = 0.441$, AUC = 0.731 (vs. 0.723 for CAPRA-S alone)
				6. Savio et al. [128] BCR; Late BCR (5 and 7 yrs post-RP) salvage RT/hormone therapy [Biopsy specimens pre-RP]	$n = 86$ ($n = 61$ no BCR, $n = 25$ BCR, $n = 75$ no salvage RT, $n = 11$ salvage RT, $n = 70$ no hormone therapy, $n = 15$ hormone therapy)	MethyLight	Median (range): 5.1 (0.1–16)	BCR-U: none; M: 4-G model [+ pre-op PSA] Late BCR-U: none; M: (1) 4-G model [+ pre-op PSA] (5 yrs), (2) 4-G model [+ pre-op PSA] (7 yrs) Salvage RT/hormone therapy: U: 4-G model; M: (1) 4-G model [+ pre-op PSA], (2) 4-G model [+ CAPRA]	BCR: U: non-sig; M: Sensitivity = 78.6%, Specificity = 64.7%, AUC = 0.714 Late BCR: U: non-sig; M: (1) Sensitivity = 80%, Specificity = 60.5%, AUC = 0.705 (vs. 0.667 for PSA alone), (2) Sensitivity = 76.9%, Specificity = 62.9%, AUC = 0.688 (vs. 0.6 for PSA alone) Salvage RT/hormone therapy-U: Sensitivity = 66.7%, Specificity = 75%, AUC = 0.699; M: (1) Sensitivity = 75%, Specificity = 61.1%, AUC = 0.699, (2) Sensitivity = 76.9%, Specificity = 58.3%, AUC = 0.797

Table 2. *Cont.*

Study [Ref] [a]	Approach (Discovery)	Cohort Size (Discovery)	Follow-Up (Discovery) [Years]	Approach (Validation)	Cohort Size (Validation)	Method (Validation)	Follow-Up (Validation) [Years]	Final Markers Identified (Validation) [c,d,e,f]	Key Results (Validation) [g]
2. Illumina GoldenGate Methylation Microarrays									
Goh et al. [129]	Low GS (6) vs. High GS (8–10) Overall survival	$n = 87$ ($n = 19$ GS6, $n = 48$ GS8–10, n = ns death)	Median (range): 4 (0–11.8)	GS (6–9) BCR	$n = 59$ ($n = 23$ GS 6, $n = 22$ GS 7, $n = 13$ GS 8–10, $n = 18$ for BCR analysis)	GoldenGate	No BCR-5 (1–13)	"PHYMA" signature: 55 probes targeting CpG loci of 46 genes, including at *ALOX12*, *PDGFRB* which were selected for functional validation GS: U: PHYMA (GS 6–8) M: not conducted BCR: U: none M: not conducted	GS: U: Logistic regression β-coefficient = 2.28, $p = 0.2$ (trend) M: NA BCR: U: non-sig M: NA
Angulo et al. 2016 Urol Int [130]	• BCR • PCa death	$n = 26$ no BCR, $n = 32$ BCR	Mean ± SD (range): 6.3 ± 3 (0.8–13.8)	No validation	NA	NA	NA	Discovery only: BCR: U: (1) Gene hypermethylation profile of cluster 3 patients (including at *GSTM2*, *GSTP1*, *RARB*, *ALOX12*, *APC*, *PDGFRB*, *SCGB3A1*, *CFTR*, *MT1A*, *PENK*, *NEU1*, *CCNA1*, *MET*, *KLK10*, *RARA*, *MFAP4*, *TERT*, *TBX1*, *TAL*, *MYCL2*, (2) *MT1A*, (3) *ALOX12*, (4) *GSTM2*, (5) *APC*, (6) *MYCL2*, (7) *RARB*, (8) *GSTM2* + *MCLY2* M: (1) Gene hypermethylation profile [+ D'Amico classification]; (2) *GSTM2* [+ ns]; (3) *MCLY2* [+ ns] PCa Death: U: *GSTM2* + *MYCL2* M: not conducted	Discovery only: BCR-U: (1) Log-rank $p = 0.0054$, Cluster 3 vs. 1 [HR 8.4 (1.86–38.46), 3 vs. 2 [HR 2.69 (1.13–5.95), 3 vs. 4 [HR 2.26 (0.89–5.72)]; (2) HR 2.14 (1.06–4.33), log-rank $p = 0.029$; (3) HR 2.21 (1.06–4.55), log-rank $p = 0.025$; (4) HR 4.59 (1.38–15.15), log-rank $p = 0.0062$; (5) HR 1.96 (0.97–3.97), log-rank $p = 0.05$; (6) HR 3.58 (1.6–8), log-rank $p = 0.0009$; (7) HR 2.5 (1.21–5.18), log-rank $p = 0.01$; (8) log-rank $p = 0.0009$; M: (1) Cox regression $p = 0.064$, Cluster 3 vs. 1 [HR 4.37 (0.94–20.41], 3 vs. 2 [HR 2.56 (1.11–5.88)], 3 vs. 4 [HR 2.26 (0.89–5.72)], C-index = 0.708 (vs. 0.679 for D'Amico alone); (2) HR 3.789 (1.11–12.83), $p = 0.03$;(3) HR 2.71 (1.21–6.09), $p = 0.016$ PCa death-U: HR 10.82 (1.96–59.67); log-rank $p = 0.006$; M: NA
3. Illumina Infinium HumanMethylation 27K Microarray									
Kobayashi et al. [131]	BCR	$n = 86$	Range: 0–5.5	No validation	NA	NA	NA	Discovery only: U: *KCNK4*, *WDR86*, *OAS2*, *TMEM179* (FDR ≤ 1%; hypermethylated) M: not conducted	Discovery only: U: ns M:

Table 2. *Cont.*

Study [Ref] [a]	Approach (Discovery)	Cohort Size (Discovery)	Follow-Up (Discovery) [Years]	Approach (Validation)	Cohort Size (Validation)	Method (Validation)	Follow-Up (Validation) [Years]	Final Markers Identified (Validation) [c,d,e,f]	Key Results (Validation) [g]
Mahapatra et al. [132]	Indolent vs. aggressive disease: No recurrence vs. recurrence BCR vs. clinical recurrence Local recurrence vs. metastatic relapse	$n = 75$ no recurrence, $n = 123$ recurrence $n = 43$ BCR, $n = 80$ clinical recurrence $n = 44$ local recurrence, $n = 36$ metastatic relapse	(Mean ± SD): No recurrence 6.2 ± 1.5 BCR: 5.9 ± 1.4 Local recurrence: 4.2 ± 1.7 Metastatic relapse: 4.4 ± 4.0	Indolent vs. aggressive disease: No recurrence vs. recurrence BCR vs. clinical recurrence Local recurrence vs. metastatic relapse	$n = 20$ no recurrence, $n = 20$ BCR, $n = 20$ local recurrence, $n = 20$ metastatic relapse	Pyro sequencing	(Mean ± SD) No recurrence-6.5 ± 1.6 BCR-5.45 ± 1.3 Local recurrence-4.5 ± 1.9 Metastatic relapse-3.5 ± 1.9	No recurrence vs. recurrence: U: (1) *CRIP1*; (2) *RUNX3*; (3) *HS3ST2*; (4) *FLNC*; (5) *RASGRF2* M: Not conducted BCR vs. clinical recurrence: U: (1) *PHILDA3*; (2) *TNFRSF10D*; (3) *RASGRF2* M: Not conducted Local vs. metastatic relapse: U: (1) *BCL11B*; (2) *POU3F3*; (3) *RASGRF2* M: Not conducted	No recurrence vs. recurrence: U: Sensitivity/Specificity, AUC, t-test (1) 65.0%/65.6%, 0.727, $p = 0.0139$; (2) 70.4%/75.3%, 0.788, $p = 0.0018$; (3) 65.0%/60.0%, 0.773, $p = 0.0115$; (4) 70.3%/60.4%, 0.660, $p = 0.0835$; (5) 75.7%/55.2%, 0.682, $p = 0.0515$ M: NA BCR vs. clinical recurrence: U: Sensitivity/Specificity, AUC, t-test (1) 65.6%/65.0%, 0.73, $p = 0.0129$; (2) 60.8%/75.6%, 0.692, $p = 0.0373$; (3) 75.4%/60.3%, 0.761, $p = 0.0047$ M: NA Local recurrence vs. metastatic relapse: U: Sensitivity/Specificity, AUC, t-test (1) 75.2%/60.0%, 0.741, $p = 0.0091$; (2) 65.5%/70.7%, 0.701, $p = 0.0295$; (3) 70.6%/75.4%, 0.748, $p = 0.0071$; M: NA
4. Illumina Infinium HumanMethylation 450K (HM450K) Microarray									
Geybels et al. [133]	Low GS (≤6) vs. High GS (8–10)	$n = 65$ Low GS, $n = 88$ High GS (TCGA)	NA	Progression	$n = 323$ no progression, $n = 108$ progression	HM450K Microarray	Mean (SD): 8.0 (4.2) years	Signature consisting of 52 CpG sites (32 unique genes) including at *RRM2, VWA3B, MFSD9, ANO7, GALNTL2, SEMA3F, ATXN7, SLC15A2, MME, USP17, KIAA0922, FOXI1, URGCP, PTPRN2, RP1, MRPS28, MKI67, CPT1A, KCNMB4, TMEM132D*. U: (1) Signature; (2) Signature (GS7 only); (3) Signature (GS7 (3 + 4) only) M: [+ GS+ pathological T-stage + pre-op PSA] (1) Signature; (2) Signature (GS7 only); (3) Signature (GS7 (3 + 4) only)	U: (1) HR 1.78 (per 25% increase) (1.48–2.16), $p = 2.05 \times 10^{-9}$; (2) HR 1.81 (1.42–2.31), $p = 1.38 \times 10^{-3}$; (3) HR 1.83 (1.36–2.45), $p = 5.64 \times 10^{-5}$ M: (1) HR 1.48 (1.21–1.81), $p = 1.38 \times 10^{-4}$, AUC = 0.78 (vs. 0.73 for GS + pathological T-stage + pre-op PSA only); (2) HR 1.59 (1.24–2.05), $p = 1.38 \times 10^{-6}$, AUC = 0.76 (vs. 0.64); (3) HR 1.65 (121–2.25), $p = 1.54 \times 10^{-3}$, AUC = 0.70 (vs. 0.62)
Zhao et al. [134]	Metastatic-lethal progression	$n = 304$ no progression vs. $n = 24$ metastatic-lethal	Mean: Metastatic relapse-8.1 Survival-12.2	1. Metastatic-lethal progression	$n = 41$ no progression, $n = 24$ metastatic-lethal	HM450K Microarray	Mean: 9	U: (1) *ALKBH5*; (2) *ATP11A*; (3) *FHAD1*; (4) *KLHL8*; (5) *PI15*; (6) Intergenic region (chr1); (7) Intergenic (chr16); (8) Intergenic (chr17) M: [+ GS] (1) *ALKBH5*; (2) *FHAD1*; (3) *KLHL8*; (4) *PI15*	U: Mean β difference (*t*-test), AUC, pAUC (1)—5% ($p = 0.037$), 0.66 ($p = 0.035$), 0.001 ($p = 0.566$); (2)—6% ($p = 0.049$), 0.66 ($p = 0.03$), 0.009 ($p = 0.022$); (3)—6% ($p = 0.007$), 0.71 ($p = 0.003$), 0.004 ($p = 0.159$); (4)—10% ($p = 0.002$), 0.75 ($p = 0.0004$), 0.002 ($p = 0.359$); (5)—7% ($p = 0.029$), 0.68 ($p = 0.014$), 0.006 ($p = 0.074$); M: AUC, pAUC, *p* (from likelihood ratio test comparing with model with GS alone: AUC = 0.816, pAUC = 0.010) (1) 0.87, 0.024, $p = 0.030$; (2) 0.86, 0.013, $p = 0.038$; (3) 0.89, 0.008, $p = 0.014$; (4) 0.89, 0.006, $p = 0.026$

Table 2. *Cont.*

Study [Ref] [a]	Approach (Discovery)	Cohort Size (Discovery)	Follow-Up (Discovery) [Years]	Approach (Validation)	Cohort Size (Validation)	Method (Validation)	Follow-Up (Validation) [Years]	Final Markers Identified (Validation) [c,d,e,f]	Key Results (Validation) [g]
				2. Zhao et al. [135] Metastatic-lethal progression	Training dataset (from Zhao et al. [134]): $n = 344$ no recurrence, $n = 48$ metastatic-lethal; Testing dataset: $n = 11$ no recurrence, 23 metastatic-lethal	Pyro sequencing	Training (Mean (minimum))—8 (5) Testing At least 5 years	Methylation score: *ALKBH5* + *ATP11A* + *FHAD1* + *KLHL8* + *PI15* [+ GS] Training-U: not conducted; M: Methylation score Testing-U: not conducted; M: Methylation score	Training-U: NA; M: Logistic regression β-coefficient-ALKBH5 [−0.75], ATP11A [−0.7], FHAD1 [−9.72], KLHL8 [−0.33], PI15 [0.70], GS [1.13] Testing-U: NA; M: Mean difference = 2.49 ($p = 6.8 \times 10^{-6}$), OR 4.0 (1.8–14.3), $p = 0.006$, AUC = 0.91 (vs. 0.87 for GS alone), pAUC = 0.037 (vs. 0.025 for GS alone), sensitivity at 95% specificity = 74% (vs. 53% for GS alone)
Mundbjerg et al. [136]	Aggressiveness (individual PCa foci vs. matched lymph node metastasis)	$n = 14$ ($n = 92$ samples: multiple tumour foci, adjacent normal tissue, lymph node metastases and normal lymph nodes)	NA	Aggressive (lymph node metastases and pathological stage T3 tumours) vs. non-aggressive	$n = 351$ (TCGA)	HM450K Microarray	Mean: 3.2 years	Aggressiveness classifier: 25 probes, including in *NXPH2, NCAPH, TRIB1, PCDHA1-PCDHA8, C3orf37, C9orf3, CPN1, TCF7L2, ROBO1, GFPT2, FBXQ47, SKI, HDAC9, CARS, SLC6A17, BCAT1, GAS1, RAI1* U: Aggressiveness classifier M: Not conducted	U: Specificity = 97.4%, Sensitivity = 96.2%, Negative predictive value = 76%, Positive predictive value = 99.7%, Lymph node metastases [Fishers exact test $p = 9.2 \times 10^{-5}$], pathological stage T3 [Fishers exact test $p = 2.2 \times 10^{-7}$] M: NA
Toth et al. [137]	Good prognosis vs. Poor prognosis	$n = 35$ good prognosis, $n = 35$ poor prognosis (80% training set, 20% testing set)	Range: 3–5	Good prognosis vs. poor prognosis (Cohort 1, 2) BCR (Cohort 1, 2, 3)	Cohort 1: $n = 222$ ($n = 63$ for prognosis analysis, n = ns BCR) (ICGC cohort [138]) Cohort 2: $n = 477$ ($n = 27$ good prognosis, 57 poor prognosis, n = ns BCR) (TCGA) Cohort 3: $n = 12{,}581$ ($n = 3612$ BCR) (for ZIC2 immunostaining analysis only)	HM450K Microarray	Cohort 1 & 2 At least 5 years Cohort 3 (Median (range)) 4 (0.08–20.08)	Signature consisting of 598 CpG sites. Top 20: *CCT8L2, NOP56, FCRL1, OR5W2, ZFP36L2, PRMT8, SLC1A6, DOK5, CCT8L2, ZFP36L2, MMP16, ESR1, ZIC2, GPR137B, NANOS1, LCE3A, C11orf87, PEG3, ZIM2, CTSC* Good prognosis vs. good prognosis: Cohort 1—U: (1) Signature, M: not conducted Cohort 2—U: Signature; M: not conducted BCR: Cohort 1—U: Signature, M: not conducted Cohort 2—U: Signature; M: Signature [+ GS] Cohort 3—U: ZIC2 protein; M: ZIC2 protein [+ GS + pathological T-stage + nodal stage + PSA]	Good vs. poor prognosis: Cohort 1—U: AUC = 0.997; M: NA Cohort 2—U: AUC = 0.775; M: NA BCR: Cohort 1—U: Log-rank $p < 0.0001$, M: NA Cohort 2—U: Log-rank $p < 0.0001$; M: Cox regression $p = 0.011$ Cohort 3—U: Log-rank $p < 0.0001$; M: ns

Abbreviations: AUC = area under the curve; av. = average, CAPRA-S = Cancer of the Prostate Risk Assessment Score; CRPC = Castration-Resistant Prostate Cancer; GS = Gleason Score; HR = hazard ratio; IDC/C = Intraductal Carcinoma and Cribriform Architecture; M = multivariate analysis; NA = not applicable; non-sig = nonsignificant; ns = not specified; OR = odds ratio; pAUC = partial area under the cure; PCa = prostate cancer; PMR = percent methylated ratio; PSA = prostate- specific antigen; RT = radiotherapy; U = univariate analysis. Definitions: BCR: Biochemical recurrence: PSA elevations ≥ 0.2n g/mL post-RP, except [130] > 0.4 ng/mL and [131] > 0.07 ng/mL; clinical recurrence = local recurrence or metastatic relapse; good prognosis: organ-confined disease (pT2) and lack of BCR for at least 5 years; local recurrence: cancer observed on prostatic bed, confirmed by histological analysis of biopsies; metastatic relapse: metastatic deposits (visceral, bony metastasis) confirmed by positive biopsies or cT/bone scans; metastatic-lethal progression = metastatic relapse or PCa death; pathological T-stage: tumour staging based on pathological examination of surgically removed prostate tissue; PCa death: prostate cancer-specific death; poor prognosis: systemic presence of metastatic disease, indicated by recurrence within 3 years and no response to local radiation therapy; progression: either of BCR, metastatic relapse or PCa death; recurrence: either of BCR, local recurrence or metastatic relapse. [a] All studies are on prostate cancer tissues from radical prostatectomy, unless specified. [b] MethylLight is a quantitative methylation-specific PCR (qMSP) platform. [c] Univariate (U) or Multivariate (M) analyses. [d] Plus (+) sign indicates variables in the same multivariate model or methylation score together. [e] Square bracket ([]) indicate the clinicopathological factors adjusted for in each multivariate model [f] The use of bracketed numbers; e.g., (1), (2), indicates different genes, sets of genes or multivariate models validated in the respective study. [g] Number in brackets following HR or OR indicate the 95% confidence interval. [h] Bolded headings within the table subdivide the different types of genome-wide platforms (restriction-based, capture-based or microarray-based) used in these studies.

2.2.1. Restriction-Based Methylation Sequencing Studies

The first genome-wide prognostic methylation biomarker discovery study in 2007 used methylation-sensitive arbitrarily primed PCR [139] and methylation CpG island amplification [140] to find markers that could distinguish between patients with high GS (8–10, $n = 5$) vs. those with low GS (2–6 with no grade 4 or 5 patterns; $n = 5$), as well as markers that could predict early BCR following RP ($n = 5$ no BCR (> 4 yrs), $n = 5$ early BCR (< 2 yrs)) [120]. In this approach, methylation-(in)sensitive restriction enzymes were used to digest DNA, and the resulting fragments were screened for methylation differences between patient groups, and sequenced if differences were found. The top 51 markers, along with 11 candidate markers, were validated in two large, independent cohorts, using a custom methylation oligonucleotide microarray (Cohort 1, $n = 304$) and MethyLight qMSP assays (Cohort 2, $n = 233$) [120]. *GRP7*, *ABHD9* and *Chr3-EST* were significantly hypermethylated in high GS patients and could distinguish between no BCR and early BCR, independent of patient GS in Cohort 1 [120]. These associations were validated in Cohort 2, where increased methylation of *ABHD9* and *Chr3-EST* correlated with high-grade disease and early BCR, even after adjusting for GS, pathological T-stage and margin status [120]. A subsequent study reported only univariate associations between *ABHD9* methylation and BCR in a larger cohort ($n = 605$) [80], whilst another saw no *ABDH9* methylation difference with BCR status ($n = 407$) [141].

A second restriction enzyme-based method used in genome-wide screening is Enhanced Reduced Representation Bisulphite Sequencing (ERRBS) platform. Similarly, ERRBS involves enzymatic digestion of DNA at CpG sites using *MspI*, followed by size selection and bisulphite sequencing, with the main advantage of enabling single base pair resolution profiling of CpG sites in GC-rich genomic regions such as promoter CpG islands [142,143]. Only one study has used this platform, profiling the methylome of a small discovery set of PCa patients, comparing indolent (localised disease with no recurrence; $n = 7$) vs. advanced cancers (aggressive castration-resistant PCa; $n = 6$) [121]. A series of differentially methylated CpG islands were identified using linear model analysis, and a prognostic panel of 13 hypermethylated CpG islands (see Table 2) was built using random forest classification. This panel successfully discriminated between indolent and advanced cancers in the validation cohort ($n = 16$ indolent, $n = 8$ advanced, MassARRAY EpiTYPER) with an AUC of 0.975 in 10-fold cross validation [121]. Of the genes included in the panel, *GSTP1* has been widely studied as a diagnostic and prognostic biomarker of PCa (see above) [44,45,144], whilst *GRASP* and *TPM4* have been previously shown to be differentially methylated in PCa compared to normal prostate tissue [132].

2.2.2. Capture-Based Methylation Sequencing Studies

Capture-based DNA methylation sequencing for PCa prognostic studies were first used in 2015. The approach involves the capture of methylated sequences by methyl-CpG binding domain (MBD) protein after shearing of genomic DNA, followed by massive parallel sequencing of enriched sequences [145,146]. A limitation of this approach is that it does not provide a single nucleotide resolution, instead identifying regions with multiple methylated CpGs. Only one study has used this method to profile and identify methylation differences between low and high GS tumours ($n = 6$ vs. 9) [122]. They reported hypermethylation of 4932 regions in high-grade disease [122]. Extensive genomic and functional characterisation of these Differentially Methylated Regions (DMRs) were conducted, including comparison with publicly available data from The Cancer Genome Atlas (TCGA) project [147]. This allowed them to validate the association between methylation and high grade disease at 101 DMRs, and show that a subset of these DMRs correlated with gene expression changes that associated with poorer survival in PCa patients, including the *CCDC8* and *HOXD4* gene [122].

2.2.3. DNA Methylation Microarray Studies

Microarrays have become the most popular technology for genome-wide DNA methylation profiling for biomarker discovery. For this method, DNA is first treated to enable later distinction between methylated and unmethylated sites (using methylated DNA immunoprecipitation, methylation-specific restriction enzymes or bisulphite-conversion). The DNA is then hybridised to unique oligonucleotide probes of CpGs on arrays, labelled with a fluorescent dye and imaged, and the signal is used to determine single nucleotide resolution CpG methylation. Several DNA methylation microarrays have been produced, including the Agilent Human CpG Island Microarray [148] (237,220 CpGs) (Figure 2) and Illumina DNA methylation microarrays, with successive array updates interrogating a broader range and number of CpG sites across the genome: GoldenGate Cancer Panel I (1505 CpGs) [149], Infinium HumanMethylation 27K Microarray (HM27K: 27,578 CpGs) [150] and Infinium HumanMethylation 450K Microarray (HM450K: 485,577 CpGs) [151] (Figure 2).

Agilent Human CpG Island Microarray

An initial genome-wide study in 2009 using the Agilent Human CpG Island Microarray [123] laid the foundation for a number of subsequent validation studies [124–128], leading to the identification of several robust methylation markers with prognostic value. The original study screened for methylation differences between patients with GS 6 (n = 10) and GS 8 (n = 10), finding 493 CpG sites (223 individual genes) that could distinguish between the patient groups. A candidate marker, *HOXD3*, was selected and assessed in an independent set of samples (n = 20 GS6 vs. n = 19 GS8), validating *HOXD3* hypermethylation in GS8 compared to GS6 patients. Further studies investigated *HOXD3* [124] and *GBX2* [126] as individual markers of progression, using BCR as their outcome of interest. *HOXD3* was associated with BCR in univariate analysis (n = 147 no BCR, n = 85 BCR), and a methylation score combining *HOXD3* with pathological T-stage was found to be an independent predictor of BCR [124]. *GBX2* methylation was assessed in methylation data from TCGA (n = 435 no BCR, n = 43 BCR), and in a second cohort (n = 202 no BCR, n = 52 BCR). In both cohorts, associations were observed between *GBX2* methylation and BCR, with *GBX2* methylation shown to have potential as an additive predictor when combined with PSA levels at diagnosis (Cohort 2) [126].

The same research team also investigated *HOXD3* in combination with other markers [125,127]. One study combined *HOXD3*, *TGFß2* (another differentially methylated gene from the original discovery study) and *APC*, an a priori candidate marker [125]. Using a cohort from an earlier study [124] (n = 219), they found that this multigene panel improved prediction of BCR over any individual markers, and was independent of existing clinicopathological variables [125]. In another study they used a penalized cox regression method to develop a 4-gene (4-G) prognostic model for BCR, consisting of *APC*, *HOXD3*, *TGFß2* and *CRIP3* [127]. The 4-G model associated with BCR as well as progression to post-surgical therapies (hormone and salvage radiotherapy) in two large cohorts (Cohort 1: n = 202 no BCR, n = 52 BCR; Cohort 2: n = 159, n = 40 BCR) [127]. Most recently, the prognostic ability of the 4-G model was investigated in presurgery prostate biopsy specimens (n = 61 no BCR, n = 25 BCR) [128]. The 4-G methylation panel was able to prognosticate BCR, late recurrence (BCR 5 & 7 yrs post-RP) and eventual progression to postsurgery treatments [127]. Additionally, a study from another team found strong evidence of *HOXD3* hypermethylation in BCR progression (n = 303 no BCR, n = 104 BCR) [141]. These studies provide strong support for *HOXD3* hypermethylation as a robust marker for BCR progression. Further studies examining the prognostic utility of *HOXD3* and other genes in the panel are warranted, particularly in cohorts with more clinically relevant endpoints for aggressive disease, such as metastatic relapse and PCa death.

GoldenGate Cancer Panel I Microarray Platform

Between 2014 and 2016, two research groups published studies using Illumina's GoldenGate Cancer Panel I Microarray platform to identify novel biomarkers for disease risk. In the first study, a Support Vector Machine was used to build a classification model, generating a signature consisting of 55 probes across 46 genes (including *ALOX12*, *PDGFRB*) [129]. The signature, termed "PHYMA", was able to distinguish between low and high GS tumours, and a high PHYMA score associated with poorer survival outcome (adjusted for clinical T-stage and GS) (n = 87). Trending associations between PHYMA score and GS, but not BCR, was observed in a separate cohort (n = 59) [129]. The second study using the GoldenGate Cancer Panel reported that a gene hypermethylation profile based on hierarchical clustering of patients (see Table 2 for details), as well as hypermethylation at individual markers *GSTM2* and *MCLY2*, independently predicted BCR risk. The concurrent methylation of the two markers was also associated with PCa death, however no further validation of the study findings in a separate independent cohort was conducted [130].

HM27K Platform

Two studies published in 2011–2012 used the HM27K Microarray platform for prognostic discovery biomarker studies of PCa. One study (n = 86) reported increased methylation at 4 CpGs (*KCNK4*, *WDR86*, *OAS2*, *TMEM179*) in patients with a shorter time to BCR, although no further validation of these markers was conducted [131]. Another study performed a number of binary comparisons of methylation levels: no recurrence (n = 75) vs. recurrence (BCR or clinical recurrence (local recurrence or metastatic relapse), n = 123); BCR (n = 43) vs. clinical recurrence (n = 80); and local (n = 44) vs. metastatic relapse (n = 36). The discovery analysis found 75, 16 and 68 genes significantly methylated in each analysis, respectively. Several markers from each group of analyses were assessed by pyrosequencing in 80 patients (n = 20 per clinical endpoint), validating many of the nominated candidate genes (see Table 2 for details), including *RUNX3*, a candidate gene previously studied in a priori prognostic biomarker studies [79,82].

HM450K Platform

The HM450K extended the HM27K probe design to provide coverage of a more diverse set of genomic categories and regions [150,151]. The platform has been widely used for prognostic biomarker discovery (since 2016) and in the generation of publicly available data, including the TCGA dataset of nearly 500 PCa methylomes, which is commonly used by researchers for biomarker discovery or validation [147]. A study by Geybels et al. used TCGA HM450K methylation data to identify methylation differences between PCa patients with low GS (≤6, n = 65) vs. high GS (8–10, n = 88) [133]. The elastic net method was used to build a signature consisting of 52 CpG sites across 32 genes, many of which were novel prognostic candidates. The signature was then tested in HM450K data from a larger validation cohort (n = 523) for its ability to predict disease progression (any of BCR, metastases and/or PCa death) and was found to be an independent predictor of progression in multivariate analysis including GS, pathological T-stage and diagnostic PSA level in all patients, and in a subset of GS 7 patients [133]. Another study from the same lab used the HM450K data from 430 primary PCa tissues, to identify 42 DNA methylation biomarkers that could predict the more serious endpoint of metastatic-lethal progression [134]. In total, eight of these CpG sites validated in a small validation cohort (n = 65, HM450K), with methylation at four of these sites observed to complement GS in discriminating between nonrecurrent and metastatic-lethal patients [134]. A follow-up study by the same research group used pyrosequencing to technically validate five of the eight differentially methylated CpG sites (in *ALKBH5*, *ATP11A*, *FHAD1*, *KLHL8*, *PI15*) [135]. They then used a training cohort (n = 392) to build a model, based on the five sites, from which they calculated a prognostic methylation score for prediction of metastatic-lethal progression. In a multivariate model with GS, a four-fold increase in risk of metastatic-lethal progression was reported in the testing cohort (n = 34), for each unit increase in the methylation score, and the methylation score outperformed prediction by GS alone [135].

A novel approach by Mundbjerg and colleagues used the HM450K to profile multiple samples per patient (different tumour foci, adjacent normal tissue, lymph node metastases and normal lymph nodes) from a cohort of patients who had undergone RP for multifocal disease (n = 14 patients, n = 92 samples). They then used a GLMnet algorithm to categorise the aggressiveness of individual PCa foci based on how well they matched the methylation profile of the lymph node metastasis. The resulting aggressiveness classifier consisted of 25 CpG sites (including in *NXPH2*, *TRIB1* and *PCDHA1-PCDHA8*), and was successfully validated in the TCGA cohort (n = 351) through accurate prediction of lymph node metastases and invasive pathological stage T3 tumours [136]. Finally, the most recent HM450K study which aligns with our criteria of prognostic discovery, used random-forest-based modelling to identify markers that could differentiate between good prognosis, defined as organ-confined disease (pT2) and no BCR for at least 5 years (n = 35), and poor prognosis, defined as systemic metastatic disease with recurrence within 3 years (n = 35) [137]. A DNA methylation-based classifier consisting of 598 sites was developed, validating in two independent cohorts of patients with publicly available methylation data, based on the same selection criteria (ICGC cohort n = 63, TCGA cohort: n = 84) [137]. Further analyses highlighted the independent prognostic value of a gene overlapping one of the 598 sites, with immunostaining analysis reporting significant association between loss of ZIC2 protein expression and poorer prognosis (adjusted for GS, pathological T- stage, nodal stage and PSA) [137].

In summary, technological advances now mean that many hundreds of thousands of CpG sites can be profiled simultaneously, which has provided a more complete view of the complexity and heterogeneity of the PCa methylome. This has enabled the discovery of more accurate and novel biomarkers for PCa prognosis that aid or outperform existing clinicopathological factors. These range from individual markers (e.g., *ABHD9*, *HOXD3*, *GBX2*, *RASGRF2*) to methylation signatures (e.g., 4-G model, PHYMA). However, with an average follow-up of just approximately 5 years across the studies, most focus on short-term clinical endpoints such as BCR. To discover and validate novel DNA methylation biomarkers for the most important clinical endpoints of metastasis and PCa specific mortality, further research needs to be conducted on large independent cohorts with extensive long-term follow-up data (≥15 years) [16]. Furthermore, the genome-wide methods described above are still limited in the number of CpGs assessed (Figure 2), and have a strong bias towards targeting methylation in CG rich regions of gene promoter and CpG islands [145]. More recent techniques, such as Illumina's EPIC microarray, cover more distal regulatory genomic regions [151], and the 'gold standard' Whole Genome Bisulphite Sequencing (WGBS) technique can profile all approximately 28 million CpGs in the methylome [152] (Figure 2). An expanded search of the methylome will enable comprehensive discovery of novel biomarkers for PCa prognosis.

3. Non-Invasive Detection of Prognostic DNA Methylation Markers in Liquid Biopsies

There is widespread interest in using 'liquid biopsies' as a minimally invasive means to improve the accuracy and safety of cancer diagnosis, risk-stratification and disease monitoring. Liquid biopsies include bodily fluids, such as blood, urine, saliva and cerebrospinal fluid, which can be sampled for the presence of circulating tumour cells, cell-free (cf) DNA (released from tumour cells by apoptosis, necrosis and active secretion) and tumour-secreted exosomes containing RNAs, DNAs and proteins. A liquid biopsy offers the opportunity to gain a more comprehensive profile of the heterogeneous molecular landscape of the tumour at diagnosis and during tumour evolution over the course of the disease and treatment. This is particularly relevant in PCa, as the majority of patients have multifocal disease, meaning that the information from a single tissue biopsy may not reflect the dynamics of all tumour foci in the prostate, which can have variable aggressiveness and progression [136].

DNA methylation biomarkers are particularly pertinent in the liquid biopsy setting. In contrast to the limited number of recurrent genetic mutations in cancer, aberrant DNA methylation events tend to be tissue and cancer-type specific and occur across larger genomic regions, allowing DNA methylation to be easily targeted for measurement [153]. The recent development of new technologies has greatly contributed to the ability to sensitively measure DNA methylation [55]. This is highly relevant in liquid biopsy samples where tumour DNA may be present at very low concentrations i.e., < 0.01% of the total DNA content [154,155]. For example, *GSTP1* hypermethylation, one of the most common epigenetic events in PCa tumour specimens, has been readily detected in liquid biopsy samples from PCa patients, such as urine, semen, blood serum and plasma samples [156].

3.1. Urine-Based Methylated Biomarkers

Early studies showed the detection of *GSTP1* methylation in urine from patients with PCa; however diagnostic sensitivity was poor (less than 30%) [157]. Expanding the panel to a three-gene signature (*GSTP1, APC* and *RARB*) improved sensitivity to 60% [158]. More recently a six-gene methylation panel has been developed, termed 'Epigenetic Cancer of the Prostate Test in Urine' (epiCaPture), which targets *GSTP1, SFRP2, IGFBP3, IGFBP7, APC* and *PTGS2* [159]. epiCaPture was applied to urine samples of men with PCa and showed significant associations between DNA methylation and disease aggressiveness, with AUC of 0.64, 0.86 and 0.83 for detecting PCa, high-grade PCa, and high-risk PCa, respectively. Overall, the study concluded that epiCaPture can accurately determine risk compared to two widely used risk stratification systems, D'Amico [26] and CAPRA [160]. In another study, a two-gene methylation panel (*HOXD3* and *GSTP1*) was developed called Prostate Cancer Urinary Epigenetic (ProCUrE) [161]. When applied to urine samples, the positive predictive value of this panel was 59.478¨C%, higher than PSA (38.2–72.1%), for all risk category comparisons. In addition, Moreira-Barbosa et al. assessed methylation of two different gene panels comprising (*miR1−93b/miR3−4b/c*) and (*APC, GSTP1, RARB*) in tissue and urine; they showed that a combination of methylation measurements from the two panels in urine independently predicted shorter disease-specific survival [162]. Hypermethylation of the *RASSF1* promoter has also been reported for its prognostic value as a urine-based methylated biomarker [93]. In this study, a multivariate model of *RASSF1* methylation together with pathological T-stage was the most significant predictor of BCR in patients (GS 6) in both tissue and urine samples [93]. Overall, these studies highlight the potential of DNA methylation as a urine-based prognostic biomarker in PCa.

3.2. Blood-Based Methylated Prognostic Biomarkers For cfDNA Testing

In cancer patients, a proportion of circulating cfDNA is derived from tumour cells, i.e., circulating tumour DNA (ctDNA). cfDNA can be isolated from blood plasma or serum and is present at very low concentrations, ranging from approximately 0–50 ng/mL in healthy individuals; in cancer patients, the proportion of ctDNA can vary between 0.01% to more that 90% of the cfDNA.

A number of studies have shown that methylated *GSTP1* in circulating cfDNA has prognostic value [163–165]; for example, Mahon and colleagues showed that *GSTP1* methylation in cfDNA was associated with overall survival and response to chemotherapy in men with advanced PCa [164]. Importantly, this study demonstrated that *GSTP1* methylation levels prior to and after one chemotherapy cycle were stronger predictors of overall survival than changes in PSA levels at 3 months post-chemotherapy. More recently, Hendriks and colleagues reported hypermethylation of *GSTP1* and *APC* in plasma cfDNA, together with the concentration of cfDNA, to be statistically significant as a prognostic biomarker for overall survival in castration-resistant PCa [166]. Further cfDNA studies report the prognostic utility of *GSTP1* methylation in combination with other frequently methylated genes; for example, *GSTP1* and *RASSF2A* methylation [59] and *GSTP1, RASSF1* and *RARB* methylation [167].

Other genes have shown promise as prognostic methylation biomarkers in cfDNA in PCa. Horning and colleagues showed that promoter hypermethylation of *SRD5A 2* and *CYP11A 1* was associated with BCR and poorer prognosis [168]. In another study, cfDNA methylation of the *APC, GSTP1, RASSFI, MDRI* and *PTGS2* genes was associated with overall survival time in men with advanced PCa [60]. Additionally, MSP on a cohort of $n = 117$ patient serum samples showed that *PCDH8* methylation was an independent predictive risk factor for BCR-free survival ($p < 0.007$) in low GS (< 7) PCa patients after surgery [169]. Overall, these studies highlight the potential value of DNA methylation biomarkers in cfDNA as prognostic indicators of relapse.

4. Conclusions and Future Directions

Research over the last two decades has shown the potential of DNA methylation as a biomarker for PCa prognosis. DNA methylation biomarker discovery has accelerated rapidly with the emergence of affordable, scalable, whole-genome profiling techniques. However, the ongoing technological advancements are bringing new analytical challenges, such as establishing the best way to aggregate methylation data across genomic regions, control for multiple tests; combine methylation with other 'omic' data types and select and prioritise the most important prognostic features from which to build predictive models [170]. A number of new analytical approaches have been made to address these issues (for example, [171–175]) Given the ever-increasing sophistication of technologies, and thus growing number of high-dimensional datasets, bioinformatic method development will continue to be a high-priority research area.

Even with the most sophisticated laboratory and bioinformatic tools for biomarker discovery, the ultimate test of whether a prospective methylation biomarker is prognostic is through validation in multiple, appropriately sized, independent cohorts. One of the obstructions to validation, and therefore translation of new DNA methylation biomarkers to the clinic, is the dearth of suitable, publicly available methylation datasets with adequate clinical follow-up data. Indeed, the flagship TCGA PCa methylation dataset has only short-term follow-up clinical data, and so cannot be used to fully assess the prognostic value of putative methylation biomarkers. For existing methylation datasets such as this, their utility for prognostic research would be increased through the continued collection of long-term follow-up data.

A notable problem is that studies frequently use the same few public cohorts for discovery and/or validation, which may be leading to biased results across the field. To advance the field, new PCa methylation public datasets need to be generated. An emphasis should be placed on using the very latest laboratory techniques which allow for full genome screening, such as the comprehensive EPIC microarray or WGBS, which will increase the likelihood of identifying novel biomarker regions. Another limitation in this field is the predominant focus on using Caucasian or European ancestry based populations, with only a handful of studies to date investigating non-Caucasian patients [96,176]. More ethnically diverse populations need to be investigated for discovery of population-specific prognostic markers, as well as examining how well promising biomarkers found in Caucasian populations translate across other ethnicities. Many of the highest impact journals now have an open data policy. Going forward, this open data ethos should be adopted by more researchers and publications, as it not only provides new resources for other researchers to use in their validation efforts, but also allows transparency in the research method, which ultimately improves the quality of research in the field overall.

Finally, we have discussed the advances in noninvasive DNA methylation prognostic biomarker research. Looking ahead, clinical translation of this research will be a priority as liquid biopsies offer a number of advantages over tissue-based methods, such as reducing side-effects like infection and surgical complications [17,18], and allowing serial collection of samples during the course of monitoring or therapy to provide opportunities for timely therapeutic interventions [177]. This should be paired with the utilisation of DNA methylation assays suitable for application in clinical settings (for example, Multiplex Bisulfite PCR Sequencing [178,179]) which are cost-effective, scalable, reproducible and capable of sensitively detecting methylated tumour DNA in limited clinical material such as liquid biopsies. In conclusion, DNA methylation shows great potential as a prognostic biomarker and could thus transform the clinical management of PCa patients. Key to the successful implementation of prognostic biomarkers is the ability to apply them in diagnostic samples, such as needle biopsy or liquid biopsy samples. Ultimately, the development of specific guidelines for clinical use still requires extensive validation of the best candidate genes in a range of tissue types in independent cohorts with long-term follow-up, for determination of methylation level cut-offs and prognostic validation.

Author Contributions: D.L., S.C., R.P. and C.S. all contributed to the writing of the manuscript. All authors have read and agreed to the published version of the manuscript.

Abbreviations

AUC	Area Under the Curve
BCR	BioChemical Recurrence
CAPRA	Cancer of the Prostate Risk Assessment
CF	Clinical Failure
cfDNA	circulating cell-free DNA
COBRAc	COmbined Bisulphite Restriction Analysis
ctDNA	circulating tumour DNA
ddPCR	Droplet Digital PCR
Df	Degrees of freedom
DMR	Differentially Methylated Regions
ERRBS	Enhanced Reduced Representation Bisulphite Sequencing
FFPET	Formalin-Fixed Paraffin-Embedded Tissue
GS	Gleason Score
HM27K	Infinium HumanMethylation 27K Microarray
WGBS	Whole Genome Bisulphite Sequencing
HM450K	Infinium HumanMethylation 450K Microarray
HR	Hazard Ratio
IQR	InterQuartile Range
LR	Likelihood Ratio
M	Multivariate
MBDCap-Seq	Methyl-CpG Binding Domain Capture sequencing
MSP	Methylation-Specific PCR
PCa	Prostate Cancer
PCR	Polymerase Chain Reaction
PSA	Prostate-Specific Antigen
qMSP	quantitative Methylation-Specific PCR
RP	Radical Prostatectomy
RRBS	Reduced Representation Bisulphite Sequencing
TCGA	The Cancer Genome Atlas
TURP	TransUrethral Resection of the Prostate
U	Univariate

References

1. Bray, F.; Me, J.F.; Soerjomataram, I.; Siegel, R.; Torre, L.A.; Jemal, A. Global cancer statistics 2018: GLOBOCAN estimates of incidence and mortality worldwide for 36 cancers in 185 countries. *CA A Cancer J. Clin.* **2018**, *68*, 394–424. [CrossRef] [PubMed]
2. WHO. GLOBOCAN 2018 Database. *Issued by World Health Organization (WHO)*. Available online: http://gco.iarc.fr/today (accessed on 1 August 2020).
3. Ferlay, J.E.; Lam, F.; Colombet, M.; Mery, L.; Pineros, M.; Znaor, A.; Soerjomataram, I.; Bray, F. Global Cancer Observatory: Cancer Tomorrow. Available online: https://gco.iarc.fr/tomorrow (accessed on 1 August 2020).
4. Rawla, P. Epidemiology of Prostate Cancer. *World J. Oncol.* **2019**, *10*, 63–89. [CrossRef] [PubMed]
5. Culp, M.B.; Soerjomataram, I.; Efstathiou, J.A.; Bray, F.; Jemal, A. Recent Global Patterns in Prostate Cancer Incidence and Mortality Rates. *Eur. Urol.* **2020**, *77*, 38–52. [CrossRef] [PubMed]

6. Litwin, M.S.; Tan, H.-J. The Diagnosis and Treatment of Prostate Cancer. *JAMA* **2017**, *317*, 2532–2542. [CrossRef] [PubMed]
7. Shao, Y.-H.; Demissie, K.; Shih, W.; Mehta, A.R.; Stein, M.N.; Roberts, C.B.; DiPaola, R.S.; Lu-Yao, G.L. Contemporary Risk Profile of Prostate Cancer in the United States. *J. Natl. Cancer Inst.* **2009**, *101*, 1280–1283. [CrossRef] [PubMed]
8. Welch, H.G.; Gorski, D.H.; Albertsen, P.C. Trends in Metastatic Breast and Prostate Cancer—Lessons in Cancer Dynamics. *N. Engl. J. Med.* **2015**, *373*, 1685–1687. [CrossRef] [PubMed]
9. Howlader, N.; Krapcho, M.; Miller, D.; Brest, A.; Yu, M.; Ruhl, J.; Tatalovich, Z.; Mariotto, A.; Lewis, D.R.; Chen, H.S.; et al. SEER Cancer Statistics Review, 1975–2016. Available online: https://seer.cancer.gov/csr/1975_2016/ (accessed on 1 August 2020).
10. Roehl, K.A.; Han, M.; Ramos, C.G.; Antenor, J.A.V.; Catalona, W.J. Cancer Progression and Survival Rates Following Anatomical Radical Retropubic Prostatectomy in 3478 Consecutive Patients: Long-Term Results. *J. Urol.* **2004**, *172*, 910–914. [CrossRef] [PubMed]
11. Eggener, S.E.; Scardino, P.T.; Walsh, P.C.; Han, M.; Partin, A.W.; Trock, B.J.; Feng, Z.; Wood, D.P.; Eastham, J.A.; Yossepowitch, O.; et al. Predicting 15-Year Prostate Cancer Specific Mortality After Radical Prostatectomy. *J. Urol.* **2011**, *185*, 869–875. [CrossRef]
12. Freedland, S.J.; Humphreys, E.B.; Mangold, L.A.; Eisenberger, M.; Dorey, F.J.; Walsh, P.C.; Partin, A.W. Risk of Prostate Cancer–Specific Mortality Following Biochemical Recurrence After Radical Prostatectomy. *JAMA* **2005**, *294*, 433–439. [CrossRef]
13. Abdollah, F.; Boorjian, S.; Cozzarini, C.; Suardi, N.; Sun, M.; Fiorino, C.; Di Muzio, N.; Karakiewicz, P.I.; Montorsi, F.; Karnes, R.J.; et al. Survival Following Biochemical Recurrence After Radical Prostatectomy and Adjuvant Radiotherapy in Patients With Prostate Cancer: The Impact of Competing Causes of Mortality and Patient Stratification. *Eur. Urol.* **2013**, *64*, 557–564. [CrossRef]
14. Valicenti, R.K.; Thompson, I.; Albertsen, P.; Davis, B.J.; Goldenberg, S.L.; Wolf, J.S.; Sartor, O.; Klein, E.; Hahn, C.; Michalski, J.; et al. Adjuvant and Salvage Radiation Therapy After Prostatectomy: American Society for Radiation Oncology/American Urological Association Guidelines. *Int. J. Radiat. Oncol.* **2013**, *86*, 822–828. [CrossRef] [PubMed]
15. Welch, H.G.; Albertsen, P.C. Prostate Cancer Diagnosis and Treatment after the Introduction of Prostate-Specific Antigen Screening: 1986–2005. *J. Natl. Cancer Inst.* **2009**, *101*, 1325–1329. [CrossRef]
16. Albertsen, P.C.; Hanley, J.A.; Fine, J. 20-Year Outcomes Following Conservative Management of Clinically Localized Prostate Cancer. *JAMA* **2005**, *293*, 2095–2101. [CrossRef] [PubMed]
17. Steineck, G.; Helgesen, F.; Adolfsson, J.; Dickman, P.W.; Johansson, J.-E.; Norlen, B.J.; Holmberg, L. Quality of Life after Radical Prostatectomy or Watchful Waiting. *N. Engl. J. Med.* **2002**, *347*, 790–796. [CrossRef]
18. Wilt, T.J.; Macdonald, R.; Rutks, I.; Shamliyan, T.; Taylor, B.C.; Kane, R.L. Systematic review: Comparative effectiveness and harms of treatments for clinically localized prostate cancer. *Ann. Intern. Med.* **2008**, *148*, 435–448. [CrossRef] [PubMed]
19. Thomsen, F.B.; Brasso, K.; Klotz, L.H.; Røder, M.A.; Berg, K.D.; Iversen, P. Active surveillance for clinically localized prostate cancer–A systematic review. *J. Surg. Oncol.* **2014**, *109*, 830–835. [CrossRef] [PubMed]
20. Cooperberg, M.R.; Carroll, P.R.; Klotz, L. Active Surveillance for Prostate Cancer: Progress and Promise. *J. Clin. Oncol.* **2011**, *29*, 3669–3676. [CrossRef]
21. Klotz, L. Active Surveillance: The Canadian Experience. *Manag. Castration Resist. Prostate Cancer* **2012**, *22*, 95–105. [CrossRef]
22. Welty, C.J.; Cooperberg, M.R.; Carroll, P.R. Meaningful end points and outcomes in men on active surveillance for early-stage prostate cancer. *Curr. Opin. Urol.* **2014**, *24*, 288–292. [CrossRef]
23. Tolkach, Y.; Kristiansen, G. The Heterogeneity of Prostate Cancer: A Practical Approach. *Pathobiology* **2018**, *85*, 108–116. [CrossRef]
24. Prensner, J.R.; Rubin, M.A.; Wei, J.T.; Chinnaiyan, A.M. Beyond PSA: The Next Generation of Prostate Cancer Biomarkers. *Sci. Transl. Med.* **2012**, *4*, 127rv3. [CrossRef] [PubMed]
25. Epstein, J.I.; Walsh, P.C.; Carmichael, M.; Brendler, C.B. Pathologic and clinical findings to predict tumor extent of nonpalpable (stage T1c) prostate cancer. *JAMA* **1994**, *271*, 368–374. [CrossRef]

26. D'Amico, A.V.; Whittington, R.; Malkowicz, S.B.; Schultz, D.; Blank, K.; Broderick, G.A.; Tomaszewski, J.E.; Renshaw, A.A.; Kaplan, I.; Beard, C.; et al. Biochemical Outcome After Radical Prostatectomy, External Beam Radiation Therapy, or Interstitial Radiation Therapy for Clinically Localized Prostate Cancer. *JAMA* **1998**, *280*, 969–974. [CrossRef]
27. Kattan, M.W.; Eastham, J.A.; Wheeler, T.M.; Maru, N.; Scardino, P.T.; Erbersdobler, A.; Graefen, M.; Huland, H.; Koh, H.; Shariat, S.F.; et al. Counseling Men With Prostate Cancer: A Nomogram for Predicting the Presence of Small, Moderately Differentiated, Confined Tumors. *J. Urol.* **2003**, *170*, 1792–1797. [CrossRef]
28. Stephenson, A.J.; Scardino, P.T.; Eastham, J.A.; Jr, F.J.B.; Dotan, Z.A.; Diblasio, C.J.; Reuther, A.; Klein, E.A.; Kattan, M.W. Postoperative Nomogram Predicting the 10-Year Probability of Prostate Cancer Recurrence After Radical Prostatectomy. *J. Clin. Oncol.* **2005**, *23*, 7005–7012. [CrossRef]
29. Chun, F.K.-H.; Haese, A.; Ahyai, S.A.; Walz, J.; Suardi, N.; Capitanio, U.; Graefen, M.; Erbersdobler, A.; Huland, H.; Karakiewicz, P.I. Critical assessment of tools to predict clinically insignificant prostate cancer at radical prostatectomy in contemporary men. *Cancer* **2008**, *113*, 701–709. [CrossRef] [PubMed]
30. Cooperberg, M.R.; Hilton, J.F.; Carroll, P.R. The CAPRA-S score. *Cancer* **2011**, *117*, 5039–5046. [CrossRef]
31. Remmers, S.; Verbeek, J.F.M.; Nieboer, D.; Van Der Kwast, T.; Roobol-Bouts, M. Predicting biochemical recurrence and prostate cancer-specific mortality after radical prostatectomy: Comparison of six prediction models in a cohort of patients with screening- and clinically detected prostate cancer. *BJU Int.* **2019**, *124*, 635–642. [CrossRef]
32. Steyerberg, E.W.; Roobol, M.; Kattan, M.; Van Der Kwast, T.; De Koning, H.; Schröder, F. Prediction of Indolent Prostate Cancer: Validation and Updating of a Prognostic Nomogram. *J. Urol.* **2007**, *177*, 107–112. [CrossRef]
33. Gandaglia, G.; Ploussard, G.; Isbarn, H.; Suardi, N.; De Visschere, P.J.; Fütterer, J.J.; Ghadjar, P.; Massard, C.; Ost, P.; Sooriakumaran, P.; et al. What is the optimal definition of misclassification in patients with very low-risk prostate cancer eligible for active surveillance? Results from a multi-institutional series. *Urol. Oncol. Semin. Orig. Investig.* **2015**, *33*, 164.e1–164.e9. [CrossRef] [PubMed]
34. Ploussard, G.; Epstein, J.I.; Montironi, R.; Carroll, P.R.; Wirth, M.; Grimm, M.-O.; Bjartell, A.S.; Montorsi, F.; Freedland, S.J.; Erbersdobler, A.; et al. The Contemporary Concept of Significant Versus Insignificant Prostate Cancer. *Eur. Urol.* **2011**, *60*, 291–303. [CrossRef] [PubMed]
35. Hughes, C.; Murphy, A.; Martin, C.M.; Sheils, O.; O'Leary, J.J. Molecular pathology of prostate cancer. *J. Clin. Pathol.* **2005**, *58*, 673–684. [CrossRef] [PubMed]
36. Kristiansen, G. Markers of clinical utility in the differential diagnosis and prognosis of prostate cancer. *Mod. Pathol.* **2018**, *31*, 143–155. [CrossRef]
37. Clinton, T.N.; Bagrodia, A.; Lotan, Y.; Margulis, V.; Raj, G.V.; Woldu, S.L. Tissue-based biomarkers in prostate cancer. *Expert Rev. Precis. Med. Drug Dev.* **2017**, *2*, 249–260. [CrossRef]
38. Fraser, M.; Berlin, A.; Bristow, R.G.; Van Der Kwast, T. Genomic, pathological, and clinical heterogeneity as drivers of personalized medicine in prostate cancer. *Urol. Oncol. Semin. Orig. Investig.* **2015**, *33*, 85–94. [CrossRef]
39. He, W.; Bishop, K.S. The potential use of cell-free-circulating-tumor DNA as a biomarker for prostate cancer. *Expert Rev. Mol. Diagn.* **2016**, *16*, 839–852. [CrossRef] [PubMed]
40. Hendriks, R.J.; Van Oort, I.M.; Schalken, J.A. Blood-based and urinary prostate cancer biomarkers: A review and comparison of novel biomarkers for detection and treatment decisions. *Prostate Cancer Prostatic Dis.* **2016**, *20*, 12–19. [CrossRef] [PubMed]
41. Cuzick, J.; Swanson, G.P.; Fisher, G.; Brothman, A.R.; Berney, D.M.; Reid, J.E.; Mesher, D.; Speights, V.; Stankiewicz, E.; Foster, C.S.; et al. Prognostic value of an RNA expression signature derived from cell cycle proliferation genes in patients with prostate cancer: A retrospective study. *Lancet Oncol.* **2011**, *12*, 245–255. [CrossRef]
42. Klein, E.A.; Cooperberg, M.R.; Magi-Galluzzi, C.; Simko, J.P.; Falzarano, S.M.; Maddala, T.; Chan, J.M.; Li, J.; Cowan, J.E.; Tsiatis, A.C.; et al. A 17-gene Assay to Predict Prostate Cancer Aggressiveness in the Context of Gleason Grade Heterogeneity, Tumor Multifocality, and Biopsy Undersampling. *Eur. Urol.* **2014**, *66*, 550–560. [CrossRef]
43. Erho, N.; Crisan, A.; Vergara, I.A.; Mitra, A.P.; Ghadessi, M.; Buerki, C.; Bergstralh, E.J.; Kollmeyer, T.; Fink, S.; Haddad, Z.; et al. Discovery and Validation of a Prostate Cancer Genomic Classifier that Predicts Early Metastasis Following Radical Prostatectomy. *PLoS ONE* **2013**, *8*, e66855. [CrossRef]

44. Chao, C.R.; Chi, M.; Preciado, M.; Black, M.H. Methylation markers for prostate cancer prognosis: A systematic review. *Cancer Causes Control* **2013**, *24*, 1615–1641. [CrossRef] [PubMed]
45. Strand, S.H.; Orntoft, T.F.; Sorensen, K.D. Prognostic DNA Methylation Markers for Prostate Cancer. *Int. J. Mol. Sci.* **2014**, *15*, 16544–16576. [CrossRef]
46. Chiam, K.; Ricciardelli, C.; Bianco-Miotto, T. Epigenetic biomarkers in prostate cancer: Current and future uses. *Cancer Lett.* **2014**, *342*, 248–256. [CrossRef] [PubMed]
47. Chan, M.F.; Liang, G.; Jones, P.A. Relationship between Transcription and DNA Methylation. *Future HIV-1 Therapeutics* **2000**, *249*, 75–86. [CrossRef]
48. Egger, G.; Liang, G.; Aparicio, A.; Jones, P.A. Epigenetics in human disease and prospects for epigenetic therapy. *Nat. Cell Biol.* **2004**, *429*, 457–463. [CrossRef] [PubMed]
49. Baylin, S.B.; Esteller, M.; Rountree, M.R.; Bachman, K.E.; Schuebel, K.; Herman, J.G. Aberrant patterns of DNA methylation, chromatin formation and gene expression in cancer. *Hum. Mol. Genet.* **2001**, *10*, 687–692. [CrossRef] [PubMed]
50. Majumdar, S.; Buckles, E.; Estrada, J.; Koochekpour, S. Aberrant DNA Methylation and Prostate Cancer. *Curr. Genom.* **2011**, *12*, 486–505. [CrossRef] [PubMed]
51. Aryee, M.J.; Liu, W.; Engelmann, J.C.; Nuhn, P.; Gurel, M.; Haffner, M.C.; Esopi, D.; Irizarry, R.A.; Getzenberg, R.H.; Nelson, W.G.; et al. DNA Methylation Alterations Exhibit Intraindividual Stability and Interindividual Heterogeneity in Prostate Cancer Metastases. *Sci. Transl. Med.* **2013**, *5*, 169ra10. [CrossRef]
52. Chan, T.A.; Glöckner, S.; Yi, J.M.; Chen, W.; Van Neste, L.; Cope, L.; Herman, J.G.; Velculescu, V.E.; Schuebel, K.E.; Ahuja, N.; et al. Convergence of Mutation and Epigenetic Alterations Identifies Common Genes in Cancer That Predict for Poor Prognosis. *PLoS Med.* **2008**, *5*, e114. [CrossRef]
53. Paziewska, A.; Dabrowska, M.; Goryca, K.; Antoniewicz, A.; Dobruch, J.; Mikula, M.; Jarosz, D.; Zapala, L.; Borówka, A.; Ostrowski, J. DNA methylation status is more reliable than gene expression at detecting cancer in prostate biopsy. *Br. J. Cancer* **2014**, *111*, 781–789. [CrossRef]
54. Issa, J.-P. DNA Methylation as a Clinical Marker in Oncology. *J. Clin. Oncol.* **2012**, *30*, 2566–2568. [CrossRef] [PubMed]
55. Bock, C.; Halbritter, F.; Carmona, F.J.; Tierling, S.; Datlinger, P.; Assenov, Y.; Berdasco, M.; Bergmann, A.K.; Booher, K.; Busato, F.; et al. Quantitative comparison of DNA methylation assays for biomarker development and clinical applications. *Nat. Biotechnol.* **2016**, *34*, 726–737. [CrossRef]
56. Stewart, G.S.; Van Neste, L.; Delvenne, P.; Delrée, P.; Delga, A.; McNeill, S.A.; O'Donnell, M.; Clark, J.; Van Criekinge, W.; Bigley, J.; et al. Clinical Utility of an Epigenetic Assay to Detect Occult Prostate Cancer in Histopathologically Negative Biopsies: Results of the MATLOC Study. *J. Urol.* **2013**, *189*, 1110–1116. [CrossRef]
57. Ellinger, J.; Müller, S.C.; Stadler, T.C.; Jung, A.; Von Ruecker, A.; Bastian, P.J. The role of cell-free circulating DNA in the diagnosis and prognosis of prostate cancer. *Urol. Oncol. Semin. Orig. Investig.* **2011**, *29*, 124–129. [CrossRef]
58. Rouprêt, M.; Hupertan, V.; Catto, J.W.; Yates, D.R.; Rehman, I.; Proctor, L.M.; Phillips, J.; Meuth, M.; Cussenot, O.; Hamdy, F.C. Promoter hypermethylation in circulating blood cells identifies prostate cancer progression. *Int. J. Cancer* **2007**, *122*, 952–956. [CrossRef]
59. Payne, S.R.; Serth, J.; Schostak, M.; Kamradt, J.; Strauss, A.; Thelen, P.; Model, F.; Day, J.K.; Liebenberg, V.; Morotti, A.; et al. DNA methylation biomarkers of prostate cancer: Confirmation of candidates and evidence urine is the most sensitive body fluid for non-invasive detection. *Prostate* **2009**, *69*, 1257–1269. [CrossRef]
60. Okegawa, T.; Nutahara, K.; Higashihara, E. Association of circulating tumor cells with tumor-related methylated DNA in patients with hormone-refractory prostate cancer. *Int. J. Urol.* **2010**, *17*, 466–475. [CrossRef]
61. Herman, J.G.; Graff, J.R.; Myohanen, S.; Nelkin, B.D.; Baylin, S.B. Methylation-specific PCR: A novel PCR assay for methylation status of CpG islands. *Proc. Natl. Acad. Sci. USA* **1996**, *93*, 9821–9826. [CrossRef]
62. Eads, C.A.; Danenberg, K.D.; Kawakami, K.; Saltz, L.B.; Blake, C.; Shibata, D.; Danenberg, P.V.; Laird, P.W. MethyLight: A high-throughput assay to measure DNA methylation. *Nucleic Acids Res.* **2000**, *28*, 32e-00. [CrossRef] [PubMed]
63. Tost, J.; Gut, I.; Sharon, M. Analysis of Gene-Specific DNA Methylation Patterns by Pyrosequencing® Technology. *Pyrosequencing Protoc.* **2007**, *373*, 89–102. [CrossRef]

64. Tost, J.; Gut, I.G. DNA methylation analysis by pyrosequencing. *Nat. Protoc.* **2007**, *2*, 2265–2275. [CrossRef] [PubMed]
65. Ehrich, M.; Nelson, M.R.; Stanssens, P.; Zabeau, M.; Liloglou, T.; Xinarianos, G.; Cantor, C.R.; Field, J.K.; Boom, D.V.D. Quantitative high-throughput analysis of DNA methylation patterns by base-specific cleavage and mass spectrometry. *Proc. Natl. Acad. Sci. USA* **2005**, *102*, 15785–15790. [CrossRef] [PubMed]
66. Perkins, G.; Lu, H.; Garlan, F.; Taly, V. Droplet-Based Digital PCR. *Int. Rev. Cytol.* **2017**, *79*, 43–91. [CrossRef]
67. Brena, R.M.; Auer, H.; Kornacker, K.; Plass, C. Quantification of DNA methylation in electrofluidics chips (Bio-COBRA). *Nat. Protoc.* **2006**, *1*, 52–58. [CrossRef]
68. Wong, E.M.; Dobrovic, A. Assessing Gene-Specific Methylation Using HRM-Based Analysis. *Recent Results Cancer Res.* **2010**, *687*, 207–217. [CrossRef]
69. Rand, K.N.; Ho, T.; Qu, W.; Mitchell, S.M.; White, R.; Clark, S.J.; Molloy, P.L. Headloop suppression PCR and its application to selective amplification of methylated DNA sequences. *Nucleic Acids Res.* **2005**, *33*, e127. [CrossRef]
70. Devaney, J.; Stirzaker, C.; Qu, W.; Song, J.Z.; Statham, A.L.; Patterson, K.I.; Horvath, L.G.; Tabor, B.; Coolen, M.W.; Hulf, T.; et al. Epigenetic Deregulation Across Chromosome 2q14.2 Differentiates Normal from Prostate Cancer and Provides a Regional Panel of Novel DNA Methylation Cancer Biomarkers. *Cancer Epidemiol. Biomark. Prev.* **2010**, *20*, 148–159. [CrossRef]
71. Montavon, C.; Gloss, B.S.; Warton, K.; Barton, C.A.; Statham, A.L.; Scurry, J.P.; Tabor, B.; Nguyen, T.V.; Qu, W.; Samimi, G.; et al. Prognostic and diagnostic significance of DNA methylation patterns in high grade serous ovarian cancer. *Gynecol. Oncol.* **2012**, *124*, 582–588. [CrossRef]
72. Xie, W.; Regan, M.M.; Buyse, M.; Halabi, S.; Kantoff, P.W.; Sartor, O.; Soule, H.; Clarke, N.W.; Collette, L.; Dignam, J.J.; et al. Metastasis-Free Survival Is a Strong Surrogate of Overall Survival in Localized Prostate Cancer. *J. Clin. Oncol.* **2017**, *35*, 3097–3104. [CrossRef]
73. Zhang, A.; Chiam, K.; Haupt, Y.; Fox, S.; Birch, S.; Tilley, W.; Butler, L.M.; Knudsen, K.; Comstock, C.; Rasiah, K.; et al. An analysis of a multiple biomarker panel to better predict prostate cancer metastasis after radical prostatectomy. *Int. J. Cancer* **2018**, *144*, 1151–1159. [CrossRef]
74. Yegnasubramanian, S.; Kowalski, J.; Gonzalgo, M.L.; Zahurak, M.; Piantadosi, S.; Walsh, P.C.; Bova, G.S.; De Marzo, A.M.; Isaacs, W.B.; Nelson, W.G. Hypermethylation of CpG islands in primary and metastatic human prostate cancer. *Cancer Res.* **2004**, *64*, 1975–1986. [CrossRef] [PubMed]
75. Rosenbaum, E.; Hoque, M.O.; Cohen, Y.; Zahurak, M.; Eisenberger, M.A.; Epstein, J.I.; Partin, A.W.; Sidransky, D. Promoter Hypermethylation as an Independent Prognostic Factor for Relapse in Patients with Prostate Cancer Following Radical Prostatectomy. *Clin. Cancer Res.* **2005**, *11*, 8321–8325. [CrossRef]
76. Woodson, K.; O'Reilly, K.J.; Ward, D.E.; Walter, J.; Hanson, J.; Walk, E.L.; Tangrea, J.A. CD44 and PTGS2 Methylation are Independent Prognostic Markers for Biochemical Recurrence Among Prostate Cancer Patients with Clinically Localized Disease. *Epigenetics* **2006**, *1*, 183–186. [CrossRef] [PubMed]
77. Henrique, R.; Ribeiro, F.R.; Fonseca, D.; Hoque, M.O.; Carvalho, A.L.; Costa, V.L.; Pinto, M.; Oliveira, J.; Teixeira, M.R.; Sidransky, D.; et al. High Promoter Methylation Levels of APC Predict Poor Prognosis in Sextant Biopsies from Prostate Cancer Patients. *Clin. Cancer Res.* **2007**, *13*, 6122–6129. [CrossRef]
78. Ellinger, J.; Bastian, P.J.; Jurgan, T.; Biermann, K.; Kahl, P.; Heukamp, L.; Wernert, N.; Müller, S.; Von Ruecker, A. CpG Island Hypermethylation at Multiple Gene Sites in Diagnosis and Prognosis of Prostate Cancer. *Urol.* **2008**, *71*, 161–167. [CrossRef] [PubMed]
79. Alumkal, J.J.; Zhang, Z.; Humphreys, E.B.; Bennett, C.; Mangold, L.A.; Carducci, M.A.; Partin, A.W.; Garrett-Mayer, E.; DeMarzo, A.M.; Herman, J.G. Effect of DNA Methylation on Identification of Aggressive Prostate Cancer. *Urology* **2008**, *72*, 1234–1239. [CrossRef] [PubMed]
80. Weiss, G.; Cottrell, S.; Distler, J.; Schatz, P.; Kristiansen, G.; Ittmann, M.; Haefliger, C.; Lesche, R.; Hartmann, A.; Corman, J.; et al. DNA Methylation of the PITX2 Gene Promoter Region is a Strong Independent Prognostic Marker of Biochemical Recurrence in Patients With Prostate Cancer After Radical Prostatectomy. *J. Urol.* **2009**, *181*, 1678–1685. [CrossRef] [PubMed]
81. Vanaja, D.K.; Ehrich, M.; Boom, D.V.D.; Cheville, J.C.; Karnes, R.J.; Tindall, D.J.; Cantor, C.R.; Young, C.Y. Hypermethylation of Genes for Diagnosis and Risk Stratification of Prostate Cancer. *Cancer Investig.* **2009**, *27*, 549–560. [CrossRef]

82. Richiardi, L.; Fiano, V.; Vizzini, L.; De Marco, L.; Delsedime, L.; Akre, O.; Tos, A.G.; Merletti, F. Promoter Methylation in APC, RUNX3, and GSTP1 and Mortality in Prostate Cancer Patients. *J. Clin. Oncol.* **2009**, *27*, 3161–3168. [CrossRef]
83. Bañez, L.L.; Sun, L.; Van Leenders, G.J.; Wheeler, T.M.; Bangma, C.H.; Freedland, S.J.; Ittmann, M.M.; Lark, A.L.; Madden, J.F.; Hartman, A.; et al. Multicenter Clinical Validation of PITX2 Methylation as a Prostate Specific Antigen Recurrence Predictor in Patients With Post-Radical Prostatectomy Prostate Cancer. *J. Urol.* **2010**, *184*, 149–156. [CrossRef]
84. Vasiljevic, N.; Wu, K.; Brentnall, A.R.; Kim, D.C.; Thorat, M.A.; Kudahetti, S.C.; Mao, X.; Xue, L.; Yu, Y.; Shaw, G.L.; et al. Absolute quantitation of DNA methylation of 28 candidate genes in prostate cancer using pyrosequencing. *Dis. Markers* **2011**, *30*, 151–161. [CrossRef] [PubMed]
85. Rosenbaum, E.; Begum, S.; Brait, M.; Zahurak, M.; Maldonado, L.; Mangold, L.A.; Eisenberger, M.A.; Epstein, J.I.; Partin, A.W.; Sidransky, D.; et al. AIM1 promoter hypermethylation as a predictor of decreased risk of recurrence following radical prostatectomy. *Prostate* **2011**, *72*, 1133–1139. [CrossRef] [PubMed]
86. Vasiljević, N.; Ahmad, A.S.; Beesley, C.; Thorat, M.A.; Fisher, G.; Berney, D.M.; Moller, H.; Yu, Y.; Lu, Y.-J.; Cuzick, J.; et al. Association between DNA methylation of HSPB1 and death in low Gleason score prostate cancer. *Prostate Cancer Prostatic Dis.* **2012**, *16*, 35–40. [CrossRef]
87. Dietrich, D.; Hasinger, O.; Bañez, L.L.; Sun, L.; Van Leenders, G.J.; Wheeler, T.M.; Bangma, C.H.; Wernert, N.; Perner, S.; Freedland, S.J.; et al. Development and Clinical Validation of a Real-Time PCR Assay for PITX2 DNA Methylation to Predict Prostate-Specific Antigen Recurrence in Prostate Cancer Patients Following Radical Prostatectomy. *J. Mol. Diagn.* **2013**, *15*, 270–279. [CrossRef] [PubMed]
88. Richiardi, L.; Fiano, V.; Grasso, C.; Zugna, D.; Delsedime, L.; Gillio-Tos, A.; Merletti, F. Methylation of APC and GSTP1 in Non-Neoplastic Tissue Adjacent to Prostate Tumour and Mortality from Prostate Cancer. *PLoS ONE* **2013**, *8*, e68162. [CrossRef]
89. Moritz, R.; Ellinger, J.; Nuhn, P.; Haese, A.; Müller, S.; Graefen, M.; Schlomm, T.; Bastian, P.-D.D.M.P.J. DNA hypermethylation as a predictor of PSA recurrence in patients with low- and intermediate-grade prostate cancer. *Anticancer. Res.* **2013**, *33*, 5249–5254.
90. Vasiljević, N.; Ahmad, A.S.; Thorat, M.A.; Fisher, G.; Berney, D.M.; Moller, H.; Foster, C.S.; Cuzick, J.; Lorincz, A.T. DNA methylation gene-based models indicating independent poor outcome in prostate cancer. *BMC Cancer* **2014**, *14*, 655. [CrossRef]
91. Vasiljević, N.; Ahmad, A.S.; Carter, P.D.; Fisher, G.; Berney, D.M.; Foster, C.S.; Cuzick, J.; Lorincz, A.T. DNA methylation ofPITX2predicts poor survival in men with prostate cancer. *Biomark. Med.* **2014**, *8*, 1143–1150. [CrossRef]
92. Maldonado, L.; Brait, M.; Loyo, M.; Sullenberger, L.; Wang, K.; Peskoe, S.B.; Rosenbaum, E.; Howard, R.; Toubaji, A.; Albadine, R.; et al. GSTP1Promoter Methylation is Associated with Recurrence in Early Stage Prostate Cancer. *J. Urol.* **2014**, *192*, 1542–1548. [CrossRef]
93. Daniunaite, K.; Jarmalaite, S.; Kalinauskaite, N.; Petroska, D.; Laurinavicius, A.; Lazutka, J.R.; Jankevicius, F. Prognostic Value of RASSF1 Promoter Methylation in Prostate Cancer. *J. Urol.* **2014**, *192*, 1849–1855. [CrossRef]
94. Litovkin, K.; Van Eynde, A.; Joniau, S.; Lerut, E.; Laenen, A.; Gevaert, T.; Gevaert, O.; Spahn, M.; Kneitz, B.; Gramme, P.; et al. DNA Methylation-Guided Prediction of Clinical Failure in High-Risk Prostate Cancer. *PLoS ONE* **2015**, *10*, e0130651. [CrossRef] [PubMed]
95. Carozzi, F.M.; Tamburrino, L.; Bisanzi, S.; Marchiani, S.; Paglierani, M.; Di Lollo, S.; Crocetti, E.; Buzzoni, C.; Burroni, E.; Greco, L.; et al. Are biomarkers evaluated in biopsy specimens predictive of prostate cancer aggressiveness? *J. Cancer Res. Clin. Oncol.* **2015**, *142*, 201–212. [CrossRef] [PubMed]
96. Rybicki, B.A.; Rundle, A.; Kryvenko, O.N.; Mitrache, N.; Do, K.C.; Jankowski, M.; Chitale, D.; Trudeau, S.; Belinsky, S.A.; Tang, D. Methylation in benign prostate and risk of disease progression in men subsequently diagnosed with prostate cancer. *Int. J. Cancer* **2016**, *138*, 2884–2893. [CrossRef]
97. Holmes, E.E.; Goltz, D.; Sailer, V.; Jung, M.; Meller, S.; Uhl, B.; Dietrich, J.; Röhler, M.; Ellinger, J.; Kristiansen, G.; et al. PITX3 promoter methylation is a prognostic biomarker for biochemical recurrence-free survival in prostate cancer patients after radical prostatectomy. *Clin. Epigenetics* **2016**, *8*, 104. [CrossRef] [PubMed]
98. Ahmad, A.S.; Vasiljević, N.; Carter, P.; Berney, D.M.; Moller, H.; Foster, C.S.; Cuzick, J.; Lorincz, A.T. A novel DNA methylation score accurately predicts death from prostate cancer in men with low to intermediate clinical risk factors. *Oncotarget* **2016**, *7*, 71833–71840. [CrossRef] [PubMed]

99. Uhl, B.; Gevensleben, H.; Tolkach, Y.; Sailer, V.; Majores, M.; Jung, M.; Meller, S.; Stein, J.; Ellinger, J.; Dietrich, D.; et al. PITX2 DNA Methylation as Biomarker for Individualized Risk Assessment of Prostate Cancer in Core Biopsies. *J. Mol. Diagn.* **2017**, *19*, 107–114. [CrossRef] [PubMed]
100. Van Neste, L.; Herman, J.G.; Otto, G.; Bigley, J.W.; Epstein, J.I.; Van Criekinge, W. The Epigenetic promise for prostate cancer diagnosis. *Prostate* **2011**, *72*, 1248–1261. [CrossRef] [PubMed]
101. Tew, K.D.; Manevich, Y.; Grek, C.; Xiong, Y.; Uys, J.; Townsend, D.M. The role of glutathione S-transferase P in signaling pathways and S-glutathionylation in cancer. *Free. Radic. Biol. Med.* **2011**, *51*, 299–313. [CrossRef]
102. Henrique, R.; Jerónimo, C. Molecular Detection of Prostate Cancer: A Role for GSTP1 Hypermethylation. *Eur. Urol.* **2004**, *46*, 660–669. [CrossRef]
103. Aoki, K.; Taketo, M.M. Adenomatous polyposis coli (APC): A multi-functional tumor suppressor gene. *J. Cell Sci.* **2007**, *120*, 3327–3335. [CrossRef]
104. Chen, Y.; Li, J.; Yu, X.; Li, S.; Zhang, X.; Mo, Z.; Hu, Y. APC gene hypermethylation and prostate cancer: A systematic review and meta-analysis. *Eur. J. Hum. Genet.* **2013**, *21*, 929–935. [CrossRef] [PubMed]
105. Moison, C.; Assemat, F.; Daunay, A.; Tost, J.; Guieysse-Peugeot, A.-L.; Arimondo, P.B. Synergistic chromatin repression of the tumor suppressor gene RARB in human prostate cancers. *Epigenetics* **2014**, *9*, 477–482. [CrossRef] [PubMed]
106. Kioussi, C.; Briata, P.; Baek, S.H.; Rose, D.W.; Hamblet, N.S.; Herman, T.; Ohgi, K.A.; Lin, C.; Gleiberman, A.; Wang, J.; et al. Identification of a Wnt/Dvl/β-Catenin → Pitx2 Pathway Mediating Cell-Type-Specific Proliferation during Development. *Cell* **2002**, *111*, 673–685. [CrossRef]
107. Harbeck, N.; Nimmrich, I.; Hartmann, A.; Ross, J.S.; Cufer, T.; Grützmann, R.; Kristiansen, G.; Paradiso, A.; Hartmann, O.; Margossian, A.; et al. Multicenter Study Using Paraffin-Embedded Tumor Tissue Testing PITX2 DNA Methylation As a Marker for Outcome Prediction in Tamoxifen-Treated, Node-Negative Breast Cancer Patients. *J. Clin. Oncol.* **2008**, *26*, 5036–5042. [CrossRef] [PubMed]
108. Goltz, D.; Holmes, E.E.; Gevensleben, H.; Sailer, V.; Dietrich, J.; Jung, M.; Röhler, M.; Meller, S.; Ellinger, J.; Kristiansen, G.; et al. CXCL12 promoter methylation and PD-L1 expression as prognostic biomarkers in prostate cancer patients. *Oncotarget* **2016**, *7*, 53309–53320. [CrossRef]
109. Gevensleben, H.; Holmes, E.E.; Goltz, D.; Dietrich, J.; Sailer, V.; Ellinger, J.; Dietrich, D.; Kristiansen, G. PD-L1 promoter methylation is a prognostic biomarker for biochemical recurrence-free survival in prostate cancer patients following radical prostatectomy. *Oncotarget* **2016**, *7*, 79943–79955. [CrossRef]
110. Meller, S.; Zipfel, L.; Gevensleben, H.; Dietrich, J.; Ellinger, J.; Majores, M.; Stein, J.; Sailer, V.; Jung, M.; Kristiansen, G.; et al. CDO1 promoter methylation is associated with gene silencing and is a prognostic biomarker for biochemical recurrence-free survival in prostate cancer patients. *Epigenetics* **2016**, *11*, 871–880. [CrossRef]
111. Nørgaard, M.; Haldrup, C.; Storebjerg, T.M.; Vestergaard, E.M.; Wild, P.J.; Høyer, S.; Borre, M.; Ørntoft, T.; Sørensen, K.D. Comprehensive Evaluation of TFF3 Promoter Hypomethylation and Molecular Biomarker Potential for Prostate Cancer Diagnosis and Prognosis. *Int. J. Mol. Sci.* **2017**, *18*, 2017. [CrossRef]
112. Haldrup, C.; Pedersen, A.L.; Ogaard, N.; Strand, S.H.; Hoyer, S.; Borre, M.; Orntoft, T.F.; Sorensen, K.D. Biomarker potential of ST6G ALNAC3 and ZNF660 promoter hypermethylation in prostate cancer tissue and liquid biopsies. *Mol. Oncol.* **2018**, *12*, 545–560. [CrossRef]
113. Haldrup, C.; Mundbjerg, K.; Vestergaard, E.M.; Lamy, P.; Wild, P.; Schulz, W.A.; Arsov, C.; Visakorpi, T.; Borre, M.; Høyer, S.; et al. DNA Methylation Signatures for Prediction of Biochemical Recurrence After Radical Prostatectomy of Clinically Localized Prostate Cancer. *J. Clin. Oncol.* **2013**, *31*, 3250–3258. [CrossRef]
114. Torres-Ferreira, J.; Ramalho-Carvalho, J.; Gomez, A.; Menezes, F.D.; Freitas, R.; Oliveira, J.; Antunes, L.; Bento, M.J.; Esteller, M.; Henrique, R.; et al. MiR1-93b promoter methylation accurately detects prostate cancer in urine sediments and miR3-4b/c or miR1-29-2 promoter methylation define subsets of clinically aggressive tumors. *Mol. Cancer* **2017**, *16*, 26. [CrossRef] [PubMed]
115. Daniunaite, K.; Dubikaityte, M.; Gibas, P.; Bakavicius, A.; Lazutka, J.R.; Ulys, A.; Jankevicius, F.; Jarmalaite, S. Clinical significance of miRNA host gene promoter methylation in prostate cancer. *Hum. Mol. Genet.* **2017**, *26*, 2451–2461. [CrossRef] [PubMed]
116. Strand, S.H.; śwítnicki, M.; Moller, M.; Haldrup, C.; Storebjerg, T.M.; Hedegaard, J.; Nordentoft, I.; Hoyer, S.; Borre, M.; Pedersen, J.S.; et al. RHCG and TCAF1 promoter hypermethylation predicts biochemical recurrence in prostate cancer patients treated by radical prostatectomy. *Oncotarget* **2016**, *8*, 5774–5788. [CrossRef]

117. Bjerre, M.T.; Strand, S.H.; Nørgaard, M.; Kristensen, H.; Rasmussen, A.K.; Mortensen, M.M.; Fredsøe, J.; Mouritzen, P.; Ulhøi, B.; Ørntoft, T.; et al. Aberrant DOCK2, GRASP, HIF3A and PKFP Hypermethylation has Potential as a Prognostic Biomarker for Prostate Cancer. *Int. J. Mol. Sci.* **2019**, *20*, 1173. [CrossRef]
118. Li, X.; Zhang, W.; Song, J.; Zhang, X.; Ran, L.; He, Y. SLCO4C1 promoter methylation is a potential biomarker for prognosis associated with biochemical recurrence-free survival after radical prostatectomy. *Clin. Epigenetics* **2019**, *11*, 99. [CrossRef]
119. Nørgaard, M.; Haldrup, C.; Bjerre, M.T.; Høyer, S.; Ulhøi, B.P.; Borre, M.; Sorensen, K.D. Epigenetic silencing of MEIS2 in prostate cancer recurrence. *Clin. Epigenetics* **2019**, *11*, 147. [CrossRef]
120. Cottrell, S.; Jung, K.; Kristiansen, G.; Eltze, E.; Semjonow, A.; Ittmann, M.; Hartmann, A.; Stamey, T.; Haefliger, C.; Weiss, G. Discovery and Validation of 3 Novel DNA Methylation Markers of Prostate Cancer Prognosis. *J. Urol.* **2007**, *177*, 1753–1758. [CrossRef]
121. Lin, P.-C.; Giannopoulou, E.G.; Park, K.; Mosquera, J.M.; Sboner, A.; Tewari, A.K.; Garraway, L.A.; Beltran, H.; Rubin, M.A.; Elemento, O. Epigenomic Alterations in Localized and Advanced Prostate Cancer. *Neoplasia* **2013**, *15*, 373-IN5. [CrossRef]
122. Bhasin, J.M.; Lee, B.H.; Matkin, L.; Taylor, M.G.; Hu, B.; Xu, Y.; Magi-Galluzzi, C.; Klein, E.A.; Ting, A.H. Methylome-wide Sequencing Detects DNA Hypermethylation Distinguishing Indolent from Aggressive Prostate Cancer. *Cell Rep.* **2015**, *13*, 2135–2146. [CrossRef]
123. Kron, K.; Pethe, V.; Briollais, L.; Sadikovic, B.; Ozcelik, H.; Sunderji, A.; Venkateswaran, V.; Pinthus, J.; Fleshner, N.; Van Der Kwast, T.; et al. Discovery of Novel Hypermethylated Genes in Prostate Cancer Using Genomic CpG Island Microarrays. *PLoS ONE* **2009**, *4*, e4830. [CrossRef]
124. Kron, K.J.; Liu, L.; Pethe, V.V.; Demetrashvili, N.; Nesbitt, M.E.; Trachtenberg, J.; Ozcelik, H.; Fleshner, N.E.; Briollais, L.; Van Der Kwast, T.H.; et al. DNA methylation of HOXD3 as a marker of prostate cancer progression. *Lab. Investig.* **2010**, *90*, 1060–1067. [CrossRef] [PubMed]
125. Liu, L.; Kron, K.J.; Pethe, V.V.; Demetrashvili, N.; Nesbitt, M.; Trachtenberg, J.; Ozcelik, H.; Fleshner, N.E.; Briollais, L.; Van Der Kwast, T.H.; et al. Association of tissue promoter methylation levels of APC, TGFβ2, HOXD3 and RASSF1A with prostate cancer progression. *Int. J. Cancer* **2011**, *129*, 2454–2462. [CrossRef] [PubMed]
126. Jeyapala, R.; Savio, A.J.; Olkhov-Mitsel, E.; Kamdar, S.; Zhao, F.; Cuizon, C.; Liu, R.S.; Zlotta, A.; Fleshner, N.; Van Der Kwast, T.; et al. GBX2 Methylation Is a Novel Prognostic Biomarker and Improves Prediction of Biochemical Recurrence Among Patients with Prostate Cancer Negative for Intraductal Carcinoma and Cribriform Architecture. *Eur. Urol. Oncol.* **2019**, *2*, 231–238. [CrossRef] [PubMed]
127. Jeyapala, R.; Kamdar, S.; Olkhov-Mitsel, E.; Savio, A.J.; Zhao, F.; Cuizon, C.; Liu, R.S.; Zlotta, A.; Fleshner, N.; Van Der Kwast, T.; et al. An integrative DNA methylation model for improved prognostication of postsurgery recurrence and therapy in prostate cancer patients. *Urol. Oncol. Semin. Orig. Investig.* **2020**, *38*, 39.e1–39.e9. [CrossRef]
128. Savio, A.J.; Kamdar, S.; Jeyapala, R.; Olkhov-Mitsel, E.; Cuizon, C.; Finelli, A.; Zlotta, A.R.; Toi, A.; Fleshner, N.E.; Van Der Kwast, T.; et al. Methylation Markers in Prostate Biopsies Are Prognosticators for Late Biochemical Recurrence and Therapy after Surgery in Prostate Cancer Patients. *J. Mol. Diagn.* **2019**, *22*, 30–39. [CrossRef]
129. Goh, L.-K.; Liem, N.; Vijayaraghavan, A.; Chen, G.; Lim, P.L.; Tay, K.J.; Chang, M.; Low, J.S.W.; Joshi, A.; Huang, H.H.; et al. Diagnostic and Prognostic Utility of a DNA Hypermethylated Gene Signature in Prostate Cancer. *PLoS ONE* **2014**, *9*, e91666. [CrossRef]
130. Angulo, J.; López, J.I.; Dorado, J.F.; Sanchez-Chapado, M.; Colas, B.; Ropero, S. A DNA Hypermethylation Profile Independently Predicts Biochemical Recurrence Following Radical Prostatectomy. *Urol. Int.* **2016**, *97*, 16–25. [CrossRef]
131. Kobayashi, Y.; Absher, D.M.; Gulzar, Z.G.; Young, S.R.; McKenney, J.K.; Peehl, D.M.; Brooks, J.D.; Myers, R.M.; Sherlock, G. DNA methylation profiling reveals novel biomarkers and important roles for DNA methyltransferases in prostate cancer. *Genome Res.* **2011**, *21*, 1017–1027. [CrossRef]
132. Mahapatra, S.; Klee, E.W.; Young, C.Y.F.; Sun, Z.; Jimenez, R.E.; Klee, G.G.; Tindall, D.J.; Donkena, K.V. Global Methylation Profiling for Risk Prediction of Prostate Cancer. *Clin. Cancer Res.* **2012**, *18*, 2882–2895. [CrossRef]
133. Geybels, M.S.; Wright, J.L.; Bibikova, M.; Klotzle, B.; Fan, J.-B.; Zhao, S.; Feng, Z.; Ostrander, E.A.; Lin, D.; Nelson, P.S.; et al. Epigenetic signature of Gleason score and prostate cancer recurrence after radical prostatectomy. *Clin. Epigenetics* **2016**, *8*, 97. [CrossRef]

134. Zhao, S.; Geybels, M.S.; Leonardson, A.; Rubicz, R.; Kolb, S.; Yan, Q.; Klotzle, B.; Bibikova, M.; Hurtado-Coll, A.; Troyer, D.; et al. Epigenome-Wide Tumor DNA Methylation Profiling Identifies Novel Prognostic Biomarkers of Metastatic-Lethal Progression in Men Diagnosed with Clinically Localized Prostate Cancer. *Clin. Cancer Res.* **2016**, *23*, 311–319. [CrossRef] [PubMed]
135. Zhao, S.; Leonardson, A.; Geybels, M.S.; McDaniel, A.S.; Yu, M.; Kolb, S.; Zong, H.; Carter, K.; Siddiqui, J.; Cheng, A.; et al. A five-CpG DNA methylation score to predict metastatic-lethal outcomes in men treated with radical prostatectomy for localized prostate cancer. *Prostate* **2018**, *78*, 1084–1091. [CrossRef] [PubMed]
136. Mundbjerg, K.; Chopra, S.; Alemozaffar, M.; Duymich, C.; Lakshminarasimhan, R.; Nichols, P.W.; Aron, M.; Siegmund, K.D.; Ukimura, O.; Aron, M.; et al. Identifying aggressive prostate cancer foci using a DNA methylation classifier. *Genome Biol.* **2017**, *18*, 3. [CrossRef] [PubMed]
137. Toth, R.; Schiffmann, H.; Hube-Magg, C.; Büscheck, F.; Höflmayer, D.; Weidemann, S.; Lebok, P.; Fraune, C.; Minner, S.; Schlomm, T.; et al. Random forest-based modelling to detect biomarkers for prostate cancer progression. *Clin. Epigenetics* **2019**, *11*, 148. [CrossRef]
138. Gerhauser, C.; Favero, F.; Risch, T.; Simon, R.; Feuerbach, L.; Assenov, Y.; Heckmann, D.; Sidiropoulos, N.; Waszak, S.M.; Hübschmann, D.; et al. Molecular Evolution of Early-Onset Prostate Cancer Identifies Molecular Risk Markers and Clinical Trajectories. *Cancer Cell* **2018**, *34*, 996–1011. [CrossRef]
139. Liang, G.; Gonzalgo, M.L.; Salem, C.; Jones, P.A. Identification of DNA methylation differences during tumorigenesis by methylation-sensitive arbitrarily primed polymerase chain reaction. *Methods* **2002**, *27*, 150–155. [CrossRef]
140. Toyota, M.; Issa, J.-P.J.; Mills, K.I.; Ramsahoye, B.H. Methylated CpG Island Amplification for Methylation Analysis and Cloning Differentially Methylated Sequences. *DNA Methylation Protoc.* **2003**, *200*, 101–110. [CrossRef]
141. Stott-Miller, M.; Zhao, S.; Wright, J.L.; Kolb, S.; Bibikova, M.; Klotzle, B.; Ostrander, E.A.; Fan, J.-B.; Feng, Z.; Stanford, J.L. Validation study of genes with hypermethylated promoter regions associated with prostate cancer recurrence. *Cancer Epidemiol. Biomark. Prev.* **2014**, *23*, 1331–1339. [CrossRef]
142. Altuna, A.; Garrett-Bakelman, F.E.; Kormaksson, M.; Busuttil, J.; Zhang, L.; Khrebtukova, I.; Milne, T.A.; Huang, Y.; Biswas, D.; Hess, J.L.; et al. Base-Pair Resolution DNA Methylation Sequencing Reveals Profoundly Divergent Epigenetic Landscapes in Acute Myeloid Leukemia. *PLoS Genet.* **2012**, *8*, e1002781. [CrossRef]
143. Garrett-Bakelman, F.; Sheridan, C.K.; Kacmarczyk, T.J.; Ishii, J.; Betel, R.; Alonso, A.; Mason, C.E.; Figueroa, M.E.; Melnick, A.M. Enhanced reduced representation bisulfite sequencing for assessment of DNA methylation at base pair resolution. *J. Vis. Exp.* **2015**, *10*, e52246. [CrossRef]
144. Hopkins, T.G.; Burns, P.A.; Routledge, M. DNA Methylation of GSTP1 as Biomarker in Diagnosis of Prostate Cancer. *Urol.* **2007**, *69*, 11–16. [CrossRef] [PubMed]
145. Stirzaker, C.; Taberlay, P.C.; Statham, A.L.; Clark, S.J. Mining cancer methylomes: Prospects and challenges. *Trends Genet.* **2014**, *30*, 75–84. [CrossRef] [PubMed]
146. Serre, D.; Lee, B.H.; Ting, A.H. MBD-isolated Genome Sequencing provides a high-throughput and comprehensive survey of DNA methylation in the human genome. *Nucleic Acids Res.* **2009**, *38*, 391–399. [CrossRef] [PubMed]
147. Abeshouse, A.; Ahn, J.; Akbani, R.; Ally, A.; Amin, S.; Andry, C.D.; Annala, M.; Aprikian, A.; Armenia, J.; Arora, A.; et al. The Molecular Taxonomy of Primary Prostate Cancer. *Cell* **2015**, *163*, 1011–1025. [CrossRef] [PubMed]
148. Agilent. Human CpG Island Microarray. Available online: https://www.agilent.com/en/product/methylation-chip-on-chip-microarray-platform/epigenetic-specialty-microarrays/dna-methylation-microarrays/human-cpg-island-microarray2$-$28444#:~{}:text=Human%20CpG%20microarrays%20enable%20comprehensive,correlated%20to%20key%20biological%20processes.&text=237%2C220%20unique%20probes%20in%20or,genome%20in%20a%20single%20experiment (accessed on 11 September 2020).
149. Illumina. High-Throughput DNA Methylation Profiling with Illumina GoldenGate Technology. Available online: https://sapac.illumina.com/content/dam/illumina-marketing/documents/products/datasheets/datasheet_goldengate_methylation.pdf (accessed on 11 September 2020).
150. Bibikova, M.; Barnes, B.; Tsan, C.; Ho, V.; Klotzle, B.; Le, J.M.; Delano, D.; Zhang, L.; Schroth, G.P.; Gunderson, K.L.; et al. High density DNA methylation array with single CpG site resolution. *Genomics* **2011**, *98*, 288–295. [CrossRef] [PubMed]

151. Pidsley, R.; Zotenko, E.; Peters, T.J.; Lawrence, M.G.; Risbridger, G.P.; Molloy, P.; Van Djik, S.; Muhlhausler, B.S.; Stirzaker, C.; Clark, S.J. Critical evaluation of the Illumina MethylationEPIC BeadChip microarray for whole-genome DNA methylation profiling. *Genome Biol.* **2016**, *17*, 208. [CrossRef]
152. Lister, R.; Pelizzola, M.; Dowen, R.H.; Hawkins, R.D.; Hon, G.; Tonti-Filippini, J.; Nery, J.R.; Lee, L.; Ye, Z.; Ngo, Q.-M.; et al. Human DNA methylomes at base resolution show widespread epigenomic differences. *Nat. Cell Biol.* **2009**, *462*, 315–322. [CrossRef]
153. Shen, S.Y.; Singhania, R.; Fehringer, G.; Chakravarthy, A.; Roehrl, M.H.A.; Chadwick, D.; Zuzarte, P.C.; Borgida, A.; Wang, T.T.; Li, T.; et al. Sensitive tumour detection and classification using plasma cell-free DNA methylomes. *Nat. Cell Biol.* **2018**, *563*, 579–583. [CrossRef]
154. Lee, T.-H.; Montalvo, L.; Chrebtow, V.; Busch, M.P. Quantitation of genomic DNA in plasma and serum samples: Higher concentrations of genomic DNA found in serum than in plasma. *Transfusion* **2001**, *41*, 276–282. [CrossRef]
155. Schwarzenbach, H.; Hoon, D.S.B.; Pantel, K. Cell-free nucleic acids as biomarkers in cancer patients. *Nat. Rev. Cancer* **2011**, *11*, 426–437. [CrossRef]
156. Wu, T.; Giovannucci, E.; Welge, J.; Mallick, P.; Tang, W.-Y.; Ho, S.-M. Measurement of GSTP1 promoter methylation in body fluids may complement PSA screening: A meta-analysis. *Br. J. Cancer* **2011**, *105*, 65–73. [CrossRef]
157. Cairns, P.; Esteller, M.; Herman, J.G.; Schoenberg, M.; Jeronimo, C.; Sanchez-Cespedes, M.; Chow, N.H.; Grasso, M.; Wu, L.; Westra, W.B.; et al. Molecular detection of prostate cancer in urine by GSTP1 hypermethylation. *Clin. Cancer Res.* **2001**, *7*, 2727–2730.
158. Baden, J.; Adams, S.; Astacio, T.; Jones, J.; Markiewicz, J.; Painter, J.; Trust, C.; Wang, Y.; Green, G. Predicting Prostate Biopsy Result in Men With Prostate Specific Antigen 2.0 to 10.0 ng/mL Using an Investigational Prostate Cancer Methylation Assay. *J. Urol.* **2011**, *186*, 2101–2106. [CrossRef] [PubMed]
159. O'Reilly, E.; Tuzova, A.V.; Walsh, A.L.; Russell, N.M.; O'Brien, O.; Kelly, S.; Ni Dhomhnallain, O.; DeBarra, L.; Dale, C.M.; Brugman, R.; et al. epiCaPture: A Urine DNA Methylation Test for Early Detection of Aggressive Prostate Cancer. *JCO Precis. Oncol.* **2019**, *2019*, 1–18. [CrossRef]
160. Cooperberg, M.R.; Pasta, D.J.; Elkin, E.P.; Litwin, M.S.; Latini, D.M.; Du Chane, J.; Carroll, P.R. The University of California, San Francisco Cancer of the Prostate Risk Assessment Score: A Straightforward and Reliable Preoperative Predictor of Disease Recurrence after Radical Prostatectomy. *J. Urol.* **2005**, *173*, 1938–1942. [CrossRef]
161. Zhao, F.; Jeyapala, R.; Olkhov-Mitsel, E.; Vesprini, D.; Fleshner, N.E.; Bapat, B. Re: Urinary DNA Methylation Biomarkers for Noninvasive Prediction of Aggressive Disease in Patients with Prostate Cancer on Active Surveillance. *J. Urol.* **2018**, *199*, 1354–1355. [CrossRef]
162. Moreira-Barbosa, C.; Barros-Silva, D.; Costa-Pinheiro, P.; Torres-Ferreira, J.; Constâncio, V.; Freitas, R.; Oliveira, J.; Antunes, L.; Henrique, R.; Jerónimo, C. Comparing diagnostic and prognostic performance of two-gene promoter methylation panels in tissue biopsies and urines of prostate cancer patients. *Clin. Epigenetics* **2018**, *10*, 132. [CrossRef] [PubMed]
163. Bastian, P.J.; Palapattu, G.S.; Lin, X.; Yegnasubramanian, S.; Mangold, L.A.; Trock, B.; Eisenberger, M.A.; Partin, A.W.; Nelson, W.G. Preoperative Serum DNA GSTP1 CpG Island Hypermethylation and the Risk of Early Prostate-Specific Antigen Recurrence Following Radical Prostatectomy. *Clin. Cancer Res.* **2005**, *11*, 4037–4043. [CrossRef]
164. Mahon, K.L.; Qu, W.; Devaney, J.; Paul, C.; Castillo, L.; Wykes, R.J.; Chatfield, M.D.; Boyer, M.J.; Stockler, M.R.; Marx, G.; et al. Methylated Glutathione S-transferase 1 (mGSTP1) is a potential plasma free DNA epigenetic marker of prognosis and response to chemotherapy in castrate-resistant prostate cancer. *Br. J. Cancer* **2014**, *111*, 1802–1809. [CrossRef]
165. Reibenwein, J.; Pils, D.; Horak, P.; Tomicek, B.; Goldner, G.; Worel, N.; Elandt, K.; Krainer, M. Promoter hypermethylation of GSTP1, AR, and 14-3-3σ in serum of prostate cancer patients and its clinical relevance. *Prostate* **2007**, *67*, 427–432. [CrossRef]
166. Hendriks, R.J.; Dijkstra, S.; Smit, F.P.; Vandersmissen, J.; Van De Voorde, H.; Mulders, P.F.A.; Van Oort, I.M.; Van Criekinge, W.; Schalken, J. Epigenetic markers in circulating cell-free DNA as prognostic markers for survival of castration-resistant prostate cancer patients. *Prostate* **2018**, *78*, 336–342. [CrossRef] [PubMed]

167. Sunami, E.; Shinozaki, M.; Higano, C.S.; Wollman, R.; Dorff, T.B.; Tucker, S.J.; Martinez, S.R.; Singer, F.R.; Hoon, D.S. Multimarker Circulating DNA Assay for Assessing Blood of Prostate Cancer Patients. *Clin. Chem.* **2009**, *55*, 559–567. [CrossRef]
168. Horning, A.M.; Awe, J.A.; Wang, C.-M.; Liu, J.; Lai, Z.; Wang, V.Y.; Jadhav, R.R.; Louie, A.D.; Lin, C.-L.; Kroczak, T.; et al. DNA methylation screening of primary prostate tumors identifies SRD5A2 and CYP11A1 as candidate markers for assessing risk of biochemical recurrence. *Prostate* **2015**, *75*, 1790–1801. [CrossRef]
169. Lin, Y.-L.; Li, Y.-L.; Ma, J.-G. Aberrant Promoter Methylation of Protocadherin8 (PCDH8) in Serum is a Potential Prognostic Marker for Low Gleason Score Prostate Cancer. *Med Sci. Monit.* **2017**, *23*, 4895–4900. [CrossRef]
170. Sung, J.; Wang, Y.; Chandrasekaran, S.; Witten, D.M.; Price, N.D. Molecular signatures from omics data: From chaos to consensus. *Biotechnol. J.* **2012**, *7*, 946–957. [CrossRef]
171. Peters, T.J.; Buckley, M.J.; Statham, A.L.; Pidsley, R.; Samaras, K.; Lord, R.V.; Clark, S.J.; Molloy, P.L. De novo identification of differentially methylated regions in the human genome. *Epigenetics Chromatin* **2015**, *8*, 6. [CrossRef] [PubMed]
172. Yosefian, I.; Farkhani, E.M.; Baneshi, M.M. Application of Random Forest Survival Models to Increase Generalizability of Decision Trees: A Case Study in Acute Myocardial Infarction. *Comput. Math. Methods Med.* **2015**, *2015*, 576413. [CrossRef]
173. Liu, C.; Wang, X.; Genchev, G.Z.; Lu, H. Multi-omics facilitated variable selection in Cox-regression model for cancer prognosis prediction. *Methods* **2017**, *124*, 100–107. [CrossRef]
174. Kvamme, H.; Borgan, Ø.; Scheel, I. Time-to-Event Prediction with Neural Networks and Cox Regression. *J. Mach. Learn. Res.* **2019**, *20*, 1–30.
175. Sanz, H.; Reverter, F.; Valim, C. Enhancing SVM for survival data using local invariances and weighting. *BMC Bioinform.* **2020**, *21*, 193. [CrossRef]
176. Li, J.; Xu, C.; Lee, H.J.; Ren, S.; Zi, X.; Zhang, Z.; Wang, H.; Yu, Y.; Yang, C.; Gao, X.; et al. A genomic and epigenomic atlas of prostate cancer in Asian populations. *Nat. Cell Biol.* **2020**, *580*, 93–99. [CrossRef] [PubMed]
177. González-Billalabeitia, E.; Conteduca, V.; Wetterskog, D.; Jayaram, A.; Attard, G. Circulating tumor DNA in advanced prostate cancer: Transitioning from discovery to a clinically implemented test. *Prostate Cancer Prostatic Dis.* **2018**, *22*, 195–205. [CrossRef] [PubMed]
178. Korbie, D.; Lin, E.; Wall, D.; Nair, S.S.; Stirzaker, C.; Clark, S.J.; Trau, M. Multiplex bisulfite PCR resequencing of clinical FFPE DNA. *Clin. Epigenetics* **2015**, *7*, 28. [CrossRef]
179. Lam, D.; Luu, P.-L.; Song, J.Z.; Qu, W.; Risbridger, G.P.; Lawrence, M.G.; Lu, J.; Trau, M.; Korbie, D.; Clark, S.J.; et al. Comprehensive evaluation of targeted multiplex bisulphite PCR sequencing for validation of DNA methylation biomarker panels. *Clin. Epigenetics* **2020**, *12*, 1–16. [CrossRef]

3

Cancer/Testis Antigens: "Smart" Biomarkers for Diagnosis and Prognosis of Prostate and Other Cancers

Prakash Kulkarni [1,*] and Vladimir N. Uversky [2,3,*]

[1] Institute for Bioscience and Biotechnology Research, University of Maryland, Rockville, MD 20850, USA
[2] Department of Molecular Medicine, Morsani College of Medicine, University of South Florida, Tampa, FL 33612, USA
[3] Laboratory of New methods in Biology, Institute for Biological Instrumentation, Russian Academy of Sciences, Pushchino 142290, Moscow Region, Russia
* Correspondence: pkulkar4@ibbr.umd.edu (P.K.); vuversky@health.usf.edu (V.N.U.)

Academic Editor: Carsten Stephan

Abstract: A clinical dilemma in the management of prostate cancer (PCa) is to distinguish men with aggressive disease who need definitive treatment from men who may not require immediate intervention. Accurate prediction of disease behavior is critical because radical treatment is associated with high morbidity. Here, we highlight the cancer/testis antigens (CTAs) as potential PCa biomarkers. The CTAs are a group of proteins that are typically restricted to the testis in the normal adult but are aberrantly expressed in several types of cancers. Interestingly, >90% of CTAs are predicted to belong to the realm of intrinsically disordered proteins (IDPs), which do not have unique structures and exist as highly dynamic conformational ensembles, but are known to play important roles in several biological processes. Using prostate-associated gene 4 (PAGE4) as an example of a disordered CTA, we highlight how IDP conformational dynamics may regulate phenotypic heterogeneity in PCa cells, and how it may be exploited both as a potential biomarker as well as a promising therapeutic target in PCa. We also discuss how in addition to intrinsic disorder and post-translational modifications, structural and functional variability induced in the CTAs by alternate splicing represents an important feature that might have different roles in different cancers. Although it is clear that significant additional work needs to be done in the outlined direction, this novel concept emphasizing (multi)functionality as an important trait in selecting a biomarker underscoring the theranostic potential of CTAs that is latent in their structure (or, more appropriately, the lack thereof), and casts them as next generation or "smart" biomarker candidates.

Keywords: biomarkers; prostate cancer; cancer/testis antigens; intrinsically disordered protein; prostate-associated gene 4 (PAGE4); nucleolar protein 4 (NOL4); centrosomal protein of 55 kDa (CEP55)

1. Introduction

Prostate cancer (PCa) is one of the most prevalent forms of cancer in older men over the age of 50. Worldwide, >1 million men are diagnosed with PCa each year and more than 300,000 die of the disease. Current US statistics show that one in five or six men will be diagnosed with PCa during their lifetime. In fact, by extrapolating statistical data from the past 40 years (1973–2013) it is estimated that in little over 100 years, one in two men will develop the disease [1]. Although these numbers appear daunting, only a fraction of those diagnosed have forms of the disease that can be considered to be "lethal" in nature.

As is true for other types of cancer, early diagnosis is believed to be crucial for the selection of the most successful and suitable PCa treatment strategy. Therefore, it follows that regular screening of men over the age 50 may be a logical thing to do. However, even today, there is no reliable test other than prostate-specific antigen (PSA), and there is no unanimous opinion in the medical community regarding the benefits of PSA screening [2,3]. Those who advocate regular screening believe that early diagnosis and treatment of PCa offers men a better chance to address the disease. On the other hand, urologists who recommend against regular screening note that because PCa is typically slow growing, the side effects of treatment would likely outweigh any benefit that might be derived from detecting the disease at a stage when it is unlikely to cause problems. Consistently, in 2012, the United States Preventive Services Task Force (USPSTF), an independent panel of experts in primary care and prevention that systematically reviews the evidence of effectiveness and develops recommendations for clinical preventive services, recommended against PCa screening in adult men of all ages. Indeed, in a roundtable discussion organized by Lee et al. to analyze studies of screening in two large randomized trials, it became obvious that the benefits of screening may not occur for 10 or more years after screening given the long natural history of the disease and that, perhaps as many as 1000 men will need to be screened and about 50 will need to be treated to save one life from PCa [4].

Many factors, including an increase in the aging population and widespread screening for PSA have contributed to the rise in the diagnoses of men who present early-stage (low or intermediate Gleason scores (GS)) or "low-risk" disease. While immediate treatment is recommended for patients with high GS ($\geq$8), the appropriate treatment for patients with low GS ($\leq$6) or intermediate GS (=7) remains ambiguous. Patients with low-risk disease are typically recommended the "wait and watch" or "active surveillance" protocol but are routinely monitored including repeat biopsies with the intention of avoiding treatment unless there is evidence of disease progression [5–7]. It is, therefore, not surprising that a staggering number of biopsies—>1 million in the US alone—are performed every year adding to the burgeoning healthcare cost and undesirable risk of serious complications requiring hospitalization [8].

While the intent of the active surveillance protocol is to minimize over-treatment, the concern is that active surveillance may miss the opportunity for early intervention of tumors that are seemingly low risk but that are actually aggressive. Indeed, despite the cautious approach, up to 40% of patients enrolled in active surveillance develop full-blown PCa [6]. Thus, a clinical dilemma today in the management of PCa is to distinguish men with aggressive disease who need definitive treatment from men whose disease does not require such intervention. Furthermore, accurate prediction of disease behavior is critical because radical treatment is associated with high morbidity.

Currently, at the time of diagnosis, most PCa cases present as localized disease and are preferentially treated by radical prostatectomy or radiation therapy with curative intent. During the last decade, a significant shift towards localized, well-differentiated tumors at radical prostatectomy (so-called stage migration) has occurred [9,10] perhaps due to the widespread use of PSA screening or a change in PCa biology [11], although, the latter would seem less likely. Therefore nowadays, PCa detected by PSA alone is often characterized by small-size and low-grade tumors in relatively younger male populations. In fact, it is reported that around 30% of cancers treated with radical prostatectomy in the US are "insignificant" tumors [12]. On the other hand, nearly 30% patients are reported to experience an isolated increase in serum PSA with long-term follow-up [13–19]. Therefore, it is important for physicians and patients to know the likelihood of disease progression following radical prostatectomy. Considered together, it follows that there is a critical need to identify reliable biomarkers that may be used for better diagnosis as well as to distinguish most of the low-GS tumors that will remain indolent from the few that are truly aggressive to better treat and manage PCa.

The advent of advanced technologies and sophisticated bioinformatics algorithms has fueled the discovery of novel biomarkers that include serum-, urine- and tissue-based assays that may supplement PSA testing, or even replace it over time (reviewed in [20–28]). These include extracellular vesicles [29], long noncoding RNAs [30,31], microRNAs [32–34] and circulating tumor cells (CTCs) [35,36], among many others. These advances have provided new insights into the individual patient's tumor biology, and several biomarkers with specific indications for disease diagnosis, prediction and prognosis, as well as risk stratification of aggressive PCa at the time of diagnosis are now commercially available.

For example, Decipher™ (GenomeDx Biosciences, Vancouver, Canada) is a tool based on 22 genes that evaluates the risk of adverse outcomes (metastasis) after radical prostatectomy [37], while Oncotype DX® (Genomics Health, Redwood City, CA, USA) was developed for use with fixed paraffin-embedded (FFPE) diagnostic prostate needle biopsies and measures expression of 12 cancer-related genes representing four biological pathways and five reference genes to calculate the Genomic Prostate Score (GPS) [38]. This assay has been analytically and subsequently clinically validated as a predictor of aggressive disease [38]. Prolaris (Myriad Genetics, Salth Lake City, UT, USA), on the other hand, is a 46-gene prognostic test that quantitatively determines the risk of recurrence in patients who have undergone prostatectomy. The assay measures the expression of 31 cell cycle progression (CCP) genes and 15 housekeeping genes that act as internal controls and normalization standards in each patient sample. The assay is also performed on FFPE samples and the results are reported as a numerical score along with accompanying interpretive information [39]. Of note, since the expression of CCP genes is likely to represent a fundamental aspect of tumor biology, the rationale for selecting these genes for prediction of outcome in PCa is based on a common biological function of the individual genes in this panel. Interestingly, the other two genomics tests also include genes associated with cell proliferation. Finally, ProMark® (Metamark Corp., Waltham, MA, USA) s based on a multiplexed proteomics assay [40] and predicts PCa aggressiveness in patients found with similar features to Oncotype DX®. These biomarkers can be helpful for post-biopsy decision-making in low-risk patients and post-radical prostatectomy in selected risk groups. These biomarkers that are intended to be used in combination with the accepted clinical criteria (i.e., GS, PSA, clinical stage) to stratify PCa according to biological aggressiveness and direct initial patient management have gained considerable popularity; however, additional studies are needed to investigate the clinical benefit of these new technologies, the financial ramifications and how they should be utilized in clinics.

2. Cancer/Testis Antigens (CTAs) as Novel PCa Biomarkers

The cancer/testis antigens (CTAs) are a group of proteins that are typically restricted to the testis in the normal adult but are aberrantly expressed in several types of cancers [41]. To date, ~250 genes encoding CTAs have been identified [42] that can be broadly divided into two groups: CT-X antigens located on the X chromosome and non-X CTAs located on various autosomes. Furthermore, members of the CT-X antigens, in particular, are typically associated with advanced disease characterized by poorer outcomes in several types of cancers, including PCa [43–48]. Because of these intriguing expression patterns, the CTAs serve as unique biomarkers for cancer diagnosis/prognosis.

A systematic study by Suyama et al. [48] using a custom DNA microarray revealed that several CT-X antigens from melanoma-associated antigen A/chondrosarcoma-associate gene (MAGE-A/CSAG) subfamilies are coordinately upregulated in castrate-resistant PCa, but not in primary PCa. Interestingly, however, the CT-X antigen prostate-associated gene 4 (PAGE4) was found to be highly upregulated in primary PCa but silent in castrate-resistant PCa, thereby raising the possibility that CTA-based "gene signature" could potentially be developed to distinguish men with aggressive PCa who need treatment from men with indolent disease not requiring immediate intervention [48].

To test this possibility, Shiraishi et al. [49] devised a multiplex real-time polymerase chain reaction (PCR) assay. From a panel of 22 CTAs that showed differential expression, they selected a subpanel of 5 CTAs that included 4 non-X CT antigens (centrosomal protein of 55 kDa—CEP55, NUF2, lymphokine-activated killer T-cell-originated protein kinase—PBK and the dual specificity protein kinase TTK) and the CT-X antigen, PAGE4 [49]. The authors found that while the non-X CTAs were upregulated, the CT-X antigen, PAGE4, was downregulated in patients with recurrent PCa after radical prostatectomy (Figure 1). Kaplan-Meier curves revealed that higher levels of expression of CEP55 and NUF2 were significantly correlated with shorter biochemical recurrence-free time [49]. In contrast, higher expression of PAGE4 was significantly correlated with longer biochemical recurrence-free time (Figure 2). Further, with the exception of TTK, the other CTAs were significantly correlated with prostatectomy GS, but none were correlated with age, preoperative PSA and tumor stage [49]. It is important note that, like in the case of the genomics tests that include several cell cycle progression genes, the five CTAs used in the study by Shiraishi et al. [49] are also associated with the cell cycle and proliferation. In fact, some of the CTAs are common to both gene sets highlighting the potential of this CTA panel.

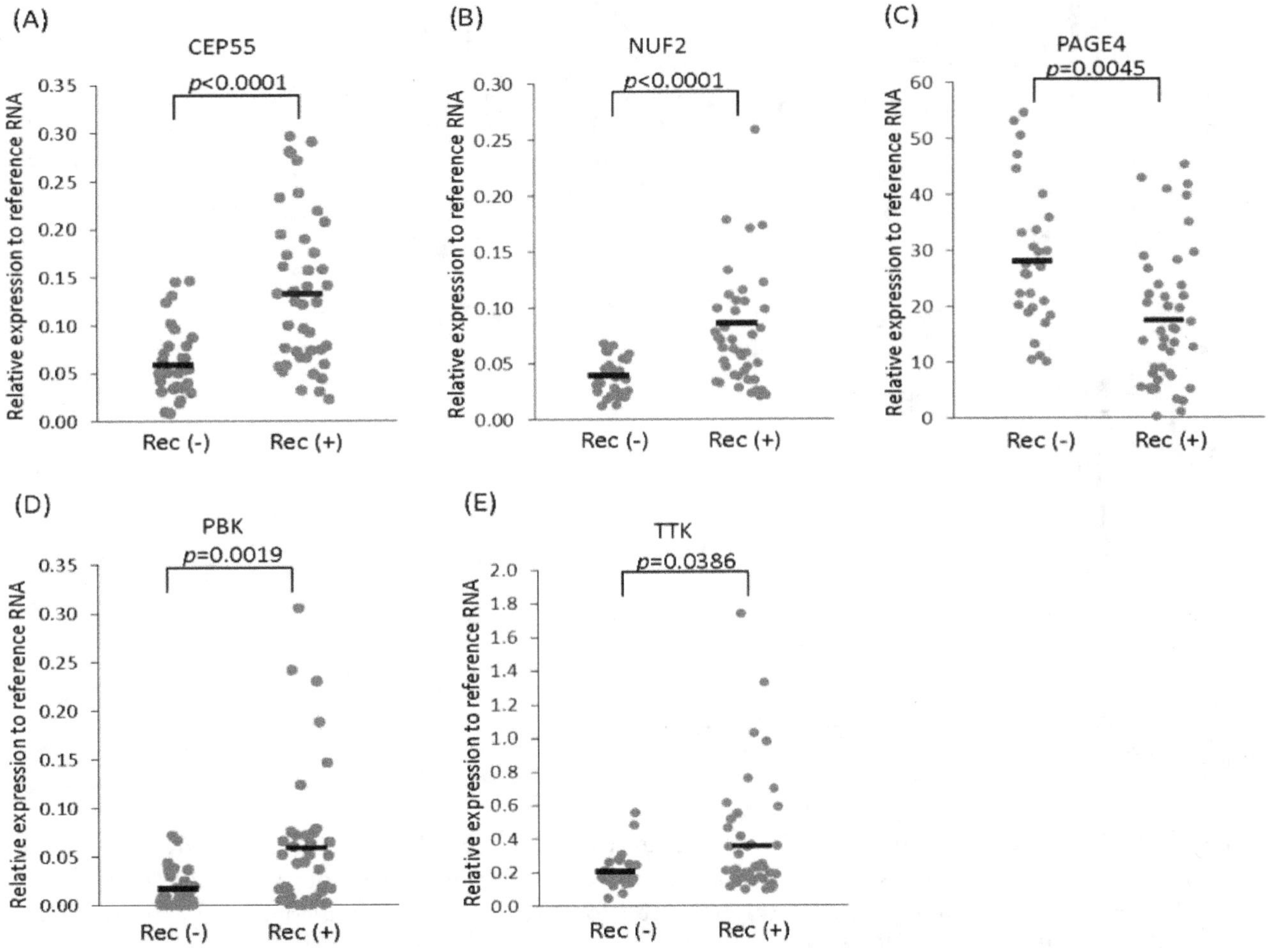

Figure 1. Cancer/Testis Antigen (CTA) expression in recurrent and non-recurrent prostate cancer. CTA expression in clinically localized prostate cancer with recurrence (Rec (+)) (n = 43) and without recurrence (Rec (−)) (n = 29). (**A**) centrosomal protein of 55 kDa (CEP55); (**B**) NDC80 kinetohore complex component NUF2; (**C**) prostate-associated gene 4 (PAGE4); (**D**) lymphokine-activated killer T-cell-originated protein kinase (PBK); (**E**) the dual specificity protein kinase TTK. Reproduced with permission from ref. [49].

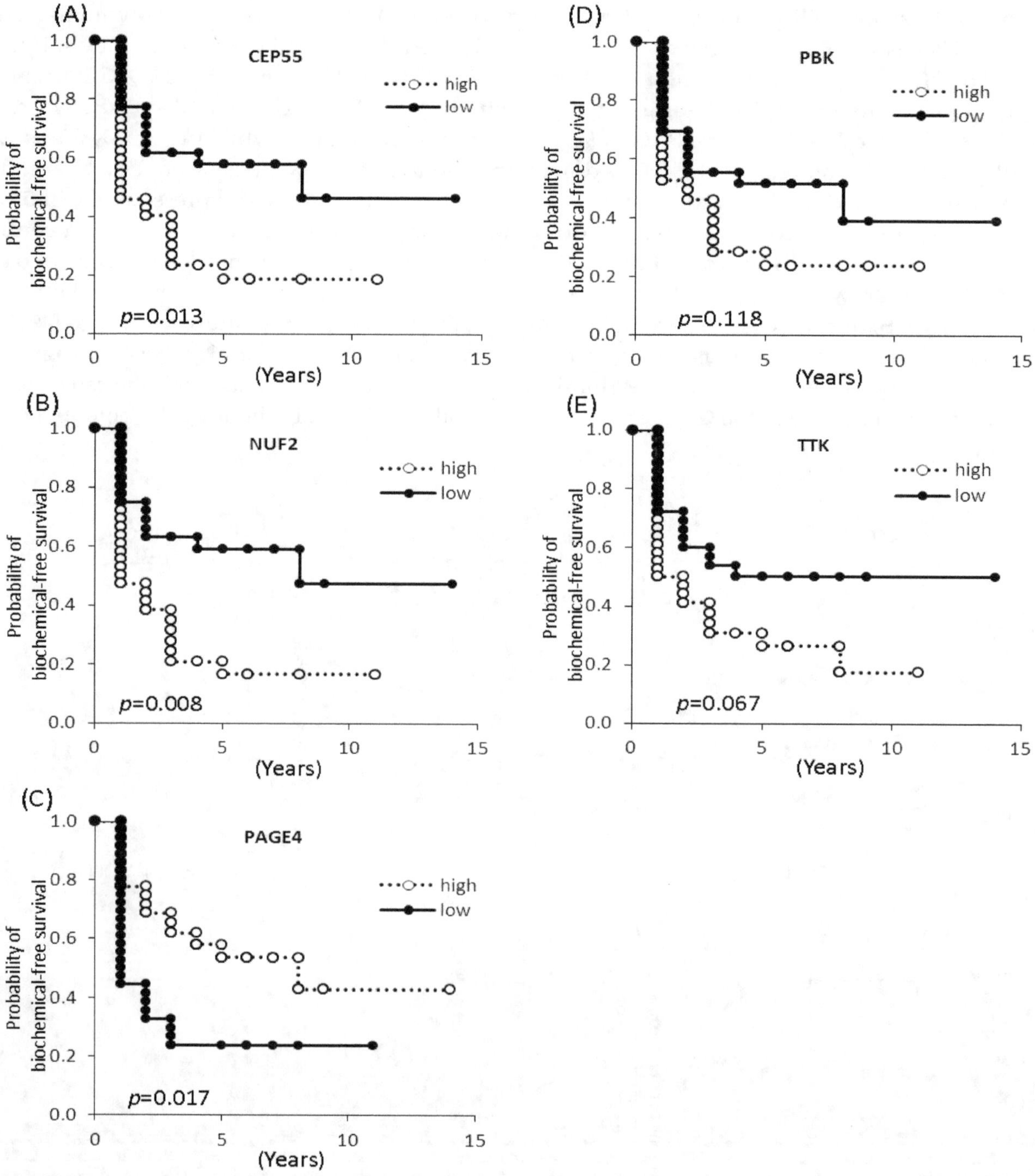

Figure 2. Kaplan-Meier analyses. Kaplan-Meier curves showing biochemical recurrence-free survival against time after radical prostatectomy stratified by the mRNA expression of (**A**) CEP55; (**B**) NUF2; (**C**) PAGE4; (**D**) PBK; and (**E**) TTK (high versus low groups dichotomized by median value). Reproduced with permission from ref. [49].

Despite the promise however, there are some limitations to the study by Shiraishi et al. [49]. First, the sample number was limited ($n = 72$), and they were not derived from patients who were consecutively and prospectively recruited for this study. Second, a high-risk cohort was used as a result of selection of specimens with large-volume tumors appropriate for frozen tissue collection, not reflecting contemporary, newly screened radical prostatectomy population. Third, there was no significant difference in the CT-X antigens (synovial sarcoma antigen X (SSX), synovial sarcoma X breakpoint 2 (SSX2), chondrosarcoma-associated gene 2/3 protein (CSAG2), melanoma-associated antigen 2 (MAGE-A2) and melanoma-associated antigen 12 (MAGE-A12)) between patients with or without recurrence [49]. However, von Boehmer et al. [50] observed that the CT-X antigen melanoma-associated antigen C2/Cancer-testis antigen 10 (MAGE-C2/CT10) may be a predictor of biochemical recurrence after radical prostatectomy, even though its expression was detected only in 3.3% of primary PCa samples.

More recently, the same research group employed the nCounter Gene Expression Assay (NanoString Technologies, Seattle, WA, USA) instead of quantitative multiplex PCR to evaluate the CTA gene signature in PCa patients [51]. The nCounter Analysis System utilizes a novel digital technology that is based on direct multiplexed measurement of gene expression and offers high levels of precision and sensitivity (<1 copy per cell). The technology uses molecular "barcodes" and single molecule imaging to detect and count hundreds of unique transcripts in a single reaction. Each color-coded barcode is attached to a single target-specific probe corresponding to a gene of interest. Mixed together with controls, they form a multiplexed CodeSet. The assay does not rely on enzymes for processing or amplification and enables highly sensitive detection and quantification of gene expression from a wide variety of sample types including direct measurement from purified total RNA, cell and tissue lysates, RNA extracted from FFPE samples and blood without globin mitigation.

The nCounter Analysis System is an integrated system comprised of a fully-automated assay and is designed to provide a sensitive, reproducible, quantitative and highly multiplexed method (up to 800 transcripts in one tube) with a wide dynamic range with superior gene expression quantification results when compared to real-time PCR without RNA purification, cDNA preparation, or amplification [51]. Of the 22 CTAs selected initially by Shiraishi et al. [49], Takahashi et al. [51] found that, in mRNA samples extracted from surgical samples, at least 5 CTAs (CEP55, NUF2, TTK, PBK, and PAGE4) appeared to be differentially expressed between metastatic and localized PCa both by quantitative PCR and the nanowire technology. As expected, CEP55 ($p < 0.01$), PBK ($p < 0.01$), NUF2 ($p < 0.01$) and sperm-associated antigen 4 (SPAG4) ($p < 0.01$) were significantly upregulated and PAGE4 ($p < 0.01$) was downregulated in metastatic PCa compared to localized disease. Further, using this assay FFPE samples, the authors found that RNA expression levels of the CTAs CSAG2 and nucleolar protein 4 (NOL4) were significantly higher in men with GS 8–10 disease than those with GS $\leq 4 + 3$ disease [51]. By contrast, the RNA expression level of PAGE4 was lower in men with GS 8–10 disease than those with GS ≤ 6 disease. Notwithstanding the slight disparity in the CTAs that appear to discriminate disease progression, this study further demonstrated the potential of the CTAs as PCa biomarkers [51] using achieved samples.

3. A Vast Majority of CTAs Are Predicted to Be Intrinsically Disordered

A bioinformatics study by Rajagopalan et al. [52] discovered that a majority of CTAs (>90%) are predicted to be intrinsically disordered proteins (IDPs). IDPs and hybrid proteins containing ordered domains and intrinsically disordered protein regions (IDPRs) are biologically active proteins that correspondingly lack rigid 3D structure either along their entire length or in localized regions, at least under physiological conditions in vitro [53–55]. Indeed, computational studies revealed that the per-proteome amounts of IDPs/IDPRs are high and increase with the increase in the organism complexity [56–58]. Indeed, all the CTAs selected by Shiraishi et al. [49] and Takahashi et al. [51] are predicted to be IDPs or as hybrid proteins containing long IDPRs (Figure 3 and Table 1). Despite the lack of unique structures, many IDPs/IDPRs can transition from disordered to ordered state upon binding to various targets [59]. The structural plasticity and conformational adaptability of IDPs/IDPRs, their ability to react and change easily and quickly in response to the changes in their environment, their capability to fold under the variety of conditions [53–55,60–69] combined with their binding promiscuity and unique capability to fold differently while interacting with different binding partners [66,70] define a wide set of functions exerted by IDPs/IDPRs in different biological systems. These same features determine the broad participation of IDPs/IDPRs in various biological processes [59,71,72] where they are involved in numerous signaling processes [73,74], regulation of different cellular pathways [75–80], cell protection [81], protein protection [82,83], cellular homeostasis [84,85] and cell cycle regulation [86–90]. Thus, biological activities of many IDPs/IDPRs are known to be precisely and tightly controlled and regulated by extensive posttranslational modifications (PTMs), such as phosphorylation, acetylation, glycosylation, etc. [59,91–93] and by alternative splicing (AS) [94–96].

Furthermore, IDPs/IDPRs are often associated with dosage sensitivity and are frequently engaged in highly promiscuous interactions, especially when concentrations of these proteins are increased [97]. Importantly, IDPs/IDPRs can interact with numerous binding partners of different natures, and many of these proteins are known to serve as essential hubs within various protein-protein interaction networks [68,98–102], where intrinsic disorder and related disorder-to-order transitions could enable one protein to interact with multiple partners (one-to-many signaling) or to enable multiple partners to bind to one protein (many-to-one signaling) [103].

Consistent with these observations, several CTAs are also predicted to bind DNA, and their forced expression appears to increase cell growth implying a potential dosage-sensitive function [52]. Furthermore, the CTAs appear to often occupy "hub" positions in protein-regulatory networks that typically adopt a "scale-free" power law distribution. Thus, the observations by Rajagopalan et al. [52] provide a novel perspective on the CTAs, implicating them in integrating and interpreting information in altered physiological states in a dosage-sensitive manner (see [52] and references therein). Considered together, these observations emphasizing the functional role of CTAs together with the development of a biomarker panel based on functionality (e.g., cell cycle progression), underscore the potential of CTAs to differentiate and discern diseased states of the prostate that is latent in their structure or lack thereof.

4. The Functional Role of Intrinsic Disorder in CTAs as Biomarkers

Here, using PAGE4 as an example, we illustrate how intrinsic disorder in CTAs may cast them as "next generation" biomarker candidates. More specifically, we discuss how conformational dynamics of this intrinsically disordered CTA may regulate the phenotype of the PCa cell and how the functionality of this IDP may be exploited as a potential biomarker in PCa.

PCa that is androgen-dependent is responsive to androgen-ablation therapy (ADT), the first line of treatment against advanced PCa, as well as an adjuvant to local treatment of high-risk disease. Although most patients initially respond to ADT, they eventually progress to a hormone-refractory state, which can prove fatal (reviewed in [104]). Yet the mechanism(s) underlying hormone resistance in PCa remains quite elusive. However, contrary to conventional wisdom, a new treatment paradigm called Bipolar ADT or BAT [105] is being tested where chemotherapy patients cycle through ADT followed by a supra-physiological dose of androgen. The results of this pilot study indicate that BAT may be more beneficial than ADT alone [105].

PAGE4 is a highly (~100%) intrinsically disordered CTA (Figure 3 and Table 1) that bears the hallmarks of a proto-oncogene; thus, it is highly expressed in the fetal human prostate, is undetectable in the normal adult gland, but is aberrantly expressed in androgen-dependent primary PCa and not in androgen-independent metastatic disease [106–108]. PAGE4 is also a strong potentiator of the transcription factor, AP-1, which is implicated in PCa [109] and is phosphorylated by two kinases namely, homeodomain-interacting protein kinase 1 (HIPK1) and CDC-like kinase 2 (CLK2). HIPK1 phosphorylates PAGE4 at predominantly T51, which is critical for its transcriptional activity [110]. In contrast, CLK2 is responsible for hyperphosphorylation of PAGE4 at multiple S/T residues. Furthermore, while HIPK1-phosphorylated PAGE4 potentiates AP-1, CLK2-phosphorylated PAGE4 attenuates its activity. Consistently, biophysical measurements indicate that HIPK1-phosphorylated PAGE4 exhibits a relatively compact conformational ensemble that binds AP-1 [111], while hyperphosphorylated PAGE4 is more expanded, resembles a random coil and is characterized by the diminished affinity for AP-1 [112].

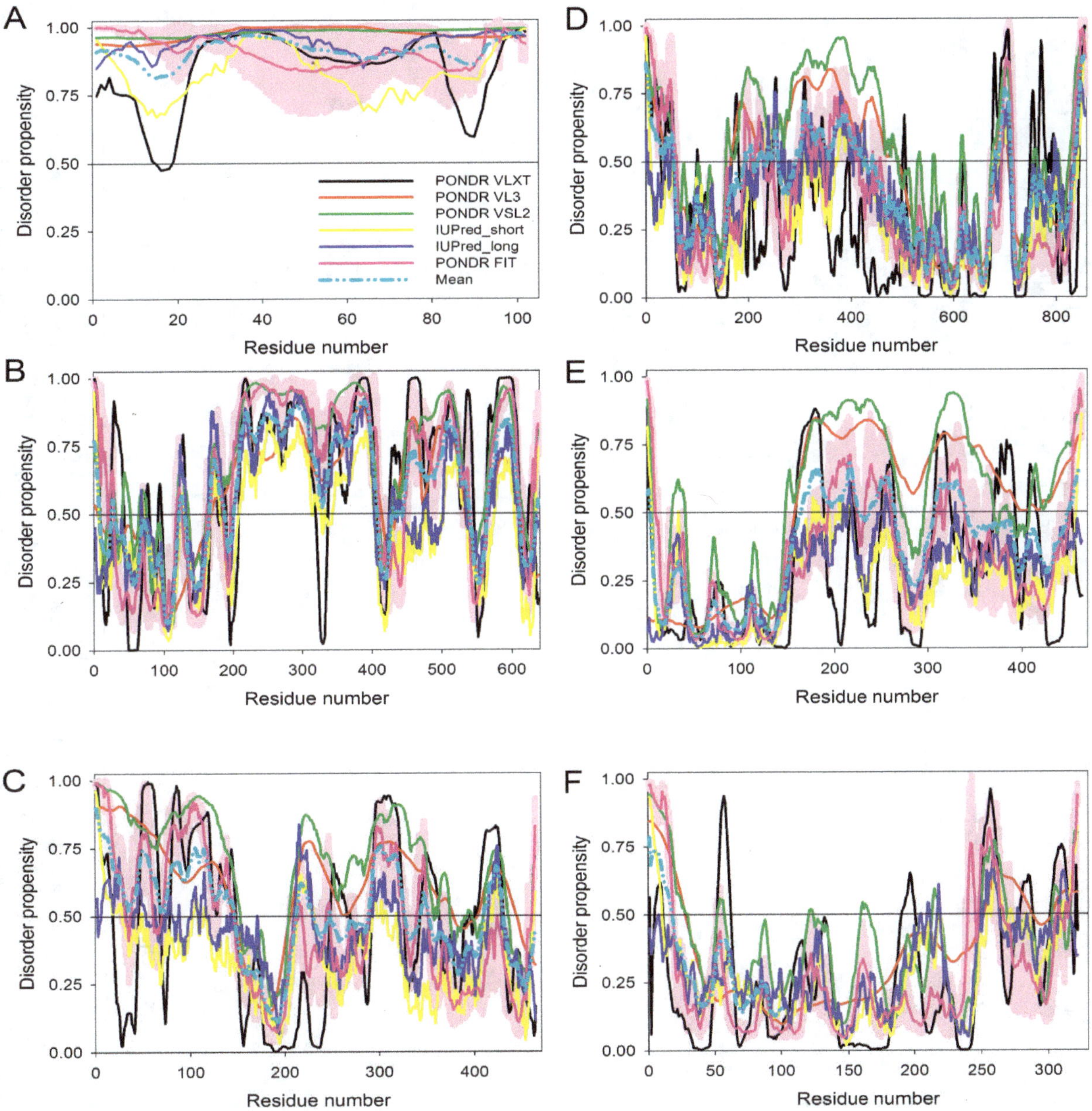

Figure 3. Variability of predicted intrinsic disorder levels and peculiarities of intrinsic disorder distributions within amino acid sequences of several CATs, PAGE4 (**A**, UniProt ID: O60829), nucleolar protein 4—NOL4 (**B**, UniProt ID: O94818), CEP55 (**C**, UniProt ID: Q53EZ4), TTK (**D**, UniProt ID: P33981), NUF2 (**E**, UniProt ID: Q9BZD4) and PBK (**F**, UniProt ID: Q96KB5). Intrinsic disorder profiles for query proteins generated by PONDR® VLXT [113], PONDR® VL3 [114], PONDR® VSL2 [114,115], PONDR® FIT [116], IUPred_short and IUPred_long [117] are shown by black, red, green, pink, yellow and blue lines, respectively. Cyan dash-dot-dotted lines show the mean disorder propensity calculated by averaging disorder profiles of individual predictors. Light pink shadow around the PONDR® FIT curve shows error distribution. In these analyses, the predicted intrinsic disorder scores above 0.5 are considered to correspond to the disordered residues/regions, whereas regions with the disorder scores between 0.2 and 0.5 are considered flexible.

Table 1. Intrinsic disorder-related characterization of some human Cancer/Testis Antigens that can be used as the prostate cancer biomarkers.

Protein	UniProt ID	Protein Length (N_{AIBS}) [a]	PONDR-FIT (%) [b]	MobiDB Consensus (%) [c]	Location (Length) of Long Disordered Regions [d]	Location (Length) of AIBSs [e]	N_{int} [f]
PAGE4, P antigen family member 4	O60829	102 (4/64.7)	100.00	100.00	1–102	1–8 (8) 14–31 (18) 53–81 (29) 92–102 (11)	N.P.
NOL4, Nucleolar protein 4	O94818	638 (13/40.1)	65.98	51.72	201–261 (61) 273–295 (23) 343–403 (61) 503–535 (33) 576–603 (28)	142–162 (21) 184–209 (26) 219–283 (65) 296–323 (28) 329–343 (15) 354–364 (11) 372–378 (7) 407–423 (17) 438–445 (8) 461–466 (6) 486–496 (11) 540–569 (30) 609–628 (20)	9
CEP55, centrosomal protein of 55 kDa	Q53EZ4	464 (8/12.1)	42.24	26.29	1–26 (26)	32–38 (7) 60–65 (6) 158–163 (6) 195–203 (9) 236–243 (8) 280–285 (6) 331–338 (8) 457–462 (6)	102
TTK, Dual specificity protein kinase TTK	P33981	857 (8/7.7)	28.70	23.64	371–410 (40) 836–857 (22)	238–244(7) 271–279 (9) 292–297 (6) 347–356 (10) 362–368 (7) 407–412 (6) 811–819 (9) 824–835 (12)	72
NUF2, Kinetochore protein Nuf2	Q9BZD4	464 (1/3.0)	23.28	5.17	N.P.	278–291 (14)	48
PBK, Lymphokine-activated killer T-cell-originated protein kinase	Q96KB5	322 (3/8.7)	16.77	13.35	N.P.	268–275 (8) 290–300 (11) 314–322 (9)	30

[a] N_{AIBS} (A/B) represents the number of potential disorder-based binding sites identified by the ANCHOR algorithm (AIBS, A) and the percentage of residues involved in disorder-based interactions (B). [b] Content of disordered residues (i.e., residues with the disorder propensity $\geq$0.5) in a protein based on the PONDR-FIT disorder prediction. [c] Content of predicted disordered residues in a protein based on the MobiDB consensus score. [d] Information on long disordered regions (i.e., disordered regions of at least 10 residues) was obtained based on the MobiDB consensus profile. [e] AIBSs are potential disorder-based binding sites identified by the ANCHOR algorithm. [f] N_{int}, number of interactions as found using the BioGRID server [118]; N.P.: not present.

AP-1 can negatively regulate AR activity [119,120], and AR inhibits CLK2 expression [112]. Furthermore, cells resistant to ADT often have enhanced AR activity (AR protein expression can increase >25 fold), suggesting a positive correlation between ADT resistance and AR activity [121]. Based on these interactions, Kulkarni et al. constructed a circuit representing the PAGE4/AP-1/AR/CLK2 interactions that drives non-genetic phenotypic heterogeneity in PCa cells and developed a mathematical model to represent the dynamics of this circuit [112]. The model predicts that this circuit can display sustained or damped oscillations; i.e., androgen dependence of a cell need not be a fixed state, but can vary temporally. Thus, the model suggests that an isogenic population of PCa cells displays a continuum of phenotypes with varying androgen-dependence. These cells can reversibly switch between androgen-dependent and androgen-independent states, without any specific genetic perturbation [112]. These findings appear to explain why BAT treatment appears more beneficial than ADT alone.

If this model is correct, then it suggests that higher levels of PAGE4 could be used as an indicator of a better PCa prognosis. Indeed, as noted by Shiraishi et al. [49], PAGE4 expression is significantly correlated with longer biochemical recurrence-free time (Figure 2). Furthermore, Sampson et al. [107] observed that in hormone-naive PCa, the median survival of patients with tumors expressing high PAGE4 levels was 8.2 years compared with 3.1 years for patients with tumors expressing negative/low levels of PAGE4 lending further credence to the model (Figure 4). Taken together, the work by Kulkarni et al. demonstrates a plausible functional link between IDP conformational dynamics and state switching in cancer [112]. Therefore, in theory, PAGE4 and its various phosphorylated variants represent novel biomarkers, as well as therapeutic targets to treat and manage PCa. For example, the detection of high levels of HIPK1-phosphorylated PAGE4 may imply that it can potentiate AP-1 and thus render the cells androgen sensitive and such patients may benefit from ADT alone. On the other hand, high levels of hyperphosphorylated PAGE4 would imply that the cells are heading towards an androgen-resistant state and thus, patients may benefit from BAT. Finally, pharmacologically targeting PAGE4 may also emerge as a viable option to treat PCa, especially low-risk disease.

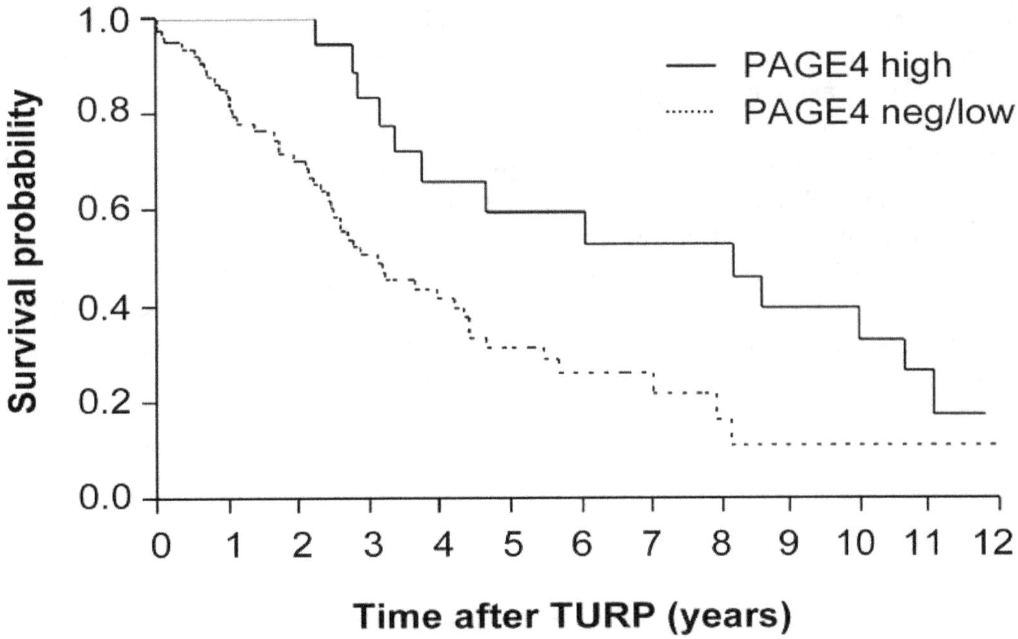

Figure 4. PAGE4 levels correlate with survival of patients with hormonenaive PCa. Overall survival of patients with hormone-naive PCa after transurethral resection of the prostate (TURP) for local advanced obstructive PCa stratified for high versus negative/low (neg/low) epithelial PAGE4 levels on the advanced PCa tissue microarray (TMA) (third quartile of mean epithelial PAGE4 intensity was set as the cut-off level). Reproduced with permission from ref. [107].

Curiously, two other highly disordered CTAs, NOL4 and CEP55, were shown to be associated with different types of cancer. For example, aberrant methylation of CpG islands in the NOL4 gene promoter was shown to be associated with cervical [122] and head and neck squamous cell carcinoma (HNSCC) [123]. These studies showed that NOL4 is methylated in 85% of cervical cancers [122] and in 91% HNSCC samples [123] and therefore the analysis of the epigenetic alteration of this gene can be used for early detection and risk prediction of cancers. Furthermore, NOL4 was recently shown to be one of the 20 aberrantly expressed genes in the most common and the most lethal primary brain tumor, glioblastoma (GBM) [124]. Although the exact biological function of NOL4 protein is not known as of yet, recent analysis revealed that different AS variants of mouse NOL4 (canonical NOL4-L, NOL4-S that lacks the N-terminal tail of NOL4-L and NOL4-SΔ, a NOL4-S with missed nuclear localization signal (NLS)) differently regulate the transactivation activities of the transcription factors Mlr1 (Mblk-1-related protein-1, where Mblk stands for mushroom body large-type kenyon cell-specific protein) and Mlr2 [125]. According to UniProt [126], human NOL4 (UniProt ID: O94818) also might exist in 4 isoforms generated by AS, such as canonical form containing the full-length polypeptide chain, isoform-2 missing 413–514 region, isoform-3, where residues 1–87 (MESERDMYRQ...KQVLYVPVKT) are changed to a shorter sequence MADLMQETFLHHA and isoform-4 with missing N-terminal residues 1–285. Analysis of the functional disorder profile generated by the D^2P^2 platform [127] (see Figure 5A) suggests that the disorder-based functionality of this protein that includes the peculiarities of the PTM distribution and presence of the molecular recognition features (which are specific binding sites that undergo disorder-to-order transition at binding to biological partners) is dramatically affected by AS, providing further support to the important idea that functionality of NOL4 can be regulated by AS (see also Table 1).

Like NOL4, CEP55 is also known to be expressed in various cancers [128,129], being barely detectable in normal tissues except for testis and thymus [130]. In fact, enhanced levels of this protein can be found in breast carcinoma, colorectal carcinoma and lung carcinoma tissues [130], as well as in human gastric carcinoma [131], urinary bladder transitional cell carcinoma [132] and in lung and liver cancers [129]. This protein is also induced at all stages of cervical cancer [133]. Furthermore, in breast cancer, CEP55 is one of the 16 genes, genomic alterations of which may be involved in tumorigenesis and in the processes of invasion and progression of disease [134]. CEP55-derived peptides were shown to serve as suitable candidates for the vaccine therapy of colorectal carcinoma [135]. Aberrant expression levels of the CEP55 genes are known to serve as prognostic marker of the estrogen receptor (ER) positive breast cancer [136]. In HNSCC, genomic instability and malignant transformation might involve CEP55 activation by aberrantly upregulated Forkhead box protein M1 (FOXM1) [137]. In gastric cancer, CEP55 plays a role in the induction of cell transformation in the RAC-alpha serine/threonine-protein kinase (AKT) signaling pathway-dependent manner [131]. CEP55 regulates cytokinesis via interaction with the peptidyl-prolyl isomerase Pin1 followed by the Polo-like kinase 1 (Plk1)-mediated phosphorylation of CEP55 needed for the function of this protein during cytokinesis.

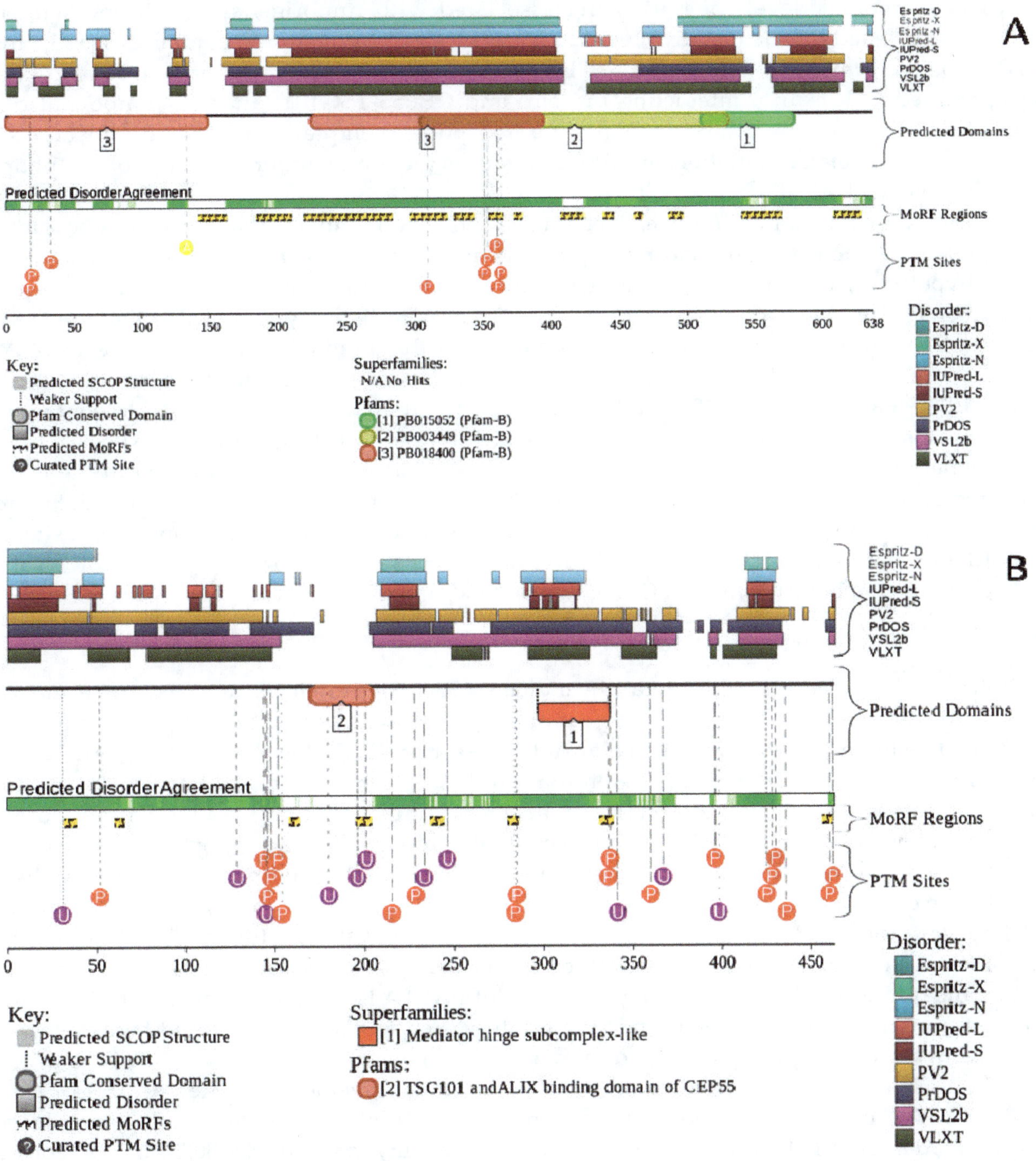

Figure 5. Intrinsic disorder propensity and some important disorder-related functional information generated for human NOL4 (**A**) and CEP55 (**B**) by the D^2P^2 database [127]. The D^2P^2 is a database of predicted disorder for a large library of proteins from completely sequenced genomes [127]. D^2P^2 database uses outputs of IUPred [117], PONDR® VLXT [113], PrDOS [138], PONDR® VSL2B [114,115], PV2 [127] and ESpritz [139] and is further supplemented by data concerning location of various curated posttranslational modifications and predicted disorder-based protein binding sites. Here, the green-and-white bar in the middle of the plot shows the predicted disorder agreement between nine predictors, with green parts corresponding to disordered regions by consensus. Yellow bar shows the location of the predicted disorder-based binding sites (molecular recognition features, MoRFs which are predicted by ANCHOR algorithm [140,141]), whereas colored circles at the bottom of the plot show location of various posttranslational modifications (PTMs).

In fact, pathologic levels of Pin1 being associated with tumorigenesis [142] and with Plk1 activity being needed for the negative regulation of the CEP55 function in cytokinesis [143]. In the BRCA2-dependent manner, CEP55 forms CEP55-ALIX (ALG-2 interacting protein X, also known as programmed cell death 6 interacting protein) and CEP55-TSG101 (another component of the ESCRT-1 (endosomal sorting complex required for transport-1) complex) complexes during abscission, whereas cancer-associated mutations in BRCA2 disrupts these interactions leading to the enhanced cytokinetic defects [144].

CEP55 is known to homodimerize, likely via its coiled-coil domains that are also responsible for protein-protein interactions, and can directly interact with centrosome components [128]. In agreement with this hypothesis, and with the emphasized ability of CEP55 to be engaged in interaction with the ALIX (which is a protein associated with the ESCRT), structural analysis revealed that the 160–217 region of CEP55 forms a non-canonical coiled-coil dimer that binds the Pro-rich sequence of ALIX (residues 797–809) [145]. Although no structural information is available for the remaining parts of human CEP55, Figures 3D and 5B and Table 1 show that this protein is predicted to contain high levels of intrinsic disorder. Furthermore, human CEP55 (UniProt ID: Q53EZ4) is expected to have two AS-generated isoforms [126], a canonical full-length form and an isoform-2 with the missing 401–464 region and the 389–400 region NQITQLESLKQL being changed to KNNTVGILETAS. Figure 5B and Table 1 show that alternative splicing causes elimination of several phosphorylation sites and one MoRF in human CEP55. In other words, it is likely that similar to NOL4, the physiological and pathological functionalities of human CEP55 can be modulated by AS.

5. Conclusions and Future Directions

Preliminary evidence in the literature indicates PAGE4 protein is detected in serum [146]. Although the authors evaluated PAGE4 as a biomarker to discern symptomatic and asymptomatic benign prostate hypertrophy (BPH), it is plausible that serum PAGE4 levels could discern PCa from normal and hence substitute for PSA given that, in the adult human male, PAGE4 is remarkably prostate-specific marker and is undetectable in the normal adult prostate [108,147]. Furthermore, it is even conceivable that a minimally invasive test could potentially also be developed to discern "good" (organ-confined/androgen-dependent disease) and "bad" (metastatic/androgen -independent disease) PCa given the positive correlation between PAGE4 and biochemical recurrence-free survival following radical prostatectomy. Additionally, monoclonal antibodies against the differentially phosphorylated forms of PAGE4 could be explored as novel tools to discern any correlation with disease prognosis. With advances in technology, estimating the levels of PAGE4 RNA and/or protein in CTCs using single-cell transcriptome (RNA-Seq) and single-cell westerns, respectively could be developed as minimally invasive tests for diagnosis and/or disease prognosis.

Although the corresponding data on the differential involvement of different AS isoforms of NOL4 and CEP55 in cancer are lacking at the moment, it is tempting to conjecture that in addition to intrinsic disorder and PTMs, structural and functional variability induced in proteins by AS represents an important feature that might have different roles in different cancers. In fact, AS was indicated as one of the cellular mechanisms (such as chromosomal translocations, altered expression, PTMs, aberrant proteolytic degradation and defective trafficking) that might cause pathogenic transformations in IDPs [148]. Furthermore, the indicated structural plasticity and multifunctionality of PAGE4, NOL4 and CEP55 are in line with the proteoform concept, according to which a functional protein product of a single gene exists in different molecular forms generated by genetic variations, alternative splicing and PTMs [149], as well as by intrinsic conformational plasticity and as a result of protein functioning [150].

Therefore, as opposed to current practice wherein any analyte such as a protein(s), RNA (structural, messenger, small interfering, long non-coding), DNA and its genetic and/or epigenetic modifications, metabolite(s) or circulating tumor cells themselves are selected as biomarkers merely based on their potential for disease diagnostics or prognostics, here we emphasize functionality as an additional trait in selecting a biomarker. For example, the standard biomarker for PCa is PSA, which is a kallikrein protease, whose function in the disease remains poorly understood. By contrast, PAGE4, which is a remarkably prostate-specific cancer/testis antigen in the adult male, is an IDP. Therefore, when overexpressed, PAGE4 can engage in promiscuous interactions resulting in pathological changes, that is, it is dosage-sensitive (see [52] and cross references therein). Furthermore, PAGE4 is a putative proto-oncogene that also appears to contribute to phenotypic heterogeneity in PCa cells due to its conformational plasticity. In other words, PAGE4 not only serves as a biomarker but also represents a therapeutic target (a theranostic). Therefore, PAGE4 and other examples of CTAs discussed here, by virtue of their functionality (for example, cell cycle progression), represent a set of "smart" biomarkers.

Considered together, these observations and considerations support an important notion: the analysis of the protein expression levels in biological fluids may not be the optimal focus of clinical proteomic research and that novel proteomic approaches are needed for the discovery of structure- and function-based next generation or smart biomarkers [151,152].

Since data presented in Figures 3 and 5 and Table 1 are the results of computational analyses used to show that some CTAs (PAGE4, NOL4 and CEP55) could be IDPs, this raises a legitimate question of whether any current biological methods can be utilized to confirm that these putative IDPs are really intrinsically disordered in cancer cells. Although earlier on there was some skepticism about the existence of disorder in proteins in the crowded cellular environment, this has been refuted by several studies that demonstrate that IDPs remain disordered in vivo both in bacterial and mammalian cells using in-cell NMR [153–155]. Clearly, conducting detailed structural and functional characterization of CTAs in vitro and in vivo represents an important future direction in this field. Another important question is related to the existence of the PAGE4-AR (androgen receptor) axis, namely, are the expression levels of PAGE4 as a PCa biomarker associated with the AR expression in the tissue specimens collected from PCa patients? Unfortunately, currently there are no direct data correlating PAGE4 and AR levels. However, as indicated in [112], one might suspect that there is an inverse correlation between the two, since PAGE4 is downregulated in metastatic disease, whereas AR is known to be upregulated at protein and/or mRNA level. Obviously, finding an exact answer to this question constitutes a very important subject for future research. Finally, it would be important to know if there is a link between PAGE4 and resistance to anti-cancer drugs, such as abiraterone or enzalutamide. Although we are not aware of any publication addressing this issue, and do not have corresponding data, we suspect an inverse correlation, since PAGE4 is downregulated in androgen-independent PCa cells. Again, careful analysis of this subject should be conducted in the future.

Author Contributions: Prakash Kulkarni and Vladimir N. Uversky conceived idea, analyzed literature data and wrote article.

References

1. Pollock, P.A.; Ludgate, A.; Wassersug, R.J. In 2124, half of all men can count on developing prostate cancer. *Curr. Oncol.* **2015**, *22*, 10–12. [CrossRef] [PubMed]
2. Dubben, H.H. Prostate-cancer screening. *N. Engl. J. Med.* **2009**, *361*, 204, author reply 204–206. [PubMed]
3. Barry, M.J. Screening for prostate cancer—The controversy that refuses to die. *N. Engl. J. Med.* **2009**, *360*, 1351–1354. [CrossRef] [PubMed]
4. Lee, T.H.; Kantoff, P.W.; McNaughton-Collins, M.F. Screening for prostate cancer. *N. Engl. J. Med.* **2009**, *360*, e18. [CrossRef] [PubMed]
5. Hayes, J.H.; Ollendorf, D.A.; Pearson, S.D.; Barry, M.J.; Kantoff, P.W.; Stewart, S.T.; Bhatnagar, V.; Sweeney, C.J.; Stahl, J.E.; McMahon, P.M. Active surveillance compared with initial treatment for men with low-risk prostate cancer: A decision analysis. *JAMA* **2010**, *304*, 2373–2380. [CrossRef] [PubMed]
6. Cooperberg, M.R.; Carroll, P.R.; Klotz, L. Active surveillance for prostate cancer: Progress and promise. *J. Clin. Oncol.* **2011**, *29*, 3669–3676. [CrossRef] [PubMed]

7. Tosoian, J.J.; Trock, B.J.; Landis, P.; Feng, Z.; Epstein, J.I.; Partin, A.W.; Walsh, P.C.; Carter, H.B. Active surveillance program for prostate cancer: An update of the Johns Hopkins experience. *J. Clin. Oncol.* **2011**, *29*, 2185–2190. [CrossRef] [PubMed]
8. Loeb, S.; Carter, H.B.; Berndt, S.I.; Ricker, W.; Schaeffer, E.M. Complications after prostate biopsy: Data from seer-medicare. *J. Urol.* **2011**, *186*, 1830–1834. [CrossRef] [PubMed]
9. Stephenson, R.A.; Stanford, J.L. Population-based prostate cancer trends in the united states: Patterns of change in the era of prostate-specific antigen. *World J. Urol.* **1997**, *15*, 331–335. [CrossRef] [PubMed]
10. Galper, S.L.; Chen, M.H.; Catalona, W.J.; Roehl, K.A.; Richie, J.P.; D'Amico, A.V. Evidence to support a continued stage migration and decrease in prostate cancer specific mortality. *J. Urol.* **2006**, *175*, 907–912. [CrossRef]
11. Polascik, T.J.; Oesterling, J.E.; Partin, A.W. Prostate specific antigen: A decade of discovery—what we have learned and where we are going. *J. Urol.* **1999**, *162*, 293–306. [CrossRef]
12. Pound, C.R.; Partin, A.W.; Eisenberger, M.A.; Chan, D.W.; Pearson, J.D.; Walsh, P.C. Natural history of progression after PSA elevation following radical prostatectomy. *JAMA* **1999**, *281*, 1591–1597. [CrossRef] [PubMed]
13. Catalona, W.J.; Smith, D.S. 5-year tumor recurrence rates after anatomical radical retropubic prostatectomy for prostate cancer. *J. Urol.* **1994**, *152*, 1837–1842. [PubMed]
14. Ohori, M.; Goad, J.R.; Wheeler, T.M.; Eastham, J.A.; Thompson, T.C.; Scardino, P.T. Can radical prostatectomy alter the progression of poorly differentiated prostate cancer? *J. Urol.* **1994**, *152*, 1843–1849. [PubMed]
15. Trapasso, J.G.; deKernion, J.B.; Smith, R.B.; Dorey, F. The incidence and significance of detectable levels of serum prostate specific antigen after radical prostatectomy. *J. Urol.* **1994**, *152*, 1821–1825. [PubMed]
16. Zincke, H.; Oesterling, J.E.; Blute, M.L.; Bergstralh, E.J.; Myers, R.P.; Barrett, D.M. Long-term (15 years) results after radical prostatectomy for clinically localized (stage T2C or lower) prostate cancer. *J. Urol.* **1994**, *152*, 1850–1857. [PubMed]
17. Pound, C.R.; Partin, A.W.; Epstein, J.I.; Walsh, P.C. Prostate-specific antigen after anatomic radical retropubic prostatectomy. Patterns of recurrence and cancer control. *Urol. Clin. N. Am.* **1997**, *24*, 395–406. [CrossRef]
18. Catalona, W.J.; Smith, D.S. Cancer recurrence and survival rates after anatomic radical retropubic prostatectomy for prostate cancer: Intermediate-term results. *J. Urol.* **1998**, *160*, 2428–2434. [CrossRef]
19. Han, M.; Partin, A.W.; Pound, C.R.; Epstein, J.I.; Walsh, P.C. Long-term biochemical disease-free and cancer-specific survival following anatomic radical retropubic prostatectomy. The 15-year Johns Hopkins experience. *Urol. Clin. N. Am.* **2001**, *28*, 555–565. [CrossRef]
20. Agell, L.; Hernandez, S.; Nonell, L.; Lorenzo, M.; Puigdecanet, E.; de Muga, S.; Juanpere, N.; Bermudo, R.; Fernandez, P.L.; Lorente, J.A.; et al. A 12-gene expression signature is associated with aggressive histological in prostate cancer: *SEC14L1* and *TCEB1* genes are potential markers of progression. *Am. J. Pathol.* **2012**, *181*, 1585–1594. [CrossRef] [PubMed]
21. Artibani, W. Landmarks in prostate cancer diagnosis: The biomarkers. *BJU Int.* **2012**, *110*, 8–13. [CrossRef] [PubMed]
22. Irshad, S.; Bansal, M.; Castillo-Martin, M.; Zheng, T.; Aytes, A.; Wenske, S.; Le Magnen, C.; Guarnieri, P.; Sumazin, P.; Benson, M.C.; et al. A molecular signature predictive of indolent prostate cancer. *Sci. Transl. Med.* **2013**, *5*, 202ra122. [CrossRef] [PubMed]
23. Klein, E.A.; Cooperberg, M.R.; Magi-Galluzzi, C.; Simko, J.P.; Falzarano, S.M.; Maddala, T.; Chan, J.M.; Li, J.; Cowan, J.E.; Tsiatis, A.C.; et al. A 17-gene assay to predict prostate cancer aggressiveness in the context of Gleason grade heterogeneity, tumor multifocality and biopsy undersampling. *Eur. Urol.* **2014**, *66*, 550–560. [CrossRef] [PubMed]
24. Qu, M.; Ren, S.C.; Sun, Y.H. Current early diagnostic biomarkers of prostate cancer. *Asian J. Androl.* **2014**, *16*, 549–554. [PubMed]
25. Sartori, D.A.; Chan, D.W. Biomarkers in prostate cancer: What's new? *Curr. Opin. Oncol.* **2014**, *26*, 259–264. [CrossRef] [PubMed]
26. Kelly, R.S.; Vander Heiden, M.G.; Giovannucci, E.; Mucci, L.A. Metabolomic biomarkers of prostate cancer: Prediction, diagnosis, progression, prognosis and recurrence. *Cancer Epidemiol. Biomark. Prev.* **2016**, *25*, 887–906. [CrossRef] [PubMed]
27. Lima, A.R.; Bastos Mde, L.; Carvalho, M.; Guedes de Pinho, P. Biomarker discovery in human prostate cancer: An update in metabolomics studies. *Transl. Oncol.* **2016**, *9*, 357–370. [CrossRef] [PubMed]

28. Tonry, C.L.; Leacy, E.; Raso, C.; Finn, S.P.; Armstrong, J.; Pennington, S.R. The role of proteomics in biomarker development for improved patient diagnosis and clinical decision making in prostate cancer. *Diagnostics* **2016**, *6*. [CrossRef] [PubMed]
29. Nawaz, M.; Camussi, G.; Valadi, H.; Nazarenko, I.; Ekstrom, K.; Wang, X.; Principe, S.; Shah, N.; Ashraf, N.M.; Fatima, F.; et al. The emerging role of extracellular vesicles as biomarkers for urogenital cancers. *Nat. Rev. Urol.* **2014**, *11*, 688–701. [CrossRef] [PubMed]
30. Mouraviev, V.; Lee, B.; Patel, V.; Albala, D.; Johansen, T.E.; Partin, A.; Ross, A.; Perera, R.J. Clinical prospects of long noncoding RNAs as novel biomarkers and therapeutic targets in prostate cancer. *Prostate Cancer Prostatic Dis.* **2015**, *19*, 14–20. [CrossRef] [PubMed]
31. Martens-Uzunova, E.S.; Bottcher, R.; Croce, C.M.; Jenster, G.; Visakorpi, T.; Calin, G.A. Long noncoding RNA in prostate, bladder and kidney cancer. *Eur. Urol.* **2014**, *65*, 1140–1151. [CrossRef] [PubMed]
32. Fendler, A.; Stephan, C.; Yousef, G.M.; Kristiansen, G.; Jung, K. The translational potential of microRNAs as biofluid markers of urological tumours. *Nat. Rev. Urol.* **2016**, *13*, 734–752. [CrossRef] [PubMed]
33. Kumar, B.; Lupold, S.E. Microrna expression and function in prostate cancer: A review of current knowledge and opportunities for discovery. *Asian J. Androl.* **2016**, *18*, 559–567. [PubMed]
34. Fabris, L.; Ceder, Y.; Chinnaiyan, A.M.; Jenster, G.W.; Sorensen, K.D.; Tomlins, S.; Visakorpi, T.; Calin, G.A. The potential of microRNAs as prostate cancer biomarkers. *Eur. Urol.* **2016**, *70*, 312–322. [CrossRef] [PubMed]
35. Gorin, M.A.; Verdone, J.E.; van der Toom, E.; Bivalacqua, T.J.; Allaf, M.E.; Pienta, K.J. Circulating tumour cells as biomarkers of prostate, bladder and kidney cancer. *Nat. Rev. Urol.* **2016**, *14*, 90–97. [CrossRef] [PubMed]
36. Hugen, C.M.; Zainfeld, D.E.; Goldkorn, A. Circulating tumor cells in genitourinary malignancies: An evolving path to precision medicine. *Front. Oncol* **2017**, *7*, 6. [CrossRef] [PubMed]
37. Erho, N.; Crisan, A.; Vergara, I.A.; Mitra, A.P.; Ghadessi, M.; Buerki, C.; Bergstralh, E.J.; Kollmeyer, T.; Fink, S.; Haddad, Z.; et al. Discovery and validation of a prostate cancer genomic classifier that predicts early metastasis following radical prostatectomy. *PLoS ONE* **2013**, *8*, e66855. [CrossRef] [PubMed]
38. Knezevic, D.; Goddard, A.D.; Natraj, N.; Cherbavaz, D.B.; Clark-Langone, K.M.; Snable, J.; Watson, D.; Falzarano, S.M.; Magi-Galluzzi, C.; Klein, E.A.; et al. Analytical validation of the oncotype Dx prostate cancer assay—A clinical RT-PCR assay optimized for prostate needle biopsies. *BMC Genom.* **2013**, *14*, 690. [CrossRef] [PubMed]
39. Cuzick, J.; Stone, S.; Fisher, G.; Yang, Z.H.; North, B.V.; Berney, D.M.; Beltran, L.; Greenberg, D.; Moller, H.; Reid, J.E.; et al. Validation of an RNA cell cycle progression score for predicting death from prostate cancer in a conservatively managed needle biopsy cohort. *Br. J. Cancer* **2015**, *113*, 382–389. [CrossRef] [PubMed]
40. Blume-Jensen, P.; Berman, D.M.; Rimm, D.L.; Shipitsin, M.; Putzi, M.; Nifong, T.P.; Small, C.; Choudhury, S.; Capela, T.; Coupal, L.; et al. Development and clinical validation of an in situ biopsy-based multimarker assay for risk stratification in prostate cancer. *Clin. Cancer Res.* **2015**, *21*, 2591–2600. [CrossRef] [PubMed]
41. Scanlan, M.J.; Simpson, A.J.; Old, L.J. The cancer/testis genes: Review, standardization and commentary. *Cancer Immun.* **2004**, *4*, 1. [PubMed]
42. Almeida, L.G.; Sakabe, N.J.; deOliveira, A.R.; Silva, M.C.; Mundstein, A.S.; Cohen, T.; Chen, Y.T.; Chua, R.; Gurung, S.; Gnjatic, S.; et al. Ctdatabase: A knowledge-base of high-throughput and curated data on cancer-testis antigens. *Nucleic Acids Res.* **2009**, *37*, D816–D819. [CrossRef] [PubMed]
43. Gure, A.O.; Chua, R.; Williamson, B.; Gonen, M.; Ferrera, C.A.; Gnjatic, S.; Ritter, G.; Simpson, A.J.; Chen, Y.T.; Old, L.J.; et al. Cancer-testis genes are coordinately expressed and are markers of poor outcome in non-small cell lung cancer. *Clin. Cancer Res.* **2005**, *11*, 8055–8062. [CrossRef] [PubMed]
44. Velazquez, E.F.; Jungbluth, A.A.; Yancovitz, M.; Gnjatic, S.; Adams, S.; O'Neill, D.; Zavilevich, K.; Albukh, T.; Christos, P.; Mazumdar, M.; et al. Expression of the cancer/testis antigen NY-ESO-1 in primary and metastatic malignant melanoma (mm)—Correlation with prognostic factors. *Cancer Immun.* **2007**, *7*, 11. [PubMed]
45. Andrade, V.C.; Vettore, A.L.; Felix, R.S.; Almeida, M.S.; Carvalho, F.; Oliveira, J.S.; Chauffaille, M.L.; Andriolo, A.; Caballero, O.L.; Zago, M.A.; et al. Prognostic impact of cancer/testis antigen expression in advanced stage multiple myeloma patients. *Cancer Immun.* **2008**, *8*, 2. [PubMed]
46. Napoletano, C.; Bellati, F.; Tarquini, E.; Tomao, F.; Taurino, F.; Spagnoli, G.; Rughetti, A.; Muzii, L.; Nuti, M.; Benedetti Panici, P. MAGE-A and NY-ESO-1 expression in cervical cancer: Prognostic factors and effects of chemotherapy. *Am. J. Obstet. Gynecol.* **2008**, *198*, e91–e97. [CrossRef] [PubMed]

47. Grigoriadis, A.; Caballero, O.L.; Hoek, K.S.; da Silva, L.; Chen, Y.T.; Shin, S.J.; Jungbluth, A.A.; Miller, L.D.; Clouston, D.; Cebon, J.; et al. CT-X antigen expression in human breast cancer. *Proc. Natl. Acad. Sci. USA* **2009**, *106*, 13493–13498. [CrossRef] [PubMed]
48. Suyama, T.; Shiraishi, T.; Zeng, Y.; Yu, W.; Parekh, N.; Vessella, R.L.; Luo, J.; Getzenberg, R.H.; Kulkarni, P. Expression of cancer/testis antigens in prostate cancer is associated with disease progression. *Prostate* **2010**, *70*, 1778–1787. [CrossRef] [PubMed]
49. Shiraishi, T.; Terada, N.; Zeng, Y.; Suyama, T.; Luo, J.; Trock, B.; Kulkarni, P.; Getzenberg, R.H. Cancer/testis antigens as potential predictors of biochemical recurrence of prostate cancer following radical prostatectomy. *J. Transl. Med.* **2011**, *9*, 153. [CrossRef] [PubMed]
50. Von Boehmer, L.; Keller, L.; Mortezavi, A.; Provenzano, M.; Sais, G.; Hermanns, T.; Sulser, T.; Jungbluth, A.A.; Old, L.J.; Kristiansen, G.; et al. MAGE-C2/CT10 protein expression is an independent predictor of recurrence in prostate cancer. *PLoS ONE* **2011**, *6*, e21366. [CrossRef] [PubMed]
51. Takahashi, S.; Shiraishi, T.; Miles, N.; Trock, B.J.; Kulkarni, P.; Getzenberg, R.H. Nanowire analysis of cancer-testis antigens as biomarkers of aggressive prostate cancer. *Urology* **2015**, *85*, e701–e707. [CrossRef] [PubMed]
52. Rajagopalan, K.; Mooney, S.M.; Parekh, N.; Getzenberg, R.H.; Kulkarni, P. A majority of the cancer/testis antigens are intrinsically disordered proteins. *J. Cell. Biochem.* **2011**, *112*, 3256–3267. [CrossRef] [PubMed]
53. Wright, P.E.; Dyson, H.J. Intrinsically unstructured proteins: Re-assessing the protein structure-function paradigm. *J. Mol. Biol.* **1999**, *293*, 321–331. [CrossRef] [PubMed]
54. Uversky, V.N.; Gillespie, J.R.; Fink, A.L. Why are "natively unfolded" proteins unstructured under physiologic conditions? *Proteins* **2000**, *41*, 415–427. [CrossRef]
55. Dunker, A.K.; Lawson, J.D.; Brown, C.J.; Williams, R.M.; Romero, P.; Oh, J.S.; Oldfield, C.J.; Campen, A.M.; Ratliff, C.M.; Hipps, K.W.; et al. Intrinsically disordered protein. *J. Mol. Graph. Model.* **2001**, *19*, 26–59. [CrossRef]
56. Xue, B.; Dunker, A.K.; Uversky, V.N. Orderly order in protein intrinsic disorder distribution: Disorder in 3500 proteomes from viruses and the three domains of life. *J. Biomol. Struct. Dyn.* **2012**, *30*, 137–149. [CrossRef] [PubMed]
57. Peng, Z.; Yan, J.; Fan, X.; Mizianty, M.J.; Xue, B.; Wang, K.; Hu, G.; Uversky, V.N.; Kurgan, L. Exceptionally abundant exceptions: Comprehensive characterization of intrinsic disorder in all domains of life. *Cell. Mol. Life Sci.* **2015**, *72*, 137–151. [CrossRef] [PubMed]
58. Walsh, I.; Giollo, M.; Di Domenico, T.; Ferrari, C.; Zimmermann, O.; Tosatto, S.C. Comprehensive large-scale assessment of intrinsic protein disorder. *Bioinformatics* **2015**, *31*, 201–208. [CrossRef] [PubMed]
59. Uversky, V.N.; Dunker, A.K. Understanding protein non-folding. *Biochim. Biophys. Acta* **2010**, *1804*, 1231–1264. [CrossRef] [PubMed]
60. Iakoucheva, L.M.; Brown, C.J.; Lawson, J.D.; Obradovic, Z.; Dunker, A.K. Intrinsic disorder in cell-signaling and cancer-associated proteins. *J. Mol. Biol.* **2002**, *323*, 573–584. [CrossRef]
61. Uversky, V.N. Natively unfolded proteins: A point where biology waits for physics. *Protein Sci.* **2002**, *11*, 739–756. [CrossRef] [PubMed]
62. Uversky, V.N. What does it mean to be natively unfolded? *Eur. J. Biochem.* **2002**, *269*, 2–12. [CrossRef] [PubMed]
63. Dunker, A.K.; Brown, C.J.; Lawson, J.D.; Iakoucheva, L.M.; Obradovic, Z. Intrinsic disorder and protein function. *Biochemistry* **2002**, *41*, 6573–6582. [CrossRef] [PubMed]
64. Tompa, P. Intrinsically unstructured proteins. *Trends Biochem. Sci.* **2002**, *27*, 527–533. [CrossRef]
65. Dyson, H.J.; Wright, P.E. Insights into the structure and dynamics of unfolded proteins from nuclear magnetic resonance. *Adv. Protein Chem.* **2002**, *62*, 311–340. [PubMed]
66. Dyson, H.J.; Wright, P.E. Intrinsically unstructured proteins and their functions. *Nat. Rev. Mol. Cell Biol.* **2005**, *6*, 197–208. [CrossRef] [PubMed]
67. Fink, A.L. Natively unfolded proteins. *Curr. Opin. Struct. Biol.* **2005**, *15*, 35–41. [CrossRef] [PubMed]
68. Uversky, V.N.; Oldfield, C.J.; Dunker, A.K. Showing your ID: Intrinsic disorder as an ID for recognition, regulation and cell signaling. *J. Mol. Recognit.* **2005**, *18*, 343–384. [CrossRef] [PubMed]
69. Dunker, A.K.; Cortese, M.S.; Romero, P.; Iakoucheva, L.M.; Uversky, V.N. Flexible nets. The roles of intrinsic disorder in protein interaction networks. *FEBS J.* **2005**, *272*, 5129–5148. [CrossRef] [PubMed]

70. Oldfield, C.J.; Meng, J.; Yang, J.Y.; Yang, M.Q.; Uversky, V.N.; Dunker, A.K. Flexible nets: Disorder and induced fit in the associations of p53 and 14-3-3 with their partners. *BMC Genom.* **2008**, *9* (Suppl. S1), S1. [CrossRef] [PubMed]
71. Ferreon, A.C.; Ferreon, J.C.; Wright, P.E.; Deniz, A.A. Modulation of allostery by protein intrinsic disorder. *Nature* **2013**, *498*, 390–394. [CrossRef] [PubMed]
72. Cozzetto, D.; Jones, D.T. The contribution of intrinsic disorder prediction to the elucidation of protein function. *Curr. Opin. Struct. Biol.* **2013**, *23*, 467–472. [CrossRef] [PubMed]
73. Mitrea, D.M.; Kriwacki, R.W. Regulated unfolding of proteins in signaling. *FEBS Lett.* **2013**, *587*, 1081–1088. [CrossRef] [PubMed]
74. Follis, A.V.; Llambi, F.; Ou, L.; Baran, K.; Green, D.R.; Kriwacki, R.W. The DNA-binding domain mediates both nuclear and cytosolic functions of p53. *Nat. Struct. Mol. Biol.* **2014**, *21*, 535–543. [CrossRef] [PubMed]
75. Galea, C.A.; Wang, Y.; Sivakolundu, S.G.; Kriwacki, R.W. Regulation of cell division by intrinsically unstructured proteins: Intrinsic flexibility, modularity and signaling conduits. *Biochemistry* **2008**, *47*, 7598–7609. [CrossRef] [PubMed]
76. Wang, Y.; Fisher, J.C.; Mathew, R.; Ou, L.; Otieno, S.; Sublet, J.; Xiao, L.; Chen, J.; Roussel, M.F.; Kriwacki, R.W. Intrinsic disorder mediates the diverse regulatory functions of the cdk inhibitor p21. *Nat. Chem. Biol.* **2011**, *7*, 214–221. [CrossRef] [PubMed]
77. Ou, L.; Waddell, M.B.; Kriwacki, R.W. Mechanism of cell cycle entry mediated by the intrinsically disordered protein p27(kip1). *ACS Chem. Biol.* **2012**, *7*, 678–682. [CrossRef] [PubMed]
78. Follis, A.V.; Galea, C.A.; Kriwacki, R.W. Intrinsic protein flexibility in regulation of cell proliferation: Advantages for signaling and opportunities for novel therapeutics. *Adv. Exp. Med. Biol.* **2012**, *725*, 27–49. [PubMed]
79. Moldoveanu, T.; Grace, C.R.; Llambi, F.; Nourse, A.; Fitzgerald, P.; Gehring, K.; Kriwacki, R.W.; Green, D.R. Bid-induced structural changes in BAK promote apoptosis. *Nat. Struct. Mol. Biol.* **2013**, *20*, 589–597. [CrossRef] [PubMed]
80. Frye, J.J.; Brown, N.G.; Petzold, G.; Watson, E.R.; Grace, C.R.; Nourse, A.; Jarvis, M.A.; Kriwacki, R.W.; Peters, J.M.; Stark, H.; et al. Electron microscopy structure of human APC/C(CDH1)-EMI1 reveals multimodal mechanism of E3 ligase shutdown. *Nat. Struct. Mol. Biol.* **2013**, *20*, 827–835. [CrossRef] [PubMed]
81. Mei, Y.; Su, M.; Soni, G.; Salem, S.; Colbert, C.L.; Sinha, S.C. Intrinsically disordered regions in autophagy proteins. *Proteins* **2014**, *82*, 565–578. [CrossRef] [PubMed]
82. Chakrabortee, S.; Tripathi, R.; Watson, M.; Schierle, G.S.; Kurniawan, D.P.; Kaminski, C.F.; Wise, M.J.; Tunnacliffe, A. Intrinsically disordered proteins as molecular shields. *Mol. BioSyst.* **2012**, *8*, 210–219. [CrossRef] [PubMed]
83. De Jonge, N.; Garcia-Pino, A.; Buts, L.; Haesaerts, S.; Charlier, D.; Zangger, K.; Wyns, L.; de Greve, H.; Loris, R. Rejuvenation of CCDB-poisoned gyrase by an intrinsically disordered protein domain. *Mol. Cell* **2009**, *35*, 154–163. [CrossRef] [PubMed]
84. Norholm, A.B.; Hendus-Altenburger, R.; Bjerre, G.; Kjaergaard, M.; Pedersen, S.F.; Kragelund, B.B. The intracellular distal tail of the Na+/H+ exchanger NHE1 is intrinsically disordered: Implications for NHE1 trafficking. *Biochemistry* **2011**, *50*, 3469–3480. [CrossRef] [PubMed]
85. Follis, A.V.; Chipuk, J.E.; Fisher, J.C.; Yun, M.K.; Grace, C.R.; Nourse, A.; Baran, K.; Ou, L.; Min, L.; White, S.W.; et al. Puma binding induces partial unfolding within Bcl-XL to disrupt p53 binding and promote apoptosis. *Nat. Chem. Biol.* **2013**, *9*, 163–168. [CrossRef] [PubMed]
86. Borriello, A.; Cucciolla, V.; Oliva, A.; Zappia, V.; Della Ragione, F. P27kip1 metabolism: A fascinating labyrinth. *Cell Cycle* **2007**, *6*, 1053–1061. [CrossRef] [PubMed]
87. Barberis, M. Sic1 as a timer of clb cyclin waves in the yeast cell cycle—Design principle of not just an inhibitor. *FEBS J.* **2012**, *279*, 3386–3410. [CrossRef] [PubMed]
88. Mitrea, D.M.; Yoon, M.K.; Ou, L.; Kriwacki, R.W. Disorder-function relationships for the cell cycle regulatory proteins p21 and p27. *Biol. Chem.* **2012**, *393*, 259–274. [CrossRef] [PubMed]
89. Yoon, M.K.; Mitrea, D.M.; Ou, L.; Kriwacki, R.W. Cell cycle regulation by the intrinsically disordered proteins p21 and p27. *Biochem. Soc. Trans.* **2012**, *40*, 981–988. [CrossRef] [PubMed]
90. Cianfanelli, V.; De Zio, D.; Di Bartolomeo, S.; Nazio, F.; Strappazzon, F.; Cecconi, F. AMBRA1 at a glance. *J. Cell Sci.* **2015**, *128*, 2003–2008. [CrossRef] [PubMed]

91. Collins, M.O.; Yu, L.; Campuzano, I.; Grant, S.G.; Choudhary, J.S. Phosphoproteomic analysis of the mouse brain cytosol reveals a predominance of protein phosphorylation in regions of intrinsic sequence disorder. *Mol. Cell. Proteom.* **2008**, *7*, 1331–1348. [CrossRef] [PubMed]
92. Pejaver, V.; Hsu, W.L.; Xin, F.; Dunker, A.K.; Uversky, V.N.; Radivojac, P. The structural and functional signatures of proteins that undergo multiple events of post-translational modification. *Protein Sci.* **2014**, *23*, 1077–1093. [CrossRef] [PubMed]
93. Kurotani, A.; Tokmakov, A.A.; Kuroda, Y.; Fukami, Y.; Shinozaki, K.; Sakurai, T. Correlations between predicted protein disorder and post-translational modifications in plants. *Bioinformatics* **2014**, *30*, 1095–1103. [CrossRef] [PubMed]
94. Romero, P.R.; Zaidi, S.; Fang, Y.Y.; Uversky, V.N.; Radivojac, P.; Oldfield, C.J.; Cortese, M.S.; Sickmeier, M.; LeGall, T.; Obradovic, Z.; et al. Alternative splicing in concert with protein intrinsic disorder enables increased functional diversity in multicellular organisms. *Proc. Natl. Acad. Sci. USA* **2006**, *103*, 8390–8395. [CrossRef]
95. Buljan, M.; Chalancon, G.; Dunker, A.K.; Bateman, A.; Balaji, S.; Fuxreiter, M.; Babu, M.M. Alternative splicing of intrinsically disordered regions and rewiring of protein interactions. *Curr. Opin. Struct. Biol.* **2013**, *23*, 443–450. [CrossRef] [PubMed]
96. Buljan, M.; Chalancon, G.; Eustermann, S.; Wagner, G.P.; Fuxreiter, M.; Bateman, A.; Babu, M.M. Tissue-specific splicing of disordered segments that embed binding motifs rewires protein interaction networks. *Mol. Cell* **2012**, *46*, 871–883. [CrossRef] [PubMed]
97. Vavouri, T.; Semple, J.I.; Garcia-Verdugo, R.; Lehner, B. Intrinsic protein disorder and interaction promiscuity are widely associated with dosage sensitivity. *Cell* **2009**, *138*, 198–208. [CrossRef] [PubMed]
98. Patil, A.; Nakamura, H. Disordered domains and high surface charge confer hubs with the ability to interact with multiple proteins in interaction networks. *FEBS Lett.* **2006**, *580*, 2041–2045. [CrossRef] [PubMed]
99. Haynes, C.; Oldfield, C.J.; Ji, F.; Klitgord, N.; Cusick, M.E.; Radivojac, P.; Uversky, V.N.; Vidal, M.; Iakoucheva, L.M. Intrinsic disorder is a common feature of hub proteins from four eukaryotic interactomes. *PLoS Comput. Biol.* **2006**, *2*, e100. [CrossRef] [PubMed]
100. Ekman, D.; Light, S.; Bjorklund, A.K.; Elofsson, A. What properties characterize the hub proteins of the protein-protein interaction network of saccharomyces cerevisiae? *Genome Biol.* **2006**, *7*, R45. [CrossRef]
101. Dosztanyi, Z.; Chen, J.; Dunker, A.K.; Simon, I.; Tompa, P. Disorder and sequence repeats in hub proteins and their implications for network evolution. *J. Proteome Res.* **2006**, *5*, 2985–2995. [CrossRef] [PubMed]
102. Singh, G.P.; Ganapathi, M.; Sandhu, K.S.; Dash, D. Intrinsic unstructuredness and abundance of pest motifs in eukaryotic proteomes. *Proteins* **2006**, *62*, 309–315. [CrossRef] [PubMed]
103. Dunker, A.K.; Garner, E.; Guilliot, S.; Romero, P.; Albrecht, K.; Hart, J.; Obradovic, Z.; Kissinger, C.; Villafranca, J.E. Protein disorder and the evolution of molecular recognition: Theory, predictions and observations. *Pac. Symp. Biocomput.* **1998**, 473–484.
104. Karantanos, T.; Corn, P.G.; Thompson, T.C. Prostate cancer progression after androgen deprivation therapy: Mechanisms of castrate resistance and novel therapeutic approaches. *Oncogene* **2013**, *32*, 5501–5511. [CrossRef] [PubMed]
105. Schweizer, M.T.; Antonarakis, E.S.; Wang, H.; Ajiboye, A.S.; Spitz, A.; Cao, H.; Luo, J.; Haffner, M.C.; Yegnasubramanian, S.; Carducci, M.A.; et al. Effect of bipolar androgen therapy for asymptomatic men with castration-resistant prostate cancer: Results from a pilot clinical study. *Sci. Transl. Med.* **2015**, *7*, 269ra262. [CrossRef] [PubMed]
106. Zeng, Y.; He, Y.; Yang, F.; Mooney, S.M.; Getzenberg, R.H.; Orban, J.; Kulkarni, P. The cancer/testis antigen prostate-associated gene 4 (PAGE4) is a highly intrinsically disordered protein. *J. Biol. Chem.* **2011**, *286*, 13985–13994. [CrossRef] [PubMed]
107. Sampson, N.; Ruiz, C.; Zenzmaier, C.; Bubendorf, L.; Berger, P. PAGE4 positivity is associated with attenuated ar signaling and predicts patient survival in hormone-naive prostate cancer. *Am. J. Pathol.* **2012**, *181*, 1443–1454. [CrossRef] [PubMed]
108. Zeng, Y.; Gao, D.; Kim, J.J.; Shiraishi, T.; Terada, N.; Kakehi, Y.; Kong, C.; Getzenberg, R.H.; Kulkarni, P. Prostate-associated gene 4 (PAGE4) protects cells against stress by elevating p21 and suppressing reactive oxygen species production. *Am. J. Clin. Exp. Urol.* **2013**, *1*, 39–52. [PubMed]

109. Rajagopalan, K.; Qiu, R.; Mooney, S.M.; Rao, S.; Shiraishi, T.; Sacho, E.; Huang, H.; Shapiro, E.; Weninger, K.R.; Kulkarni, P. The stress-response protein prostate-associated gene 4, interacts with c-Jun and potentiates its transactivation. *Biochim. Biophys. Acta* **2014**, *1842*, 154–163. [CrossRef] [PubMed]

110. Mooney, S.M.; Qiu, R.; Kim, J.J.; Sacho, E.J.; Rajagopalan, K.; Johng, D.; Shiraishi, T.; Kulkarni, P.; Weninger, K.R. Cancer/testis antigen PAGE4, a regulator of c-jun transactivation, is phosphorylated by homeodomain-interacting protein kinase 1, a component of the stress-response pathway. *Biochemistry* **2014**, *53*, 1670–1679. [CrossRef] [PubMed]

111. He, Y.; Chen, Y.; Mooney, S.M.; Rajagopalan, K.; Bhargava, A.; Sacho, E.; Weninger, K.; Bryan, P.N.; Kulkarni, P.; Orban, J. Phosphorylation-induced conformational ensemble switching in an intrinsically disordered cancer/testis antigen. *J. Biol Chem.* **2015**, *290*, 25090–25102. [CrossRef] [PubMed]

112. Kulkarni, P.; Jolly, M.K.; Jia, D.; Mooney, S.M.; Bhargava, A.; Kagohara, L.T.; Chen, Y.; Hao, P.; He, Y.; Veltri, R.W.; et al. Phosphorylation-induced conformational dynamics in an intrinsically disordered protein and potential role in phenotypic heterogeneity. *Proc. Natl. Acad. Sci. USA* **2017**. [CrossRef] [PubMed]

113. Romero, P.; Obradovic, Z.; Li, X.; Garner, E.C.; Brown, C.J.; Dunker, A.K. Sequence complexity of disordered protein. *Proteins* **2001**, *42*, 38–48. [CrossRef]

114. Peng, K.; Radivojac, P.; Vucetic, S.; Dunker, A.K.; Obradovic, Z. Length-dependent prediction of protein intrinsic disorder. *BMC Bioinform.* **2006**, *7*, 208. [CrossRef] [PubMed]

115. Obradovic, Z.; Peng, K.; Vucetic, S.; Radivojac, P.; Dunker, A.K. Exploiting heterogeneous sequence properties improves prediction of protein disorder. *Proteins* **2005**, *61*, 176–182. [CrossRef] [PubMed]

116. Xue, B.; Dunbrack, R.L.; Williams, R.W.; Dunker, A.K.; Uversky, V.N. PONDR-FIT: A meta-predictor of intrinsically disordered amino acids. *Biochim. Biophys. Acta* **2010**, *1804*, 996–1010. [CrossRef] [PubMed]

117. Dosztanyi, Z.; Csizmok, V.; Tompa, P.; Simon, I. IUPred: Web server for the prediction of intrinsically unstructured regions of proteins based on estimated energy content. *Bioinformatics* **2005**, *21*, 3433–3434. [CrossRef] [PubMed]

118. Chatr-Aryamontri, A.; Oughtred, R.; Boucher, L.; Rust, J.; Chang, C.; Kolas, N.K.; O'Donnell, L.; Oster, S.; Theesfeld, C.; Sellam, A.; et al. The BioGRID interaction database: 2017 Update. *Nucleic Acids Res.* **2017**, *45*, 369–379. [CrossRef] [PubMed]

119. Sato, N.; Sadar, M.D.; Bruchovsky, N.; Saatcioglu, F.; Rennie, P.S.; Sato, S.; Lange, P.H.; Gleave, M.E. Androgenic induction of prostate-specific antigen gene is repressed by protein-protein interaction between the androgen receptor and AP-1/c-Jun in the human prostate cancer cell line lncap. *J. Biol. Chem.* **1997**, *272*, 17485–17494. [CrossRef] [PubMed]

120. Tillman, K.; Oberfield, J.L.; Shen, X.Q.; Bubulya, A.; Shemshedini, L. C-fos dimerization with c-Jun represses c-Jun enhancement of androgen receptor transactivation. *Endocrine* **1998**, *9*, 193–200. [CrossRef]

121. Isaacs, J.T.; D'Antonio, J.M.; Chen, S.; Antony, L.; Dalrymple, S.P.; Ndikuyeze, G.H.; Luo, J.; Denmeade, S.R. Adaptive auto-regulation of androgen receptor provides a paradigm shifting rationale for bipolar androgen therapy (BAT) for castrate resistant human prostate cancer. *Prostate* **2012**, *72*, 1491–1505. [CrossRef] [PubMed]

122. Wang, S.S.; Smiraglia, D.J.; Wu, Y.Z.; Ghosh, S.; Rader, J.S.; Cho, K.R.; Bonfiglio, T.A.; Nayar, R.; Plass, C.; Sherman, M.E. Identification of novel methylation markers in cervical cancer using restriction landmark genomic scanning. *Cancer Res.* **2008**, *68*, 2489–2497. [CrossRef] [PubMed]

123. Demokan, S.; Chuang, A.Y.; Pattani, K.M.; Sidransky, D.; Koch, W.; Califano, J.A. Validation of nucleolar protein 4 as a novel methylated tumor suppressor gene in head and neck cancer. *Oncol. Rep.* **2014**, *31*, 1014–1020. [PubMed]

124. Stangeland, B.; Mughal, A.A.; Grieg, Z.; Sandberg, C.J.; Joel, M.; Nygard, S.; Meling, T.; Murrell, W.; Vik Mo, E.O.; Langmoen, I.A. Combined expressional analysis, bioinformatics and targeted proteomics identify new potential therapeutic targets in glioblastoma stem cells. *Oncotarget* **2015**, *6*, 26192–26215. [CrossRef] [PubMed]

125. Takayanagi-Kiya, S.; Misawa-Hojo, K.; Kiya, T.; Kunieda, T.; Kubo, T. Splicing variants of NOL4 differentially regulate the transcription activity of MLR1 and MLR2 in cultured cells. *Zool. Sci.* **2014**, *31*, 735–740. [CrossRef] [PubMed]

126. Pundir, S.; Martin, M.J.; O'Donovan, C. Uniprot protein knowledgebase. *Methods Mol. Biol.* **2017**, *1558*, 41–55. [PubMed]

127. Oates, M.E.; Romero, P.; Ishida, T.; Ghalwash, M.; Mizianty, M.J.; Xue, B.; Dosztanyi, Z.; Uversky, V.N.; Obradovic, Z.; Kurgan, L.; et al. D(2)p(2): Database of disordered protein predictions. *Nucleic Acids Res.* **2013**, *41*, D508–D516. [CrossRef] [PubMed]
128. Martinez-Garay, I.; Rustom, A.; Gerdes, H.H.; Kutsche, K. The novel centrosomal associated protein CEP55 is present in the spindle midzone and the midbody. *Genomics* **2006**, *87*, 243–253. [CrossRef] [PubMed]
129. Jeffery, J.; Sinha, D.; Srihari, S.; Kalimutho, M.; Khanna, K.K. Beyond cytokinesis: The emerging roles of CEP55 in tumorigenesis. *Oncogene* **2016**, *35*, 683–690. [CrossRef] [PubMed]
130. Inoda, S.; Hirohashi, Y.; Torigoe, T.; Nakatsugawa, M.; Kiriyama, K.; Nakazawa, E.; Harada, K.; Takasu, H.; Tamura, Y.; Kamiguchi, K.; et al. CEP55/C10ORF3, a tumor antigen derived from a centrosome residing protein in breast carcinoma. *J. Immunother.* **2009**, *32*, 474–485. [CrossRef] [PubMed]
131. Tao, J.; Zhi, X.; Tian, Y.; Li, Z.; Zhu, Y.; Wang, W.; Xie, K.; Tang, J.; Zhang, X.; Wang, L.; et al. CEP55 contributes to human gastric carcinoma by regulating cell proliferation. *Tumour Biol.* **2014**, *35*, 4389–4399. [CrossRef] [PubMed]
132. Singh, P.K.; Srivastava, A.K.; Rath, S.K.; Dalela, D.; Goel, M.M.; Bhatt, M.L. Expression and clinical significance of centrosomal protein 55 (CEP55) in human urinary bladder transitional cell carcinoma. *Immunobiology* **2015**, *220*, 103–108. [CrossRef] [PubMed]
133. Koch, M.; Wiese, M. Gene expression signatures of angiocidin and darapladib treatment connect to therapy options in cervical cancer. *J. Cancer Res. Clin. Oncol.* **2013**, *139*, 259–267. [CrossRef] [PubMed]
134. Colak, D.; Nofal, A.; Albakheet, A.; Nirmal, M.; Jeprel, H.; Eldali, A.; Al-Tweigeri, T.; Tulbah, A.; Ajarim, D.; Malik, O.A.; et al. Age-specific gene expression signatures for breast tumors and cross-species conserved potential cancer progression markers in young women. *PLoS ONE* **2013**, *8*, e63204. [CrossRef] [PubMed]
135. Inoda, S.; Morita, R.; Hirohashi, Y.; Torigoe, T.; Asanuma, H.; Nakazawa, E.; Nakatsugawa, M.; Tamura, Y.; Kamiguchi, K.; Tsuruma, T.; et al. The feasibility of CEP55/C10ORF3 derived peptide vaccine therapy for colorectal carcinoma. *Exp. Mol. Pathol.* **2010**, *90*, 55–60. [CrossRef] [PubMed]
136. Martin, K.J.; Patrick, D.R.; Bissell, M.J.; Fournier, M.V. Prognostic breast cancer signature identified from 3D culture model accurately predicts clinical outcome across independent datasets. *PLoS ONE* **2008**, *3*, e2994. [CrossRef] [PubMed]
137. Gemenetzidis, E.; Bose, A.; Riaz, A.M.; Chaplin, T.; Young, B.D.; Ali, M.; Sugden, D.; Thurlow, J.K.; Cheong, S.C.; Teo, S.H.; et al. FOXM1 upregulation is an early event in human squamous cell carcinoma and it is enhanced by nicotine during malignant transformation. *PLoS ONE* **2009**, *4*, e4849. [CrossRef] [PubMed]
138. Ishida, T.; Kinoshita, K. Prdos: Prediction of disordered protein regions from amino acid sequence. *Nucleic Acids Res.* **2007**, *35*, W460–W464. [CrossRef] [PubMed]
139. Walsh, I.; Martin, A.J.; Di Domenico, T.; Tosatto, S.C. Espritz: Accurate and fast prediction of protein disorder. *Bioinformatics* **2012**, *28*, 503–509. [CrossRef] [PubMed]
140. Meszaros, B.; Simon, I.; Dosztanyi, Z. Prediction of protein binding regions in disordered proteins. *PLoS Comput. Biol.* **2009**, *5*, e1000376. [CrossRef] [PubMed]
141. Dosztanyi, Z.; Meszaros, B.; Simon, I. ANCHOR: Web server for predicting protein binding regions in disordered proteins. *Bioinformatics* **2009**, *25*, 2745–2746. [CrossRef] [PubMed]
142. van der Horst, A.; Khanna, K.K. The peptidyl-prolyl isomerase pin1 regulates cytokinesis through CEP55. *Cancer Res.* **2009**, *69*, 6651–6659. [CrossRef] [PubMed]
143. Bastos, R.N.; Barr, F.A. Plk1 negatively regulates CEP55 recruitment to the midbody to ensure orderly abscission. *J. Cell Biol.* **2010**, *191*, 751–760. [CrossRef] [PubMed]
144. Mondal, G.; Rowley, M.; Guidugli, L.; Wu, J.; Pankratz, V.S.; Couch, F.J. BRCA2 localization to the midbody by filamin a regulates CEP55 signaling and completion of cytokinesis. *Dev. Cell* **2012**, *23*, 137–152. [CrossRef] [PubMed]
145. Lee, H.H.; Elia, N.; Ghirlando, R.; Lippincott-Schwartz, J.; Hurley, J.H. Midbody targeting of the escrt machinery by a noncanonical coiled coil in CEP55. *Science* **2008**, *322*, 576–580. [CrossRef] [PubMed]
146. Cannon, G.W.; Mullins, C.; Lucia, M.S.; Hayward, S.W.; Lin, V.; Liu, B.C.; Slawin, K.; Rubin, M.A.; Getzenberg, R.H. A preliminary study of JM-27: A serum marker that can specifically identify men with symptomatic benign prostatic hyperplasia. *J. Urol.* **2007**, *177*, 610–614, discussion 614. [CrossRef] [PubMed]
147. Prakash, K.; Pirozzi, G.; Elashoff, M.; Munger, W.; Waga, I.; Dhir, R.; Kakehi, Y.; Getzenberg, R.H. Symptomatic and asymptomatic benign prostatic hyperplasia: Molecular differentiation by using microarrays. *Proc. Natl. Acad. Sci. USA* **2002**, *99*, 7598–7603. [CrossRef] [PubMed]

148. Uversky, V.N. Wrecked regulation of intrinsically disordered proteins in diseases: Pathogenicity of deregulated regulators. *Front. Mol. Biosci.* **2014**, *1*, 6. [CrossRef] [PubMed]
149. Smith, L.M.; Kelleher, N.L. Proteoform: A single term describing protein complexity. *Nat. Methods* **2013**, *10*, 186–187. [CrossRef] [PubMed]
150. Uversky, V.N. P53 proteoforms and intrinsic disorder: An illustration of the protein structure-function continuum concept. *Int. J. Mol. Sci.* **2016**, *17*, 1874. [CrossRef] [PubMed]
151. Zaslavsky, B.Y.; Uversky, V.N.; Chait, A. Analytical applications of partitioning in aqueous two-phase systems: Exploring protein structural changes and protein-partner interactions in vitro and in vivo by solvent interaction analysis method. *Biochim. Biophys. Acta* **2016**, *1864*, 622–644. [CrossRef] [PubMed]
152. Zaslavsky, B.Y.; Uversky, V.N.; Chait, A. Solvent interaction analysis as a proteomic approach to structure-based biomarker discovery and clinical diagnostics. *Expert Rev. Proteom.* **2016**, *13*, 9–17. [CrossRef] [PubMed]
153. Felli, I.C.; Gonnelli, L.; Pierattelli, R. In-cell ^{13}C-NMR spectroscopy for the study of intrinsically disordered proteins. *Nat. Protoc.* **2014**, *9*, 2005–2016. [CrossRef] [PubMed]
154. Theillet, F.X.; Binolfi, A.; Frembgen-Kesner, T.; Hingorani, K.; Sarkar, M.; Kyne, C.; Li, C.; Crowley, P.B.; Gierasch, L.; Pielak, G.J.; et al. Physicochemical properties of cells and their effects on intrinsically disordered proteins (IDPS). *Chem. Rev.* **2014**, *114*, 6661–6714. [CrossRef] [PubMed]
155. Ikeya, T.; Hanashima, T.; Hosoya, S.; Shimazaki, M.; Ikeda, S.; Mishima, M.; Guntert, P.; Ito, Y. Improved in-cell structure determination of proteins at near-physiological concentration. *Sci. Rep.* **2016**, *6*, 38312. [CrossRef] [PubMed]

4

Wisteria floribunda Agglutinin and its Reactive-Glycan-Carrying Prostate-Specific Antigen as a Novel Diagnostic and Prognostic Marker of Prostate Cancer

Kazuhisa Hagiwara [1], Yuki Tobisawa [1], Takatoshi Kaya [2], Tomonori Kaneko [2], Shingo Hatakeyama [1], Kazuyuki Mori [1], Yasuhiro Hashimoto [3], Takuya Koie [1], Yoshihiko Suda [2], Chikara Ohyama [1,3] and Tohru Yoneyama [1,3,*]

1 Department of Urology, Hirosaki University Graduate School of Medicine, Hirosaki 036-8562, Japan; hagiwara.kazuhisa@gmail.com (K.H.); tobisawa@hirosaki-u.ac.jp (Y.T.); shingoh@hirosaki-u.ac.jp (S.H.); moribio@hirosaki-u.ac.jp (K.M.); goodwin@hirosaki-u.ac.jp (T.K.); coyama@hirosaki-u.ac.jp (C.O.)

2 Corporate R&D Headquarters, Konica Minolta, Inc., Hino-shi, Tokyo 191-8511, Japan; takatoshi.kaya@konicaminolta.com (T.K.); tomonori.kaneko1@konicaminolta.com (T.K.); yoshihiko.suda@konicaminolta.com (Y.S.)

3 Department of Advanced Transplant and Regenerative Medicine, Hirosaki University Graduate School of Medicine, Hirosaki 036-8562, Japan; bikkuri@opal.plala.or.jp

* Correspondence: tohruyon@hirosaki-u.ac.jp

Academic Editor: Carsten Stephan

Abstract: *Wisteria floribunda* agglutinin (WFA) preferably binds to LacdiNAc glycans, and its reactivity is associated with tumor progression. The aim of this study to examine whether the serum LacdiNAc carrying prostate-specific antigen–glycosylation isomer (PSA-Gi) and WFA-reactivity of tumor tissue can be applied as a diagnostic and prognostic marker of prostate cancer (PCa). Between 2007 and 2016, serum PSA-Gi levels before prostate biopsy (Pbx) were measured in 184 biopsy-proven benign prostatic hyperplasia patients and 244 PCa patients using an automated lectin-antibody immunoassay. WFA-reactivity on tumor was analyzed in 260 radical prostatectomy (RP) patients. Diagnostic and prognostic performance of serum PSA-Gi was evaluated using area under the receiver-operator characteristic curve (AUC). Prognostic performance of WFA-reactivity on tumor was evaluated via Cox proportional hazards regression analysis and nomogram. The AUC of serum PSA-Gi detecting PCa and predicting Pbx Grade Group (GG) 3 and GG $\geq$ 3 after RP was much higher than those of conventional PSA. Multivariate analysis showed that WFA-reactivity on prostate tumor was an independent risk factor of PSA recurrence. The nomogram was a strong model for predicting PSA-free survival provability with a *c*-index $\geq$0.7. Serum PSA-Gi levels and WFA-reactivity on prostate tumor may be a novel diagnostic and pre- and post-operative prognostic biomarkers of PCa, respectively.

Keywords: prostate-specific antigen; *N*-glycan; LacdiNAc; *Wisteria floribunda* agglutinin (WFA) lectin; biomarker

1. Introduction

Prostate cancer (PCa) is a common cancer in men worldwide [1,2]. The most important issues regarding PCa is overdiagnosis and overtreatment [3,4]. Although the majority of patients diagnosed as clinically localized PCa, 30%–40% of patients who receive aggressive treatment such as radical prostatectomy (RP) experience biochemical recurrence [5,6]. Although, active surveillance (AS) is also proposed for low-risk PCa patients who meet the Prostate Cancer Research International Active Surveillance (PRIAS) criteria, 10%–30% of AS patients experience extraprostatic extension, and 42%–80% of AS patients experience an upgrade of the Gleason score after RP (ope GS) [7–10]. Pre-operative prostate-specific antigen (PSA) levels and biopsy GS are also powerful indicators of biological outcomes after RP [11]. Nevertheless, these indicators are not sufficient to prevent the overtreatment of PCa, and there is a need for more accurate diagnostic and prognostic indicators to select an appropriate treatment option for localized PCa.

N- and *O*-glycosylation plays important roles in disease progression. The nonreducing terminal GalNAcβ1-4GlcNAc-(LacdiNAc) structure is found in *N*- and *O*-glycans of many mammalian glycoproteins though in very small amounts [12]. *Wisteria floribunda* agglutinin (WFA) is a good probe for LacdiNAc glycan [12]. Several researchers reported about LacdiNAc expression in cancer using WFA. They stated that LacdiNAc in *N*-glycans significantly decreases during progression of human breast cancer [13,14]. In contrast, the enhanced expression of LacdiNAc has been shown to be associated with the progression of human prostate, ovarian, colon, and liver cancers [12,15–17]. Therefore, the quantification of LacdiNAc glycan carrying glycoproteins or tissue-specific expression of LacdiNAc glycan detected by the WFA has shown promise as cancer glycobiomarkers [17–19]. In particular, regarding PCa, there are only three papers about LacdiNAc distribution in prostate biopsy (Pbx) and RP specimens using WFA [15,16,20], and they did not report the relation between WFA-reactivity in tissues and PCa prognosis. Although there are only a few reports including our group's about PCa-associated aberrant LacdiNAc carrying PSA-glycosylation isomer (PSA-Gi) (Figure 1) [21,22], we demonstrate a pilot study of serum PSA-Gi as a diagnostic biomarker by using an automated two-step WFA–anti-PSA antibody sandwich immunoassay using high-sensitivity surface plasmon field-enhanced fluorescence spectrometry (SPFS) (Figure 2) [22]. Therefore, in this study, we retrospectively evaluated diagnostic and pre-operative prognostic performance of serum PSA-Gi and examined the association between WFA-reactivity on PCa tissues and PSA recurrence after RP.

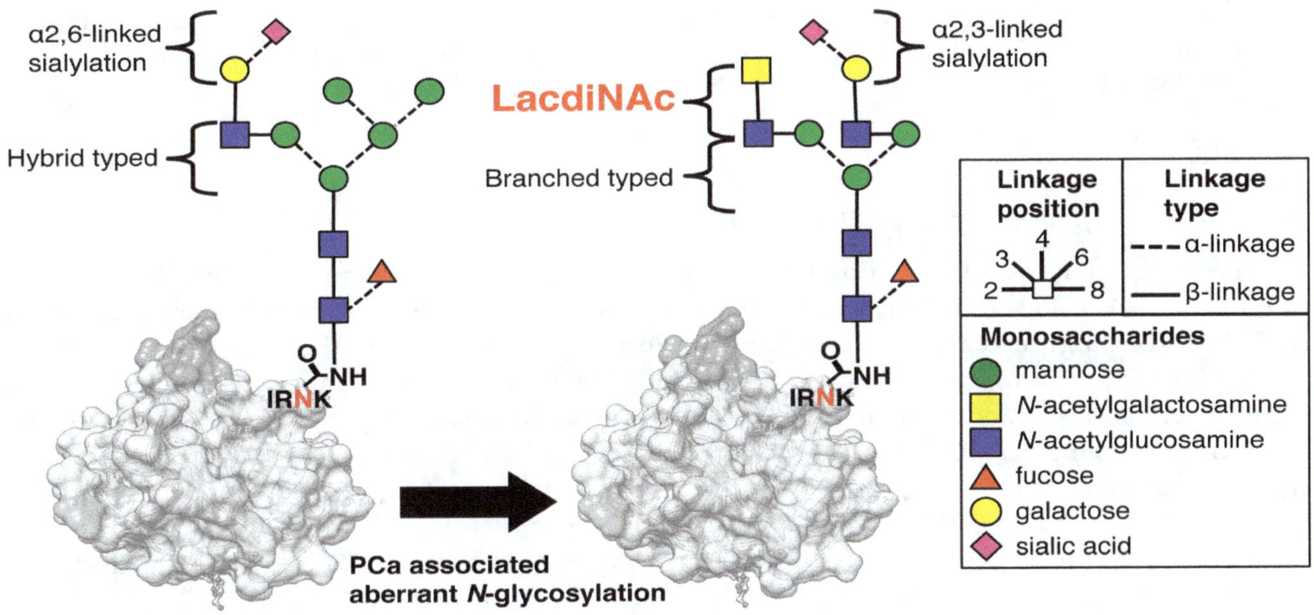

Figure 1. Prostate cancer (PCa)-associated aberrant *N*-glycosylation of prostate-specific antigen (PSA). PSA derived from PCa serum and culture supernatant of LNCaP carries *Wisteria floribunda* agglutinin (WFA)-reactive LacdiNAc glycans; this is not the case for PSA derived from benign prostatic hyperplasia (BPH) serum. PCa-associated aberrant LacdiNAc carrying PSA glycosylation isomer designated as PSA–glycosylation isomer (PSA-Gi) [21]. Carbon linkage positions are denoted by the bond position drawn on each monosachharide. IRNK indicate *N*-glycosylation site of PSA.

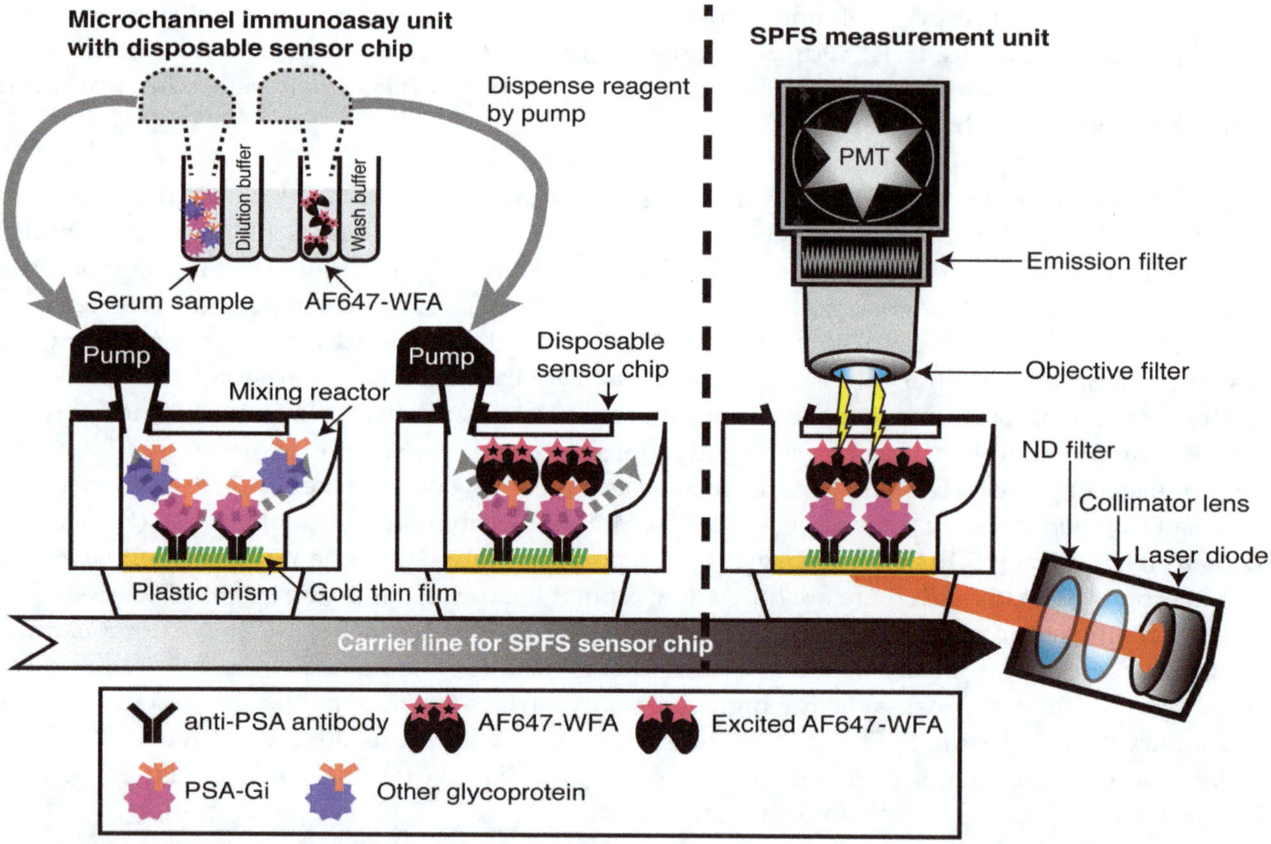

Figure 2. The schematic representation of serum PSA-Gi detection using a two-step surface plasmon field-enhanced fluorescence spectrometry (SPFS)-based WFA lectin-anti-PSA antibody immunoassay. Gray line arrows indicated that reagent dispense from reagent container to mixing reactor using pump. Gray dotted line arrows indicated mixing the content of mixing reactor by pump.

2. Results

2.1. Diagnostic Performance of Serum PSA-Gi before Pbx Much Superior to Total PSA

Serum PSA-Gi levels before Pbx was measured in patients with benign prostatic hyperplasia (BPH) (n = 184) or PCa (n = 244) to evaluate diagnostic performance. Patients' characteristics in the BPH and PCa groups are shown in Table 1. Serum PSA-Gi levels in the both total PSA range ≤20 ng/mL (Figure 3a,b) and ≤10 ng/mL (Figure 3d,e) were significantly higher in patients with PCa (median: 0.1680 U/mL and median: 0.1140 U/mL, respectively) than in patients with BPH (median: 0.0715 U/mL and median: 0.0670 U/mL, respectively), $p < 0.0001$. The area under the receiver-operator characteristic curve (AUC) of PSA-Gi predicting PCa in any concentration range of total PSA (0.795, 95% CI; 0.753–0.837 and 0.752, 95% CI; 0.690–0.813, respectively) was much higher than those of PSA-Gi/total PSA (0.734, 95% CI; 0.686–0.782 and 0.718, 95% CI; 0.659–0.779, respectively) and total PSA (0.638, 95% CI; 0.586–0.691 and 0.550, 95% CI; 0.483–0.618, respectively) (Table 2, Figure 3c,f). At the cutoff PSA-Gi levels (0.0495 U/mL) for the prediction of PCa, the specificity at 90% sensitivity was 36.8%—much higher than the specificity of total PSA (18.8%). Furthermore, we found that higher PSA-Gi levels (≥0.1140 U/mL) in patients with BPH at first Pbx moderately predicted a diagnosis of PCa within 1–4 years after the first Pbx (Figure 3a,d). The nonparametric spearman correlation coefficient between the PSA-Gi level in BPH and total PSA in BPH was 0.3294 (95% CI, 0.1989–0.4559, $p < 0.0001$) and that between the PSA-Gi level in PCa and total PSA in PCa was 0.4613 (95% CI, 0.3531–0.5573, $p < 0.0001$) (Figure 3g). This means the PSA-Gi level was positively correlated with total PSA in BPH and PCa patients.

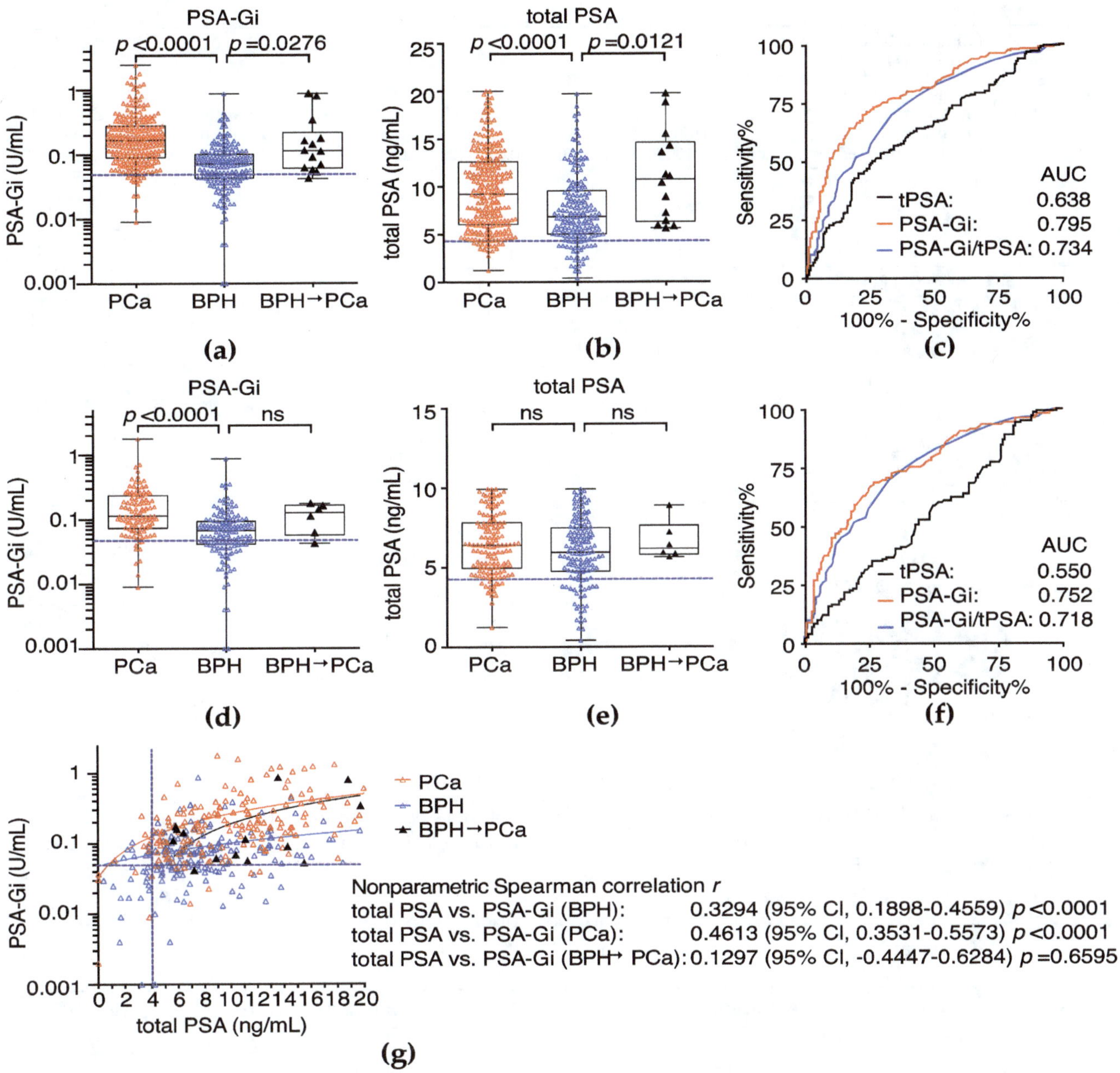

Figure 3. Serum levels of the PSA-Gi at Pbx in the patients who diagnosed as BPH or PCa by an SPFS-based lectin-antibody immunoassay. (**a**) PSA-Gi and (**b**) total PSA levels in patients with a diagnosis of BPH or PCa at a total PSA $\leq$ 20 ng/mL; (**c**) receiver-operator characteristic (ROC) curve analysis of total PSA, PSA-Gi, and PSA-Gi/total PSA in patients who had a diagnosis of BPH or PCa at a total PSA $\leq$ 20 ng/mL. The areas under the ROC curve (AUCs) for the prediction of PCa of PSA-Gi, total PSA, and PSA-Gi/total PSA were 0.795, 0.638, and 0.734, respectively; (**d**) PSA-Gi and (**e**) total PSA levels in patients with BPH or PCa at total PSA $\leq$ 10 ng/mL; (**f**) ROC curve analysis of total PSA, PSA-Gi, and PSA-Gi/total PSA in patients with BPH or PCa at a total PSA $\leq$ 10 ng/mL. The AUCs for the prediction of PCa by means of PSA-Gi, total PSA, and PSA-Gi/total PSA were 0.752, 0.550, and 0.718, respectively; (**g**) correlation between PSA-Gi and total PSA. Correlation coefficient was analyzed by non-parametric Spearman's *r*-test. (**a–g**) The cutoff level at 90% sensitivity of PSA-Gi and/or total PSA is presented as a blue dotted line.

Table 1. Characteristics of BPH patients and PCa patients.

Characteristics n = 442	BPH [a] 184	PCa [b] 244	BPH-> PCa 14	p ([a] vs. [b])
Age, median (range)	69 (30–87)	68 (44–85)	69 (52–80)	ns [1]
PSA [2], ng/mL, median (range)	6.8 (0.4–19.7)	9.0 (1.2–62.6)	6.3 (5.9–19.7)	<0.001
PSA-Gi, U/mL, median (range)	0.0715 (0.001–0.86)	0.165 (0.002–2.43)	0.113 (0.04–0.87)	<0.001
PSA-Gi/total PSA, U/ng, median (range)	0.0100 (0.00–0.1150)	0.0200 (0.002–0.1980)	0.0135 (0.003–0.0640)	<0.001
Clinical T stage, n (%)		n = 244		
cT1		144 (59.3)		
cT2		46 (18.5)		
cT3		55 (22.2)		
Pbx GS [3], n (%) Pbx GG [4]		n = 244		
3 + 3 [1]		6 (2.4)		
3 + 4 [2]		79 (32.4)		
4 + 3 [3]		29 (11.9)		
4 + 4 [4]		30 (12.3)		
3 + 5 [4]		3 (1.2)		
4 + 5 [5]		72 (29.5)		
5 + 4 [5]		20 (8.2)		
5 + 5 [5]		5 (2.0)		
Pathological T stage, n (%)		n = 92	n = 8	
pT1		4 (4.3)	0 (0)	
pT2		53 (57.6)	5 (62.5)	
pT3		38 (41.3)	3 (37.5)	
Ope GS [5], n (%) Ope GG [6]		n = 92	n = 8	
3 + 3 [1]		1 (1.1)		
3 + 4 [2]		13 (14.1)	2 (25.0)	
4 + 3 [3]		14 (15.2)		
3 + 5 [4]		3 (3.2)	1 (12.5)	
4 + 4 [4]		9 (9.8)	1 (12.5)	
5 + 3 [4]		1 (1.1)		
4 + 5 [5]		37 (40.2)	3 (37.5)	
5 + 4 [5]		12 (13.0)	1 (12.5)	
5 + 5 [5]		2 (2.2)		

[1] not significantly difference; [2] total PSA; [3] prostate biopsy Gleason score; [4] prostate biopsy grade group; [5] Gleason score after radical prostatectomy; [6] grade group after radical prostatectomy. Pbx: prostate biopsy; [a] BPH; [b] PCa.

Table 2. Comparison of areas under the receiver-operator characteristic curve (AUCs) of PSA, PSA-Gi, and PSA-Gi/total PSA for the detection of PCa.

Test Name	PSA Range	AUC	95% CI	p (vs. [a])	p (vs. [b])	p (vs. [c])
Total PSA [a]	-	0.638	0.586–0.691	-	<0.0001	0.0376
PSA-Gi [b]	20 ng/mL	0.795	0.753–0.837	<0.0001	-	0.0003
PSA-Gi/total PSA[c]	-	0.734	0.586–0.691	0.0376	0.0003	-
Total PSA [a]	-	0.550	0.483–0.618	-	<0.0001	<0.0001
PSA-Gi [b]	10 ng/mL	0.752	0.690–0.813	<0.0001	-	0.567
PSA-Gi/total PSA [c]	-	0.719	0.659–0.779	0.0009	0.0009	-

[a] Total PSA test; [b] PSA-Gi test; [c] PSA-Gi/total PSA test.

2.2. *Serum PSA-Gi before Pbx Can Discriminate between Pbx Grade Group 2 and 3*

Serum PSA-Gi levels before Pbx was measured in 244 PCa patients to evaluate the pre-operative predictor for a prostate biopsy. PSA-Gi levels were significantly correlated with Pbx grade group (GG) [23] (Figure 4a,b). Although total PSA could not discriminate between Pbx GG 2 and 3, serum PSA-Gi levels were significantly higher at ope GG 3 (median: 0.2500 U/mL, p = 0.0118) than at ope GG 2 (median: 0.1280 U/mL, Figure 4a,b). The AUC of PSA-Gi predicting Pbx GG 3 tumors was 0.649 (95% CI, 0.5221–0.7735) in contrast to the total PSA AUC of 0.520 (95% CI, 0.4091–0.6312; p = 0.162; Figure 4c). At the cutoff PSA-Gi level (0.1930 U/mL) for the prediction of GG 3 tumors at

Pbx, sensitivity was 57.1%, and specificity was 80.8%—muchhigher than the specificity of the total PSA test (47.4%).

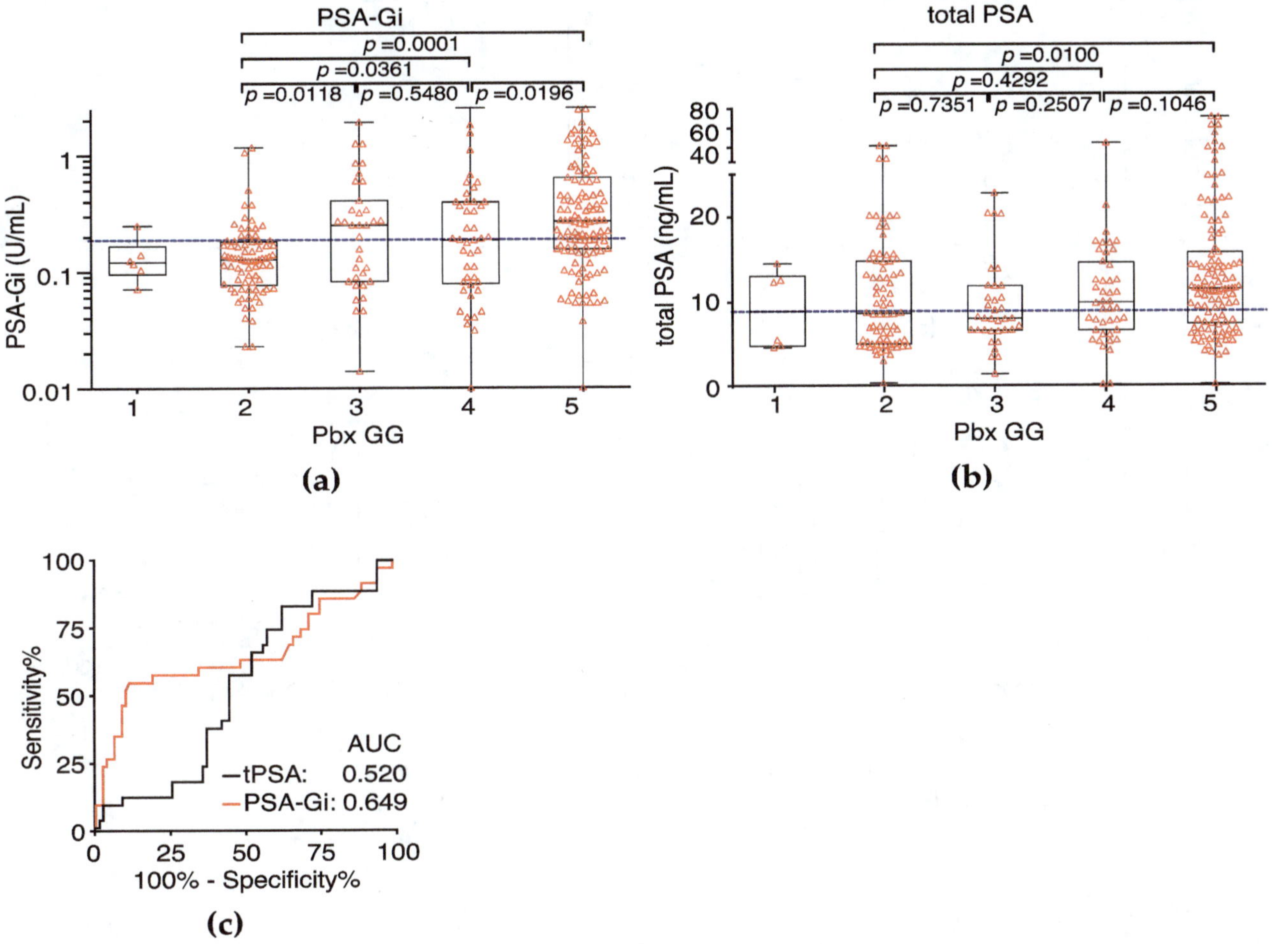

Figure 4. The serum PSA-Gi levels at Pbx in PCa patients who underwent radical prostatectomy (RP). (**a**) PSA-Gi levels before Pbx among PCa patients classified by the Pbx grade group (Pbx GG); (**b**) total PSA level before Pbx of PCa patients classified by the Pbx GG. Cutoff levels at 57.1% sensitivity of PSA-Gi and/or total PSA is presented as a blue dotted line; (**c**) ROC curve analysis of total PSA and PSA-Gi in PCa patients with Pbx GG 2 and Pbx GG 3. The AUCs for the prediction of patients with Pbx GG 3 of PSA-Gi and total PSA were 0.649 and 0.520, respectively.

2.3. Serum PSA-Gi before Pbx Can Discriminate between Ope Grade Group ≤2 and ≥3

Serum PSA-Gi levels before Pbx was measured in 92 PCa patients who underwent RP to evaluate the pre-operative prognostic performance. PSA-Gi levels were moderately correlated with grade group after RP (ope GG) [23] (Figure 5a,b). Although total PSA could not discriminate tumors with ope GG $\geq$ 3, serum PSA-Gi levels was significantly higher at ope GG $\geq$ 3 (median: 0.1885 U/mL, $p = 0.0068$) than at ope GG $\leq$ 2 (median: 0.0985 U/mL, Figure 5c,d). The AUC of PSA-Gi predicting ope GG $\geq$ 3 tumors was 0.724 (95% CI, 0.603–0.845) in contrast to the total PSA AUC of 0.618 (95% CI, 0.442–0.794; $p = 0.202$; Figure 5e). Furthermore, the PSA-Gi levels tended to be higher in patients with a GG upgrade from 2 at Pbx to ope GG $\geq$ 3 and were associated with a GG downgrade from ≥3 at Pbx to ope GG $\leq$ 2 (Figure 5f,g). At the cutoff PSA-Gi level (0.1445 U/mL) for the prediction of GG $\geq$ 3 tumors, sensitivity was 60.3%, and specificity was 78.6%—much higher than the specificity of the total PSA test (50.0%).

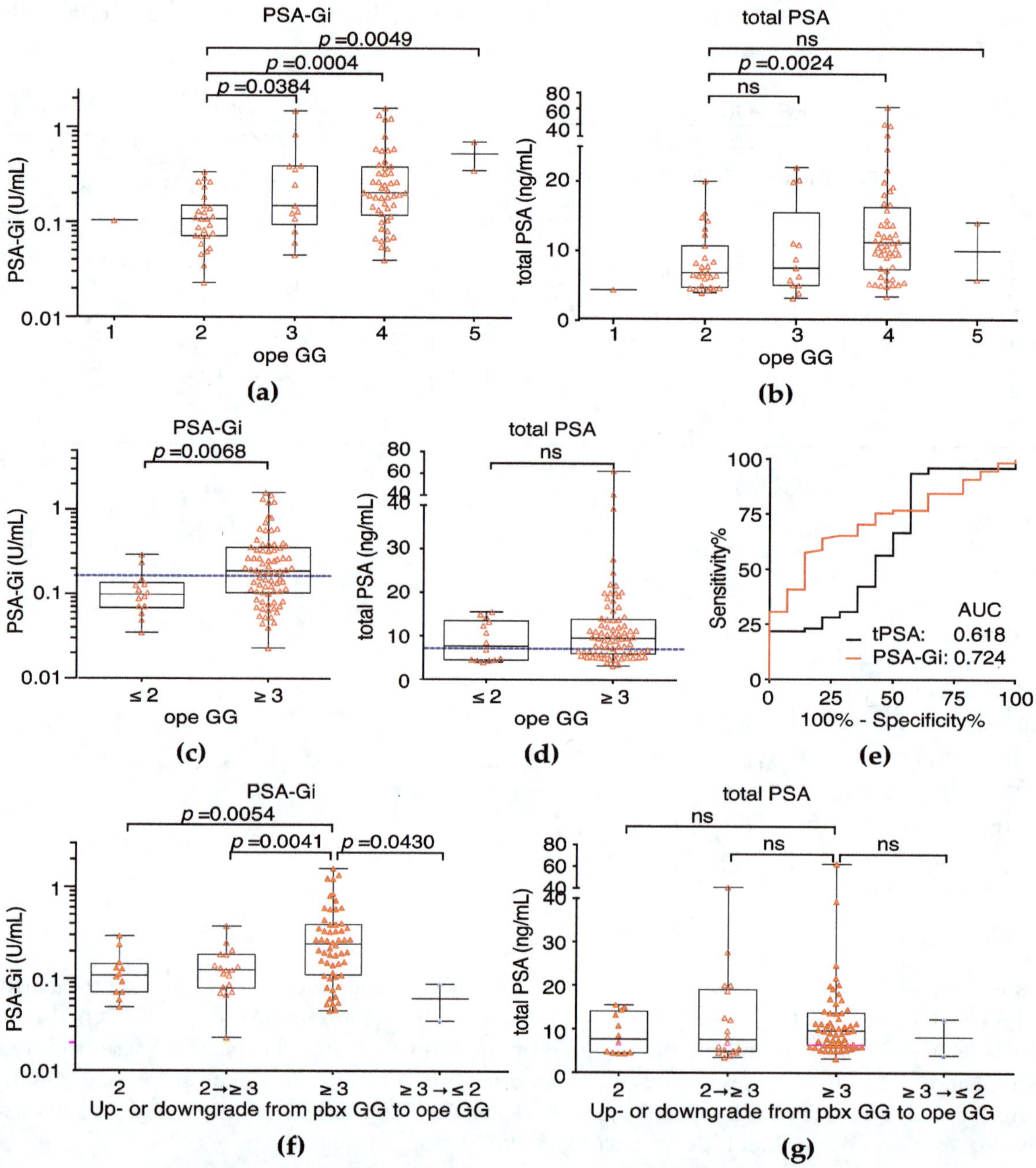

Figure 5. The serum PSA-Gi levels at Pbx in PCa patients who underwent RP. (**a**) PSA-Gi levels before Pbx among PCa patients classified by the grade group after RP (ope GG); (**b**) total PSA level before Pbx of PCa patients classified by the ope GG; (**c**,**d**) PSA-Gi and total PSA levels before Pbx between patients with ope GG ≤ 2 and ope GG ≥ 3. Cutoff levels at 60% sensitivity of PSA-Gi and/or total PSA is presented as a blue dotted line; (**e**) ROC curve analysis of total PSA and PSA-Gi in PCa patients with ope GG ≤ 2 and ope GG ≥ 3. The AUCs for the prediction of patients with ope GG ≥ 3 of PSA-Gi and total PSA were 0.724 and 0.618, respectively; (**f**,**g**) PSA-Gi and total PSA levels in patients with a GG upgrade from 2 at Pbx to ope GG ≥ 3 and a GG downgrade from ≥ 3 at Pbx to ope GG ≤ 2.

2.4. Tumors Strongly and Moderately Positive for WFA Is an Independent Risk Factor of PSA Recurrence

Immunohistochemical staining of RP specimens by WFA was performed to examine the association between WFA-reactivity of tumor site and clinicopathological status. Patients' characteristics in the 260 RP patients are shown in Table 3. WFA-reactive glycan was expressed in both benign prostate glands and tumors. On the basis of the reciprocal intensity of a tumor site [24], the WFA-reactivity was classified into three groups: weakly positive (median 78.5, range 74–85), moderately positive (median 98.5, range 86–104), and strongly positive (median 132, range 105–170; Figures 6a and A1). When collated with these criteria, tumors strongly and moderately positive for WFA were significantly associated with a higher ope GS, pathological stage (≥pT3), and perineural invasion (pn)-positive status (Figure 6b and Table 3). As shown in Figure 5c, patients with tumors strongly and moderately positive for WFA had a much shorter period of PSA recurrence after RP than patients with tumors weakly positive for WFA (log-rank test, $p = 0.0044$). Multivariate Cox regression analysis revealed that WFA-reactivity was an independent risk factor of PSA recurrence (Table 4) and developed post-operative nomogram including WFA-reactivity, age, grade group, pT, RM, and pn status for prediction of PSA-free survival provability (Figure 6d). The c-index of nomogram was 0.754 (95% CI, 0.697–0.812) [25].

Table 3. Characteristics of PCa patients who underwent RP categorized by WFA-reactivity.

Characteristics		WFA-Reactivity						p
		Weakly Positive [a]		Moderately Positive [b]		Strongly Positive [c]		[a] vs. [b + c]
n, Total = 260		51		95		112		
Age, median (range)		68 (48–75)		68 (56–76)		68 (52–78)		0.555
PSA [1], ng/mL, median (range)		7.5 (2.3–18.4)		7.4 (0.6–27.6)		7.5 (0.5–35.9)		0.473
Pathological T stage, n (%)								0.008 [2]
pT2, $n = 163$		41	(26.4)	48	(29.4)	72	(44.2)	0.002
pT3, $n = 96$		10	(10.4)	47	(49.0)	39	(40.6)	0.002
pT4, $n = 1$		0	(0)	0	(0)	1	(100)	0.612
Ope GS [3], n (%)	Ope GG [4]							0.045 [2]
3 + 3, $n = 11$	Ope GG 1	5	(45.4)	3	(27.3)	3	(27.3)	0.035
3 + 4, $n = 112$	Ope GG 2	28	(26.5)	34	(27.9)	50	(44.6)	0.108
4 + 3, $n = 63$	Ope GG 3	13	(19.3)	28	(45.2)	22	(35.5)	0.955
4 + 4, $n = 9$	Ope GG 4	2	(22.3)	3	(33.3)	4	(44.4)	0.889
3 + 5, $n = 9$	Ope GG 4	1	(11.1)	3	(33.3)	5	(55.6)	0.482
4 + 5, $n = 42$	Ope GG 5	4	(9.5)	17	(40.5)	21	(50.0)	0.056
5 + 4, $n = 14$	Ope GG 5	0	(0)	7	(50.0)	7	(50.0)	0.052
pn [5], n (%)								
pn−, $n = 56$		21	(37.5)	18	(32.1)	17	(30.4)	<0.001
pn+, $n = 204$		32	(15.7)	77	(37.7)	95	(46.6)	<0.001
RM [6], n (%)								
RM−, $n = 188$		43	(22.9)	65	(34.6)	80	(42.5)	0.108
RM+, $n = 72$		10	(13.9)	30	(41.7)	32	(44.4)	0.108
PSA failure, n (%)								
−, $n = 194$		49	(25.3)	66	(34.0)	79	(40.7)	<0.001
+, $n = 66$		4	(6.1)	29	(43.9)	33	(50.0)	<0.001

[1] total PSA; [2] χ^2 test; [3] Ope GS, Gleason score after radical prostatectomy; [4] Ope GG, grade group after radical prostatectomy; [5] pn, perineural invasion; [6] RM, resection margin; [a] weakly positive; [b] moderately positive; [c] strongly positive.

Table 4. Multivariate analysis to determine an independent predictor of PSA recurrence.

Variable	Hazard Ratio	Standard Error	p
Age	1.046	0.027	0.099
WFA-reactivity	2.831	0.529	0.049
pT [1]	1.589	0.336	0.168
Grade group	1.246	0.099	0.027
RM [2]	2.424	0.319	0.006
pn [3]	1.715	0.447	0.227

[1] pathological T stage; [2] resection margin; [3] perineural invasion.

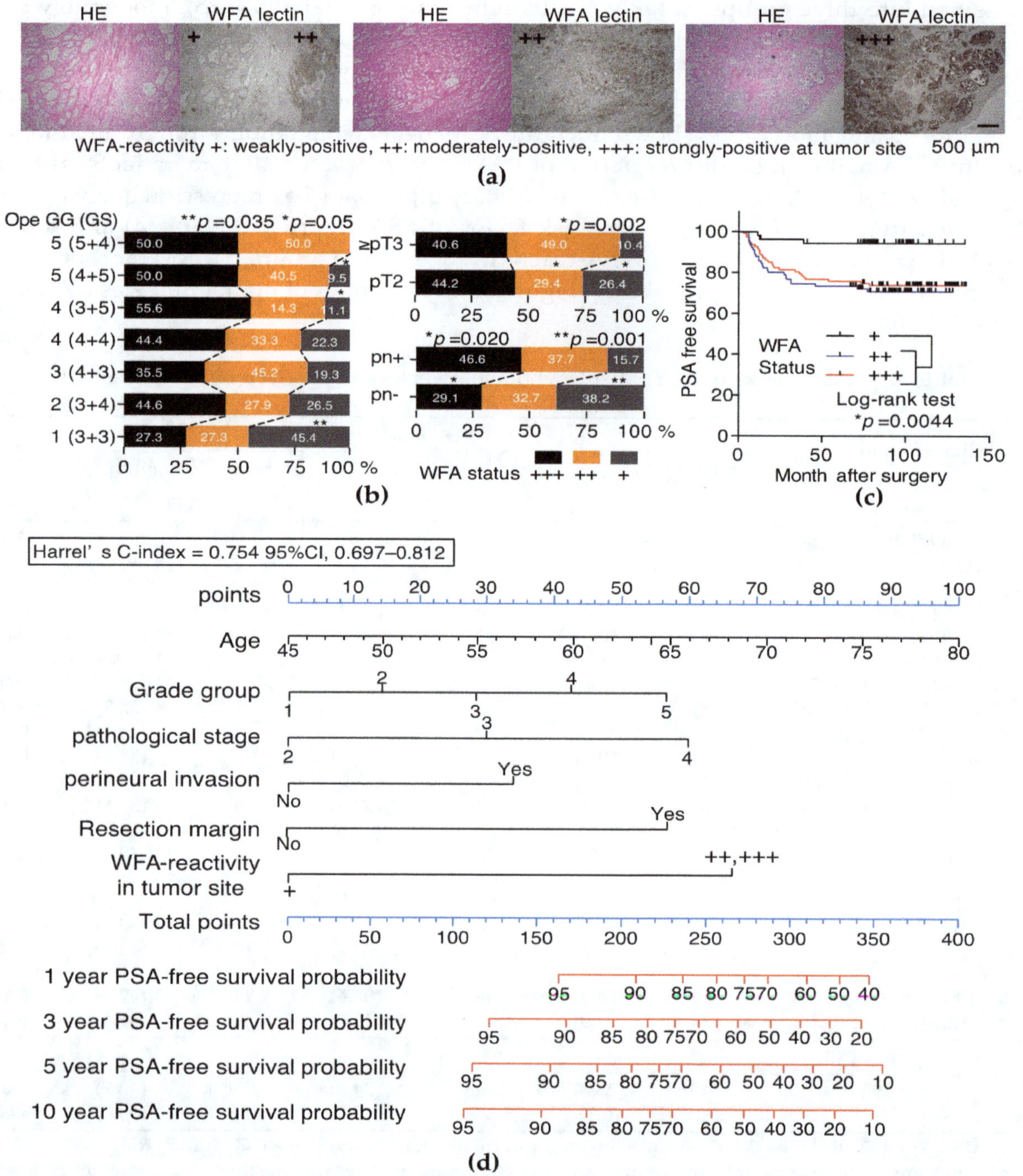

Figure 6. Immunohistochemical analysis of RP specimens using WFA lectin and post-operative nomogram predicting PSA-free survival probability. (**a**) Representative hematoxylin-eosin (HE) staining and WFA reactive-glycan expression of tumors of RP specimens. WFA-reactivity was classified into three groups: weakly positive, moderately positive, and strongly positive at a tumor site, respectively. Scale bar indicated 500 μm; (**b**) association between with WFA-reactive glycan expression and ope GG (ope GS), pathological stage, and perineural invasion-status; (**c**) PSA-free survival was evaluated using Kaplan–Meier curves and differences between three groups were assessed using the log-rank test. Patients with tumors strongly or moderately positive for WFA had a much shorter period of PSA recurrence after RP than did patients with tumors weakly positive for WFA; (**d**) Cox hazard regression analysis-based post-operative nomogram predicting PSA-free survival probability after RP. The c-index (0.754, 95% CI, 0.697–0.812), which is similar to the area under a receiver operating characteristic curve, was used to estimate the discrimination ability of the nomogram [25].

3. Discussion

One of the most important problems with PCa is overdiagnosis [3]. PSA-based screening has become controversial due to false positive results of total PSA in the PSA gray zone [4]. Overtreatment is also a major problem among certain segments of PCa patients [3] such as localized PCa and active surveillance patients [7–10]. Current biomarkers are not sufficient to prevent the overtreatment of PCa. Several serum-based testing (Phi, %p2PSA, and 4KScore), urine-based testing (PCA3) and MRI imaging has shown promising results in terms of diagnosis, localization, risk stratification, and staging of clinically significant PCa [26,27]. However, these promising biomarkers and imaging data are not yet cost-effective enough for routine clinical practice [28]. Therefore, there is a need for more accurate and cost-effective diagnostic and prognostic biomarkers. PCa-associated aberrant glycosylation of PSA is one of the candidate biomarkers. Fukushima et al. demonstrated that PSA derived from PCa serum and culture supernatant of LNCaP carries WFA-reactive LacdiNAc glycans; this is not the case for PSA derived from BPH serum [21] (Figure 1).

In the present study, we evaluated the diagnostic and pre-operative prognostic performance of WFA-reactive glycan-carrying PSA-Gi by using an SPFS-based automated immunoassay system [22]. We demonstrated that the AUC of PSA-Gi predicting PCa was much higher than that of the total PSA and PSA-Gi/total PSA (Figure 3c,f). We also demonstrated that a higher PSA-Gi level in BPH patients was moderately associated with a diagnosis of PCa within 1–4 years after first biopsy (Figure 3a,d). These results suggested that the diagnostic performance of a PSA-Gi single marker was much superior to conventional total PSA.

Furthermore, we showed that PSA-Gi before Pbx significantly higher in patients with Pbx GG 3 than that of patients with Pbx GG 2 and specificity for prediction of Pbx GG 3 was much higher than PSA (Figure 4a–c). This suggests that PSA-Gi can discriminate between GG 2 and GG 3 tumors and may be used as a predictor for a prostate biopsy to discriminate between non-aggressive and aggressive tumors in the active surveillance program. We also showed that the AUC of PSA-Gi predicting ope GG ≥ 3 tumors was higher than that of the total PSA and specificity for prediction of ope GG ≥ 3 was much higher than PSA (Figure 5e). The PSA-Gi levels before Pbx tends to be higher in patients with GG upgraded from 2 at Pbx to ope GG ≥ 3. A similar result was reported that pre-operative fucosylated haptoglobin (Fuc-Hpt) levels is significantly higher in patients with GS ≥ 7 than those with GS ≥ 6 [29]. Nevertheless, the serum Fuc-Hpt levels is also higher in patients with pancreatic, ovarian, and hepatocellular cancers [30,31]. In addition, Li et al. reported that the serum fucosylated PSA (Fuc-PSA) levels is significantly higher in patients with GS ≥ 7 than those with GS ≥ 6 [32]. It is well-known that PSA is a prostate-specific protein, and aberrant glycosylation of PSA including Fuc-PSA and PSA-Gi was thus found to be a more specific glycobiomarker of PCa than Fuc-Hpt. Although our sample size is small and retrospective, these results suggest that aberrant glycosylation of PSA is associated with PCa aggressiveness. Stark et al. demonstrated that GG 3 tumors are associated with a three-fold increase in lethal PCa compared with GG 2 tumors in RP specimens [33]. More recently, Epstein et al. also demonstrated that there are large differences in 5-year recurrence rates between both the GG 2 and GG 3 in a large multi-institutional surgical cohort and hazard ratios for GG 3 disease were generally threefold higher than for GG 2 [34]. Therefore, discrimination between GG 2 and GG 3 is an important task for the reduction of overtreatment of PCa. Thus, our PSA-Gi may be a promising pre-operative prognostic biomarker predicting Pbx GG 3 tumors and ope GG ≥ 3 tumors, particularly in very low-risk PCa patients who have met PRIAS criteria and PCa patients at an intermediate risk.

Moreover, we examined WFA-reactivity of prostate tumors showed that tumors strongly and moderately positive for WFA are significantly associated with higher ope GG, pT, and pn-positive status (Figure 6b) and worse PSA-free survival as compared to patients with weakly positive tumors for WFA (Figure 6c). Cox regression analysis here provided WFA-reactivity in tumors was an independent risk factor of PSA recurrence (Table 4). Thus, nomogram developed in this study including WFA-reactivity in the tumor site combined with clinocopathological parameters seemed to be a strong model for predicting PSA-free survival provability with a c-index (0.754) (Figure 6d). Further internal and external validation study was required for the evaluation of predictive performance in this nomogram.

Our results reveal that serum PSA-Gi levels before Pbx is useful for the discrimination of PCa as well as Pbx GG 3 and ope GG $\geq$ 3 patients and the WFA-reactivity of tumors is also useful for the prediction of PSA recurrence. Thus, both PSA-Gi and WFA-reactivity of tumors may reduce overdiagnosis and overtreatment of PCa.

4. Materials and Methods

This study was performed in accordance with the ethical standards of the Declaration of Helsinki and was approved by the Ethics Committee of Hirosaki University Graduate School of Medicine ("The Study about Carbohydrate Structure Change in Urological Disease"; approval number: 2014-195; approval date: 22 December 2014). Informed consent was obtained from all patients.

4.1. Serum Samples from Patients with BPH and PCa

A total of 442 patients with benign prostatic hyperplasia (BPH) and PCa were treated at our hospital between June 2007 and August 2016. Serum samples from patients with BPH (n = 184), PCa (n = 244 of whom 92 patients underwent RP), or PCa who diagnosed as BPH at first Pbx (n = 14) were obtained before the first Pbx. The final diagnoses of BPH or PCa were confirmed using the histopathological findings of prostate biopsies. Staging and grading information of the tumors for RP patients was obtained from medical charts. The grade group of prostate biopsy and prostatectomy specimens were evaluated according to the International Society of Urological Pathology (ISUP) guidelines [23]. Patient demographics are shown in Table 1. All samples were stored at −80 °C until use.

4.2. Detection of Serum PSA-Gi and Total PSA

The serum PSA-Gi was detected by using an SPFS-based two-step WFA–anti-PSA antibody sandwich immunoassay with a disposable sensor chip as described previously [22]. The system was developed by Konica Minolta Inc. (Figure 1). Two-step sandwich SPFS immunoassays of PSA-Gi were carried out automatically by moving a cylindrical pump between the anti-total-PSA monoclonal antibody (No. 72, Mikuri Immunological Laboratories Co., Ltd., Osaka, Japan) immobilized on a thin gold film in a disposable sensor chip and a reagent container in a self-developed assay machine. The reagent container already contained a number of separate reagents, including wash buffer (TBS 0.05% Tween 20, 10× TBS (Nippon Gene Co., Ltd., Tokyo, Japan) and polysorbate 20 (MP Biomedicals, LLC., Santa Ana, CA, USA)), AF647-WFA (WFA (vector laboratories, Inc., Burlingame, CA, USA) labeled using an Alexa Fluor 647-labeling kit (A20186, Thermo Fisher Scientific Inc., Waltham, MA, USA)) and the sample for measurement. The 20 µL of serum was diluted by 100 µL of a PBS-based dilution buffe. Then the 100 µL diluted serum samples and AF647-WFA solution (10.0 µg/mL in 1% BSA in PBS) were allowed to react for 10 min, and unreacted lectins were removed with washing buffer (four washes) after the WFA lectin reaction. After four washes, the final washing buffer was kept for SPFS optical measurement in the microchannel of each disposable sensor chips. After the final washing step, AF647 in the microchannel of disposable sensor chips were sequentially excited by laser light, which was applied on the backside of a thin gold film through the plastic prism. The laser light was already p-polarized and collimated by the internal laser diode system. A laser diode (635 nm, 0.95 mW; Edmund Optics Japan, Ltd., Tokyo, Japan) was used as a light source with a Neutral Density filter (AND20C-10 (10%), Sigmakoki Co., Ltd., Saitama, Japan). The fluorescent signal of AF647 that passed through the emission filter (DIF-BP-1 (half width: 668 ± 5 nm), Optical Coatings Japan, Tokyo, Japan) was detected by a photomultiplier tube (H7421-40, Hamamatsu Photonics K.K., Shizuoka, Japan), which was located at the end of a light-converging optical system (numerical aperture, NA = 0.6; Edmund Optics Japan Ltd., Tokyo, Japan). All assays were conducted automatically at 25 °C; four immunoassays were carried out simultaneously. Standard PSA-Gi sample was obtained from culture supernatant of LNCaP cells (RCB2144, RIKEN Bio-resource Center through the National Bio-Resource Project of the MEXT, Tsukuba, Japan), as reported previously [22]. In brief, LNCaP cells were cultured in the RPMI 1640 medium (Thermo Fisher Scientific Inc., Waltham, MA, USA) supplemented with 10% fetal calf serum (FCS) at 5% CO_2 at 37 °C. PSA secreted into the medium by the human PCa cell line, LNCaP cells, was used as a standard material of PSA-Gi in this study. The standard PSA-Gi concentration in the medium of the human LNCaP cell line was measured by WFA agarose column chromatography combined with a total-PSA enzyme-linked immunosorbent assay, as reported previously [22]. Fifty-five percent of total PSA in the medium of the LNCaP cell line possessed PSA-Gi (data not shown) [22]. Serum total PSA was measured by Architect i1000 system (Abbott Japan, Tokyo, Japan) and special reagents for total PSA (Abbott Japan) in a PSA range from 0.001 to 100 ng/mL.

4.3. Immunohistochemical Analysis of RP Specimens by WFA

A total of 260 paraffin-embedded RP specimens were obtained from PCa patients who underwent RP without neoadjuvant therapy between June 2007 and August 2016 in Hirosaki University Hospital. Patient demographics are shown in Table 3. Staging and grading information regarding the tumors and patient follow-up have been described previously [35]. In brief, PSA recurrence after RP was defined by two consecutive PSA values of >0.2 ng/mL with a 1-month interval and after a postoperative decrease below the detection limit (<0.001 ng/mL). Time zero was defined as the day of surgical treatment. Patients with constantly undetectable PSA levels (<0.001 ng/mL as the detection limit) after surgery were considered as patients without biochemical recurrence. Follow-up intervals were calculated from the date of the operation to the last recorded follow-up. Information on patients with PCa and tumor characteristics was obtained from medical charts. The grade group of prostate biopsy and prostatectomy specimens were evaluated according to the International Society of Urological Pathology (ISUP) guidelines [23]. Deparaffinized RP specimens were incubated with the biotinylated-WFA (Vector Laboratories, Burlingame, CA, USA) in PBS containing 5% of bovine serum albumin (1:500 dilution) at 4 °C, overnight. Biotinylated-WFA was detected by Vectastain Elite ABC kit (Vector Laboratories). WFA-reactivity was classified into three groups according to the reciprocal intensity scale as described previously [24]. Representative images of each Gleason grade tumor are shown in Figure A1.

4.4. Statistical Analysis

All calculations for clinical data were performed in the SPSS software, ver. 21.0 (SPSS, Inc., Chicago, IL, USA) and in GraphPad Prism 6.03 (GraphPad Software, San Diego, CA, USA). Intergroup differences were statistically analyzed by a Student's t-test for normally distributed variables or by the Mann–Whitney U-test for non-normally distributed models. Data with $p < 0.05$ were considered significant. ROC curves developed using the library "rms" in R (available on: http://www.r-project.org/) [25] and the statistical difference of AUCs were calculated by the same program. The χ^2 test was used to analyze the association of the WFA-reactivity status with clinicopathological parameters. PSA-free survival was evaluated using Kaplan–Meier curves, and differences between groups were assessed by the log-rank test. Multivariate test by Cox proportional hazards regression analysis was performed to detect significant and independent parameters with which PSA recurrence after RP can be predicted. Post-operative nomogram predicting PSA-free survival provability after RP was developed using the library "rms" in R (available on: http://www.r-project.org/), and the c-index was also calculated by same program [25].

5. Conclusions

At present, the majority of promising markers such as Phi, 4KScore, and tissue-based markers [26] are used in multiplex testing to improve diagnostic and prognostic accuracy. PSA-Gi is used as a single marker and yields results comparable to the diagnostic and prognostic performance of multiplex markers. PCA3 was also a promising urine marker for repeat biopsy decision-making [26]. However, there are a few cumbersome procedures for sample handling for avoiding RNA degradation. In this study, although we used frozen serum samples stored from 2007 to 2016, diagnostic and prognostic performance of PSA-Gi was substantially superior to total PSA. The serum sample handling of PSA-Gi was almost the same as the PSA test. Therefore, serum PSA-Gi is a promising pre-operative marker for detecting PCa and assessing the aggressiveness of PCa and has an advantage of cost-effectiveness and sample handling for routine clinical practice. Furthermore, the nomogram developed in this study is also a promising predictive tool for determining PSA-free survival probability. Larger clinical trials are warranted to confirm our findings.

Acknowledgments: All of the authors thank Katsuko Yamashita, Ph.D. for providing basically information about PSA-Gi and Yukie Nishizawa, Kaname Higuchi, and Satomi Sakamoto, technical assistant of Hirosaki University Graduate School of Medicine, for their invaluable help with sample collection and patient data management. This study was supported by the Japan Agency for Medical Research and Development-SENTAN KEISOKU BUNSEKIGIJYUTU KAIHATSU program (AMED)-SENTAN project from Japan Agency for Medical Research and Development (AMED), and also supported by the Japan Society for the Promotion of Science (JSPS) KAKENHI grant no. 15K15579 and grant no. 15H02563.

Author Contributions: Tohru Yoneyama and Yuki Tobisawa conceived and designed the experiments; Kazuhisa Hagiwara, Takatoshi Kaya, Tomonori Kaneko, and Tohru Yoneyama performed the experiments; Takatoshi Kaya and Tohru Yoneyama analyzed the data; Takatoshi Kaya, Tomonori Kaneko, and Yoshihiko Suda developed the SPFS-based automated immunoassay system; Shingo Hatakeyama, Yasuhiro Hashimoto, Takuya Koie, and Chikara Ohyama diagnosed BPH and PCa, and performed biopsy and radical prostatectomy; Chikara Ohyama and Yoshihiko Suda obtained funding. Chikara Ohyama and Tohru Yoneyama supervised. Yuki Tobisawa and Kazuyuki Mori critically revised the manuscript for intellectual content; Tohru Yoneyama wrote the paper.

Abbreviations

SPFS	surface plasmon field-enhanced fluorescence spectrometry
WFA	*Wisteria floribunda* agglutinin
PSA	prostate-specific antigen
PCa	prostate cancer
BPH	benign prostatic hyperplasia
LacdiNAc	GalNAcβ1-4GlcNAc-
Gal	galactose
Man	mannose
Fuc	fucose
Sia	sialic acid
GalNAc	*N*-acetylgalactosamine
GlcNAc	*N*-acetylglucosamine
Pbx GS	prostate biopsy Gleason Score
Pbx GG	prostate biopsy grade group
cT	clinical T stage
pT	pathological T stage
Ope GS	gleason score after radical prostatectomy
Ope GG	grade group after radical prostatectomy
RP	radical prostatectomy
pn	perineural invasion
RM	resection margin

Appendix A

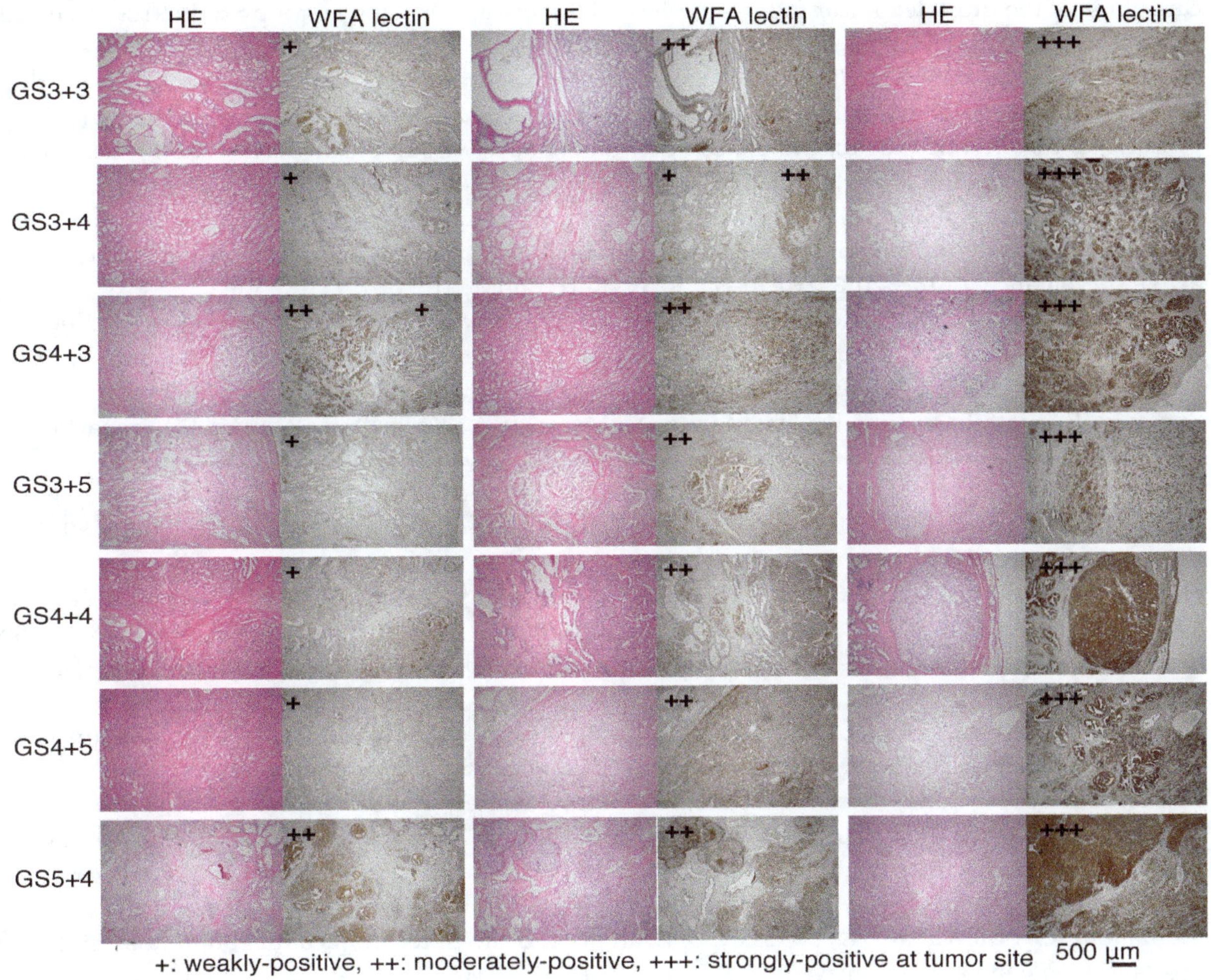

Figure A1. Representative hematoxylin-eosin (HE) staining and WFA reactive-glycan expression of tumors of each Gleason grade among RP specimens. WFA staining intensity was classified into three groups: weakly positive, moderately positive, and strongly positive at a tumor site, respectively. Scale bar indicated 500 μm.

References

1. Torre, L.A.; Bray, F.; Siegel, R.L.; Ferlay, J.; Lortet-Tieulent, J.; Jemal, A. Global cancer statistics, 2012. *CA: Cancer J. Clin.* **2015**, *65*, 87–108. [CrossRef] [PubMed]
2. Ferlay, J.; Steliarova-Foucher, E.; Lortet-Tieulent, J.; Rosso, S.; Coebergh, J.W.; Comber, H.; Forman, D.; Bray, F. Cancer incidence and mortality patterns in Europe: Estimates for 40 countries in 2012. *Eur. J. Cancer* **2013**, *49*, 1374–1403. [CrossRef] [PubMed]
3. Klotz, L. Prostate cancer overdiagnosis and overtreatment. *Curr. Opin. Endocrinol. Diabetes Obes.* **2013**, *20*, 204–209. [CrossRef] [PubMed]
4. Kim, E.H.; Andriole, G.L. Prostate-specific antigen-based screening: Controversy and guidelines. *BMC Med.* **2015**, *13*, 61. [CrossRef] [PubMed]
5. Ward, J.F.; Blute, M.L.; Slezak, J.; Bergstralh, E.J.; Zincke, H. The long-term clinical impact of biochemical recurrence of prostate cancer 5 or more years after radical prostatectomy. *J. Urol.* **2003**, *170*, 1872–1876. [CrossRef] [PubMed]

6. Powell, I.J.; Tangen, C.M.; Miller, G.J.; Lowe, B.A.; Haas, G.; Carroll, P.R.; Osswald, M.B.; deVere White, R.; Thompson, I.M., Jr.; Crawford, E.D. Neoadjuvant therapy before radical prostatectomy for clinical T3/T4 carcinoma of the prostate: 5-Year followup, phase II Southwest Oncology Group Study 9109. *J. Urol.* **2002**, *168*, 2016–2019. [CrossRef]
7. Mitsuzuka, K.; Narita, S.; Koie, T.; Kaiho, Y.; Tsuchiya, N.; Yoneyama, T.; Kakoi, N.; Kawamura, S.; Tochigi, T.; Habuchi, T.; et al. Pathological and biochemical outcomes after radical prostatectomy in men with low-risk prostate cancer meeting the Prostate Cancer International: Active surveillance criteria. *Br. J. Urol. Int.* **2013**, *111*, 914–920. [CrossRef] [PubMed]
8. Satkunasivam, R.; Kulkarni, G.S.; Zlotta, A.R.; Kalnin, R.; Trachtenberg, J.; Fleshner, N.E.; Hamilton, R.J.; Jewett, M.A.; Finelli, A. Pathological, oncologic and functional outcomes of radical prostatectomy following active surveillance. *J. Urol.* **2013**, *190*, 91–95. [CrossRef] [PubMed]
9. Maurice, M.J.; Sundi, D.; Schaeffer, E.M.; Abouassaly, R. Risk of pathological upgrading and upstaging among men with low-risk prostate cancer varies by race: Results from the National Cancer Data Base. *J. Urol.* **2016**. [CrossRef] [PubMed]
10. Sussman, R.; Staff, I.; Tortora, J.; Champagne, A.; Meraney, A.; Kesler, S.S.; Wagner, J.R. Impact of active surveillance on pathology and nerve sparing status. *Can. J. Urol.* **2014**, *21*, 7299–7304. [PubMed]
11. Kattan, M.W.; Eastham, J.A.; Stapleton, A.M.; Wheeler, T.M.; Scardino, P.T. A preoperative nomogram for disease recurrence following radical prostatectomy for prostate cancer. *J. Natl. Cancer Inst.* **1998**, *90*, 766–771. [CrossRef] [PubMed]
12. Haji-Ghassemi, O.; Gilbert, M.; Spence, J.; Schur, M.J.; Parker, M.J.; Jenkins, M.L.; Burke, J.E.; van Faassen, H.; Young, N.M.; Evans, S.V. Molecular basis for recognition of the cancer glycobiomarker LacdiNAc (GalNAc(β1–4)GlcNAc) by *Wisteria floribunda* agglutinin. *J. Biol. Chem.* **2016**, *291*, 24085–24095. [CrossRef] [PubMed]
13. Kitamura, N.; Guo, S.; Sato, T.; Hiraizumi, S.; Taka, J.; Ikekita, M.; Sawada, S.; Fujisawa, H.; Furukawa, K. Prognostic significance of reduced expression of β-*N*-acetylgalactosaminylated *N*-linked oligosaccharides in human breast cancer. *Int. J. Cancer* **2003**, *105*, 533–541. [CrossRef] [PubMed]
14. Hirano, K.; Matsuda, A.; Kuji, R.; Nakandakari, S.; Shirai, T.; Furukawa, K. Enhanced expression of the β4-*N*-acetylgalactosaminyltransferase 4 gene impairs tumor growth of human breast cancer cells. *Biochem. Biophys. Res. Commun.* **2015**, *461*, 80–85. [CrossRef] [PubMed]
15. McMahon, R.F.; McWilliam, L.J.; Mosley, S. Evaluation of three techniques for differential diagnosis of prostatic needle biopsy specimens. *J. Clin. Pathol.* **1992**, *45*, 1094–1098. [CrossRef] [PubMed]
16. McMahon, R.F.; McWilliam, L.J.; Clarke, N.W.; George, N.J. Altered saccharide sequences in two groups of patients with metastatic prostatic carcinoma. *Br. J. Urol.* **1994**, *74*, 80–85. [CrossRef] [PubMed]
17. Yamaguchi, T.; Yokoyama, Y.; Ebata, T.; Matsuda, A.; Kuno, A.; Ikehara, Y.; Shoda, J.; Narimatsu, H.; Nagino, M. Verification of WFA-sialylated MUC1 as a sensitive biliary biomarker for human biliary tract cancer. *Ann. Surg. Oncol.* **2016**, *23*, 671–677. [CrossRef] [PubMed]
18. Iio, E.; Ocho, M.; Togayachi, A.; Nojima, M.; Kuno, A.; Ikehara, Y.; Hasegawa, I.; Yatsuhashi, H.; Yamasaki, K.; Shimada, N.; et al. A novel glycobiomarker, *Wisteria floribunda* agglutinin macrophage colony-stimulating factor receptor, for predicting carcinogenesis of liver cirrhosis. *Int. J. Cancer* **2016**, *138*, 1462–1471. [CrossRef] [PubMed]
19. Sogabe, M.; Nozaki, H.; Tanaka, N.; Kubota, T.; Kaji, H.; Kuno, A.; Togayachi, A.; Gotoh, M.; Nakanishi, H.; Nakanishi, T.; et al. Novel glycobiomarker for ovarian cancer that detects clear cell carcinoma. *J. Proteome Res.* **2014**, *13*, 1624–1635. [CrossRef] [PubMed]
20. Khabaz, M.N.; McClure, J.; McClure, S.; Stoddart, R.W. Glycophenotype of prostatic carcinomas. *Folia Histochem. Cytobiol.* **2010**, *48*, 637–645. [PubMed]
21. Fukushima, K.; Satoh, T.; Baba, S.; Yamashita, K. α1,2-Fucosylated and β-*N*-acetylgalactosaminylated prostate-specific antigen as an efficient marker of prostatic cancer. *Glycobiology* **2010**, *20*, 452–460. [CrossRef] [PubMed]
22. Kaya, T.; Kaneko, T.; Kojima, S.; Nakamura, Y.; Ide, Y.; Ishida, K.; Suda, Y.; Yamashita, K. High-sensitivity immunoassay with surface plasmon field-enhanced fluorescence spectroscopy using a plastic sensor chip: Application to quantitative analysis of total prostate-specific antigen and GalNAcβ1–4GlcNAc-linked prostate-specific antigen for prostate cancer diagnosis. *Anal. Chem.* **2015**, *87*, 1797–1803. [PubMed]

23. Humphrey, P.A.; Moch, H.; Cubilla, A.L.; Ulbright, T.M.; Reuter, V.E. The 2016 WHO classification of tumours of the urinary system and male genital organs-part B: Prostate and bladder tumours. *Eur. Urol.* **2016**, *70*, 106–119. [CrossRef] [PubMed]
24. Nguyen, D. Quantifying chromogen intensity in immunohistochemistry via reciprocal intensity. *Protoc. Exchange* **2013**. [CrossRef]
25. Harrell, F.E., Jr.; Lee, K.L.; Mark, D.B. Multivariable prognostic models: Issues in developing models, evaluating assumptions and adequacy, and measuring and reducing errors. *Stat. Med.* **1996**, *15*, 361–387. [CrossRef]
26. Hatakeyama, S.; Yoneyama, T.; Tobisawa, Y.; Ohyama, C. Recent progress and perspectives on prostate cancer biomarkers. *Int. J. Clin. Oncol.* **2016**. [CrossRef] [PubMed]
27. Haider, M.A.; Yao, X.; Loblaw, A.; Finelli, A. Multiparametric magnetic resonance imaging in the diagnosis of prostate cancer: A systematic review. *Clin. Oncol.* **2016**, *28*, 550–567. [CrossRef] [PubMed]
28. Nicholson, A.; Mahon, J.; Boland, A.; Beale, S.; Dwan, K.; Fleeman, N.; Hockenhull, J.; Dundar, Y. The clinical effectiveness and cost-effectiveness of the PROGENSA (R) prostate cancer antigen 3 assay and the prostate health index in the diagnosis of prostate cancer: A systematic review and economic evaluation. *Health Technol. Assess.* **2015**, *19*, 1–191. [CrossRef] [PubMed]
29. Fujita, K.; Shimomura, M.; Uemura, M.; Nakata, W.; Sato, M.; Nagahara, A.; Nakai, Y.; Takamatsu, S.; Miyoshi, E.; Nonomura, N. Serum fucosylated haptoglobin as a novel prognostic biomarker predicting high-Gleason prostate cancer. *Prostate* **2014**, *74*, 1052–1058. [CrossRef] [PubMed]
30. Okuyama, N.; Ide, Y.; Nakano, M.; Nakagawa, T.; Yamanaka, K.; Moriwaki, K.; Murata, K.; Ohigashi, H.; Yokoyama, S.; Eguchi, H.; et al. Fucosylated haptoglobin is a novel marker for pancreatic cancer: A detailed analysis of the oligosaccharide structure and a possible mechanism for fucosylation. *Int. J. Cancer* **2006**, *118*, 2803–2808. [CrossRef] [PubMed]
31. Thompson, S.; Dargan, E.; Turner, G.A. Increased fucosylation and other carbohydrate changes in haptoglobin in ovarian cancer. *Cancer Lett.* **1992**, *66*, 43–48. [CrossRef]
32. Li, Q.K.; Chen, L.; Ao, M.H.; Chiu, J.H.; Zhang, Z.; Zhang, H.; Chan, D.W. Serum fucosylated prostate-specific antigen (PSA) improves the differentiation of aggressive from non-aggressive prostate cancers. *Theranostics* **2015**, *5*, 267–276. [CrossRef] [PubMed]
33. Stark, J.R.; Perner, S.; Stampfer, M.J.; Sinnott, J.A.; Finn, S.; Eisenstein, A.S.; Ma, J.; Fiorentino, M.; Kurth, T.; Loda, M.; et al. Gleason score and lethal prostate cancer: Does 3 + 4 = 4 + 3? *J. Clin. Oncol.* **2009**, *27*, 3459–3464. [CrossRef] [PubMed]
34. Epstein, J.I.; Zelefsky, M.J.; Sjoberg, D.D.; Nelson, J.B.; Egevad, L.; Magi-Galluzzi, C.; Vickers, A.J.; Parwani, A.V.; Reuter, V.E.; Fine, S.W.; et al. A contemporary prostate cancer grading system: A validated alternative to the gleason score. *Eur. Urol.* **2016**, *69*, 428–435. [CrossRef] [PubMed]
35. Koie, T.; Ohyama, C.; Hatakeyama, S.; Imai, A.; Yoneyama, T.; Hashimoto, Y.; Yoneyama, T.; Tobisawa, Y.; Hosogoe, S.; Yamamoto, H.; et al. Significance of preoperative butyrylcholinesterase as an independent predictor of biochemical recurrence-free survival in patients with prostate cancer treated with radical prostatectomy. *Int. J. Clin. Oncol.* **2016**, *21*, 379–383. [CrossRef] [PubMed]

5

Early Prediction of Therapy Response to Abiraterone Acetate Using PSA Subforms in Patients with Castration Resistant Prostate Cancer

Katrin Schlack [1,*], Laura-Maria Krabbe [1,2], Manfred Fobker [3], Andres Jan Schrader [1], Axel Semjonow [1] and Martin Boegemann [1]

1 Department of Urology, Prostate Center, University Hospital Muenster, Albert-Schweitzer-Campus 1, GB A1, Muenster D-48149, Germany; laura-maria.krabbe@ukmuenster.de (L.-M.K.); andresjan.schrader@ukmuenster.de (A.J.S.); axel.semjonow@ukmuenster.de (A.S.); martin.boegemann@ukmuenster.de (M.B.)

2 Department of Urology, University of Texas Southwestern Medical Center, Dallas, TX 75390-9110, USA

3 Center for Laboratory Medicine, University Hospital Muenster, Albert-Schweitzer-Campus 1, GB A1, Muenster D-48149, Germany; manfred.fobker@ukmuenster.de

* Correspondence: katrin.schlack@ukmuenster.de

Academic Editor: Carsten Stephan

Abstract: The purpose of this study was to evaluate the prognostic ability of early changes of total prostate specific antigen (tPSA), free PSA (fPSA), [−2]proPSA and the Prostate Health Index (PHI) following initiation of Abiraterone-therapy in men with castration resistant prostate cancer (mCRPC). In 25 patients, PSA-subforms were analyzed before and at 8–12 weeks under therapy as prognosticators of progression-free-survival (PFS) and overall survival (OS). Comparing patients with a PFS < vs. ≥12 months by using Mann–Whitney–Wilcoxon Tests, the relative-median-change of tPSA (−0.1% vs. −86.8%; p = 0.02), fPSA (12.1% vs. −55.3%; p = 0.03) and [−2]proPSA (8.1% vs. −59.3%; p = 0.05) differed significantly. For men with ≤ vs. >15 months of OS there was a non-significant trend for a difference in the relative-median-change of fPSA (17.0% vs. −46.3%; p = 0.06). In Kaplan–Meier analyses, declining fPSA and [−2]proPSA were associated with a longer median PFS (13 months, 95% confidence interval (CI): 9.6–16.4 vs. 10 months, 95% CI: 3.5–16.5; p = 0.11), respectively. Correspondingly, decreasing fPSA and [−2]proPSA values indicated an OS of 32 months (95% CI: not reached (NR)) compared to 21 months in men with rising values (95% CI: 7.7–34.3; p = 0.14), respectively. We concluded that the addition of fPSA- and [−2]proPSA-changes to tPSA-information might be further studied as potential markers of early Abiraterone response in mCRPC patients.

Keywords: mCRPC; surrogate biomarker; abiraterone acetate; prognosticators; prostate cancer; [−2]proPSA; fPSA; PHI; tPSA

1. Introduction

During the past few years, there has been significant progress in treatment options for metastatic castration resistant prostate cancer (mCRPC). After prostate cancer develops, resistance to androgen-deprivation therapy (ADT), patients can be treated with different agents including chemotherapy, next generation ADT drugs, Sipuleucel-T or Radium-223 [1–8]. Amongst these, Abiraterone acetate (Abiraterone), a selective CYP450 17A1 inhibitor, is available in the pre- and post-chemotherapy setting and is broadly accepted as a standard of care due to its life-prolonging potential and generally low toxicity [1,2,9].

A challenging aspect for clinicians in this setting is the early determination of treatment success, particularly the early identification of response or failure in patients whose lack of symptoms makes a clinical decision difficult. Except a decline in total prostate specific antigen (tPSA), there are no easily available prognostic biomarkers besides clinical parameters to determine therapeutic success. Therefore, the decision whether to continue or to change a therapy regime is mainly based on clinical factors (e.g., eastern cooperative oncology group performance status (ECOG)) and tPSA, which is still the most commonly used therapy control marker in mCRPC.

However, there are several limitations concerning tPSA, especially in mCRPC. The parameter does not always decline right away even though patients might still benefit from therapy. Thus, in the registration trials, tPSA could not be validated as an independent prognosticator for therapy response [1,2]. Furthermore, an early rise of tPSA during the first 12 weeks of therapy followed by a delayed decline (PSA-flare) during Abiraterone-therapy was recently found to be a prognosticator for an improved median progression free survival (PFS) [10]. PSA-flare occurs in about 10% of the patients treated with Abiraterone. A larger proportion of patients with initial increase of tPSA (nearly 50%), however, will suffer a continuous rise of tPSA over time followed by clinical progression [10]. In clinical routines, the differentiation between PSA-flare and continuous rise is difficult, resulting in either early, sometimes premature, interruption of therapy or waiting for the potential benefit of a delayed tPSA-decline with, in many cases, a treatment beyond true progression. Therefore, additional biomarkers to distinguish between true progression and a delayed tPSA response are desperately needed for these situations.

Several biomarkers, including circulating tumor cells (CTCs) and lactate dehydrogenase (LDH), have recently been discussed as response-indicators [11,12].

CTC counts at baseline are considered to be prognostic for the duration of treatment with a resulting shorter time of treatment for $\geq$5 CTCs [11]. However, the sensitivity of detection of CTCs is limited in patients with low tumor load and differs depending on the site of metastasis [13]. Additionally, CTC-assays are expensive and not broadly available.

Similar data show that the combination of $\geq$5 CTC count and an elevated LDH level after 12 weeks of therapy may be a surrogate for poor overall survival (OS) [12]. However, for broad acceptance and use, more easily available as well as more sensitive, validated and non-expensive assays are required [14].

In 1991, the low specificity of PSA for the detection of prostate cancer was improved by the identification of two major molecular subforms of PSA, an unbound proportion (free PSA, fPSA) and a form complexed with the protease inhibitor alpha-1-antichimotrypsin [15]. It was shown that the chance of detecting prostate cancer was lower with increasing proportion of fPSA (%fPSA) [16,17]. Following the detection of precursor forms of fPSA (proPSA), further investigation concluded that proPSA was associated with prostate cancer with a higher probability of cancer as the percentage of proPSA in fPSA increases [18,19]. Within the proPSA fraction, further discrimination could be made by the detection of truncated forms which are more resistant to activation to mature PSA, with [−2]proPSA being the most consistent of these [20]. According to recent investigations, the ratio of [−2]proPSA to fPSA (%[−2]proPSA) and the Prostate Health Index (PHI = ([−2]proPSA/fPSA) $\times \sqrt{\text{tPSA}}$) seem to be the strongest predictors of prostate cancer compared to tPSA and its subforms [21,22]. In addition, there was evidence for a correlation with more aggressive variants of prostate cancer since the variables increased with increasing Gleason-Score [23,24].

In this study, we aimed to investigate whether PSA subforms could be helpful for predicting treatment response and prognosticating survival outcomes in patients with mCRPC treated with Abiraterone. When added to tPSA in the setting of organ confined prostate cancer, the Supplementary Materials of fPSA, [−2]proPSA and PHI help to diagnose and identify more aggressive forms of prostate cancer [25,26]. Therefore, we assumed that these markers could also be useful to facilitate decision making in the treatment of mCRPC.

2. Results

2.1. Characteristics of the Study Group

For the patients alive at the time of analysis, the median follow-up was 25 months (Interquartile range (IQR) 14.5–28.0) in July 2015. The median time on Abiraterone-therapy was 13 months (IQR 10.5–19.0) with six (24%) patients on therapy at the time of last data acquisition. No dose modifications were necessary for any patients. Descriptive characteristics of the cohort are given in Table 1. The median age of the patients was 71 years (IQR 63–74). Bone metastases were present in 76%, lymphonodal metastases in 64% and visceral metastases in 8% of patients at the beginning of Abiraterone-therapy. An unfavorable Gleason-Score of ≥8 at initial diagnosis of PCa was found in 60%. Median baseline levels were 61.7 ng/mL for tPSA (IQR 29.0–299.5), 11.2 ng/mL for fPSA (IQR 5.2–29.1), 485.3 pg/mL for [−2]proPSA (IQR 272.8–1107.9) and 327.3 for PHI (IQR 212.5–612.0). No patient showed elevated liver enzyme- or creatinine-concentrations during the course of the study.

Antiresorptive therapy (Zoledronic acid or Denosumab) was administered in 12 patients (48%). All of these remained on a stable dose of the drug during the course of Abiraterone-therapy.

Table 1. Baseline characteristics of patients with mCRPC under therapy with Abiraterone IQR, interquartile range; ECOG, eastern cooperative oncology group performance status.

Variable	Number
Patients (*n*) (%)	25 (100)
Age, median (years) (IQR)	71.0 (62.5–74.0)
Median follow-up (months) (IQR)	25.0 (14.5–28.0)
Median duration of therapy (months) (IQR)	13.0 (10.5–19.0)
Presence of lymphnode metastases (*n*) (%)	16 (64.0)
Presence of bone metastases (*n*) (%)	19 (76.0)
Presence of visceral metastases (*n*) (%)	2 (8.0)
Pre chemotherapy (*n*) (%)	20 (80.0)
Post chemotherapy (*n*) (%)	5 (20.0)
Antiresorptive therapy (*n*) (%)	12 (48.0)
Zoledronic acid (*n*) (%)	7 (28.0)
Denosumab (*n*) (%)	5 (20.0)
ECOG (all) (*n*) (%)	
0–1	22 (88.0)
>1	3 (12.0)
Gleason Score ≥ 8 (*n*) (%)	15 (60.0)
Median tPSA baseline (ng/mL) (IQR)	61.7 (29.0–299.5)
Median fPSA baseline (ng/mL) (IQR)	11.2 (5.2–29.1)
Median [−2]proPSA baseline (pg/mL) (IQR)	485.3 (272.8–1107.9)
Median PHI baseline (IQR)	327.3 (212.5–612.0)
Best clinical outcome (*n*) (%)	
Complete remission	1 (4.0)
Partial remission	10 (40.0)
Stable disease	10 (40.0)
Progressive disease	4 (16.0)
tPSA decrease ≥ 50% (*n*) (%)	12 (48.0)
tPSA decrease ≥ 90% (*n*) (%)	7 (28.0)
Patients died (*n*) (%)	11 (44.0)

2.2. Value of PSA Subforms as Prognostic Markers

Alterations of the baseline values are presented as relative change of median values in percent (Figure 1). The definition of progressive disease is explained in paragraph 4 (Materials and Methods). For patients with shorter response to therapy (PFS < 12 months and OS ≤ 15 months) the median fPSA and [−2]proPSA increased at 8–12 weeks. In contrast to these two subforms, the median tPSA showed stable values at the same time for these patients. The other parameters (PHI, %[−2]proPSA and %fPSA) seem to play a minor role, considering the scope of our study, since changes did not differ between the groups (Table 2).

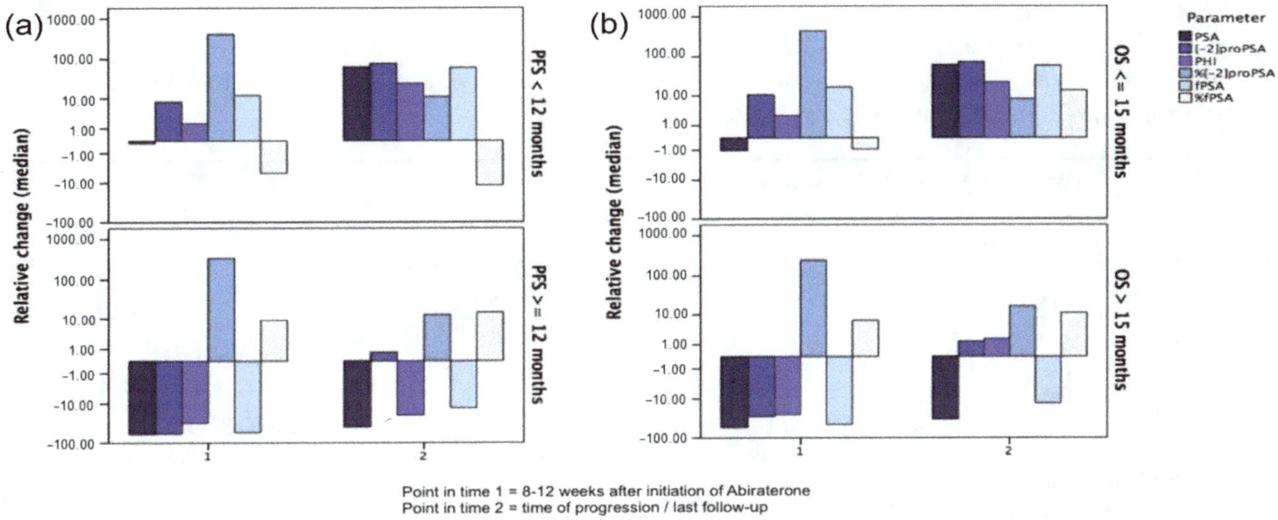

Figure 1. Relative median changes of PSA subforms at 8–12 weeks and at progression or last follow-up compared to baseline for (**a**) PFS < 12 months vs. ≥12 months; and (**b**) OS ≤ 15 months vs. >15 months.

Table 2. Relative changes of median PSA-subform values (%) in 25 patients at 8–12 weeks for OS and PFS OS, overall survival; PFS, progression free survival.

Variable	OS ≤ 15 Months	OS > 15 Months	p
tPSA	−1.1 (−54.5–66.3)	−55.1 (−74.6–13.2)	0.20
[−2]proPSA	10.5 (−50.7–62.0)	−29.1 (−66.9–19.9)	0.15
PHI	2.6 (−42.9–39.0)	−25.9 (−41.4–19.0)	0.32
%[−2]proPSA	449.0 (260.6–588.4)	242.1 (149.5–577.7)	0.27
fPSA	17.0 (−41.8–50.3)	−46.3 (−72.0–8.1)	0.06
%fPSA	−0.9 (−19.6–28.1)	7.0 (−27.6–41.3)	0.61
	PFS < 12 Months	**PFS ≥ 12 Months**	
tPSA	−0.1 (−0.1–71.3)	−86.8 (−60.9–9.4)	0.02
[−2]proPSA	8.1 (−21.2–60.1)	−59.3 (−74.0–18.5)	0.05
PHI	1.7 (−24.4–63.6)	−32.1 (−47.8–4.1)	0.12
%[−2]proPSA	416.0 (159.8–754.2)	335.5 (163.2–550.7)	0.73
fPSA	12.1 (−22.7–43.8)	−55.3 (−83.3–13.6)	0.03
%fPSA	−5.2 (−28.3–16.7)	9.1 (−17.3–42.0)	0.15

In patients with < vs. ≥12 months of PFS, the relative change of median tPSA values (−0.1% vs. −86.8%; p = 0.02 (Mann–Whitney–Wilcoxon Test)) at 8–12 weeks compared to baseline differed significantly. Similar results were shown for decreasing [−2]proPSA- (8.1% vs. −59.3%; p = 0.05) and fPSA values (12.1% vs. −55.3%; p = 0.03), respectively.

For men with ≤ vs. >15 months of OS, there was a non-significant trend for a difference in relative changes of median fPSA values (17.0% vs. −46.3%; p = 0.06). Considering OS, no conclusive change of median values was seen for the other parameters (tPSA, [−2]proPSA, PHI, %[−2]proPSA and %fPSA).

In univariate Cox-regression analysis, rising [−2]proPSA and fPSA were non-significant prognosticators of shorter PFS (Hazard ratio (HR): 2.0, (95% confidence interval (CI): 0.8–4.8); $p = 0.14$ for both parameters). Analogously, the results for OS showed a non-significant trend for rising [−2]proPSA and fPSA regarding the prognostication of poor OS (HR: 2.5 (95% CI: 0.7–9.1); $p = 0.16$ for both parameters). In this analysis, PHI also showed a trend towards shortened PFS in case of an early increase (HR: 2.0 (95% CI: 0.9–5.0); $p = 0.11$). For OS, however, PHI did not show any trend for shortened survival (HR: 1.5 (95% CI: 0.4–5.4); $p = 0.49$). Of note, rising tPSA changes did not prove to be a prognosticator for worse PFS (HR: 1.6 (95% CI: 0.6–4.0); $p = 0.29$) or OS (HR: 1.3 (95% CI: 0.4–4.5); $p = 0.72$) (Table 3).

Table 3. Changes of median PSA-subform values in univariate analysis OS, overall survival; PFS, progression; HR, hazard ratio; CI, confidence interval.

Univariate Analysis for OS			Univariate Analysis for PFS		
Variable	**HR (95% CI)**	***p***	**Variable**	**HR (95% CI)**	***p***
tPSA increase yes vs. no	1.3 (0.4–4.5)	0.72	tPSA increase yes vs. no	1.6 (0.6–4.0)	0.29
fPSA increase yes vs. no	2.5 (0.7–9.1)	0.16	fPSA increase yes vs. no	2.0 (0.8–4.8)	0.14
[−2]proPSA increase yes vs. no	2.5 (0.7–9.1)	0.16	[−2]proPSA increase yes vs. no	2.0 (0.8–4.8)	0.14
PHI increase yes vs. no	1.5 (0.4–5.4)	0.49	PHI increase yes vs. no	2.0 (0.9–5.0)	0.11
%[−2]proPSA increase yes vs. no	23.1 (0–∞)	0.57	%[−2]proPSA increase yes vs. no	1.8 (0.2–13.5)	0.57
%fPSA increase no vs. yes	0.4 (0.1–1.7)	0.23	%fPSA increase no vs. yes	1.2 (0.5–2.8)	0.73

2.3. Kaplan–MEIER Survival Analysis

The Kaplan–Meier analyses for PFS and OS are presented in Figures 2–4. Here, the strongest marker for longer PFS in Mann–Whitney–Wilcoxon comparison of median values, declining fPSA, also showed better survival outcomes. A declining fPSA value at 8–12 weeks was associated with a median PFS of 13 months (95% CI: 9.6–16.4 months) compared to 10 months (95% CI: 3.5–16.5 months) in patients with increasing values (log-rank $p = 0.11$).

Correspondingly, in the analysis of OS, a decreasing fPSA at 8–12 weeks of therapy indicated a median OS of 32 months (95% CI: not reached (NR)) compared to 21 months (95% CI: 7.7–34.3 months) in men with rising fPSA ($p = 0.14$) (Figure 2).

The Kaplan–Meier analysis of PFS and OS with declining and rising [−2]proPSA showed similar results (Figure 3).

In contrast, in the analysis of PFS for tPSA, there was less difference between rising and declining values. A tPSA decrease was associated with a median PFS of 12 months (95% CI: 8.4–15.6 months) compared to 10 months (95% CI: 7.1–13.0 months) in the case of increasing values ($p = 0.26$). Correspondingly, the evaluation of OS did not show differences between tPSA values in both groups with 32 months (95% CI: NR) vs. 28 months (95% CI: 17.2–38.8 months, $p = 0.72$) (Figure 4).

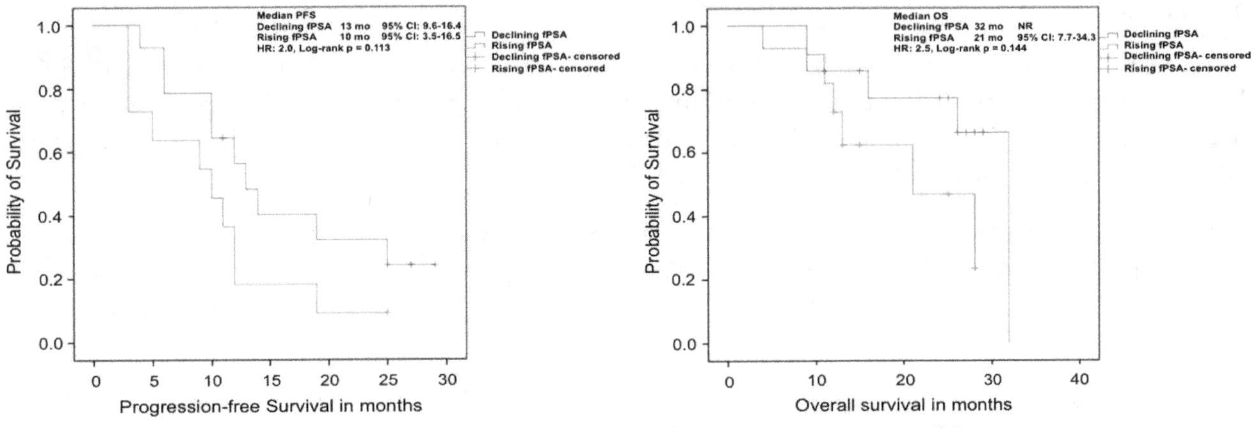

(a) (b)

Figure 2. Kaplan–Meier analyses of (**a**) progression free survival; and (**b**) overall survival of mCRPC patients treated with Abiraterone with rising or declining fPSA values after 8–12 weeks of therapy.

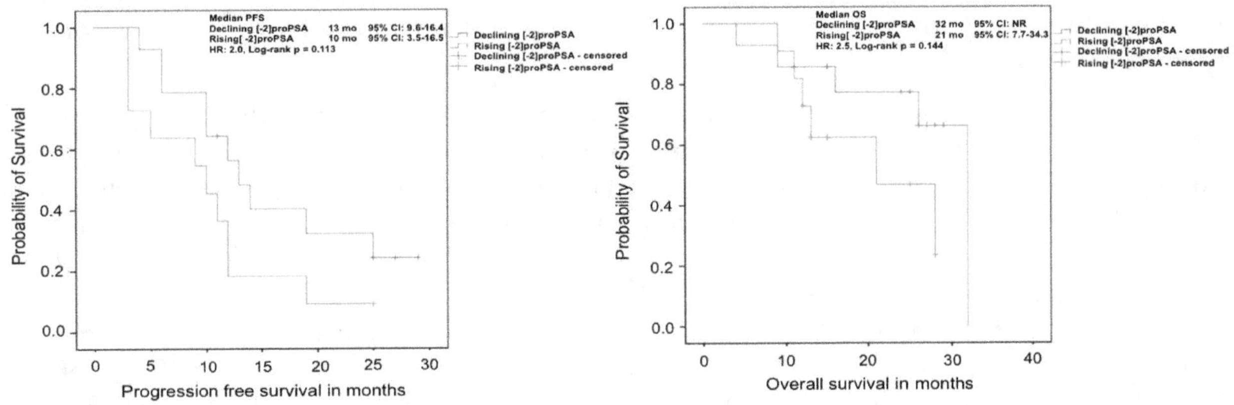

(a) (b)

Figure 3. Kaplan–Meier analyses of (**a**) progression free survival; and (**b**) overall survival of mCRPC patients treated with Abiraterone with rising or declining [−2]proPSA values after 8–12 weeks of therapy.

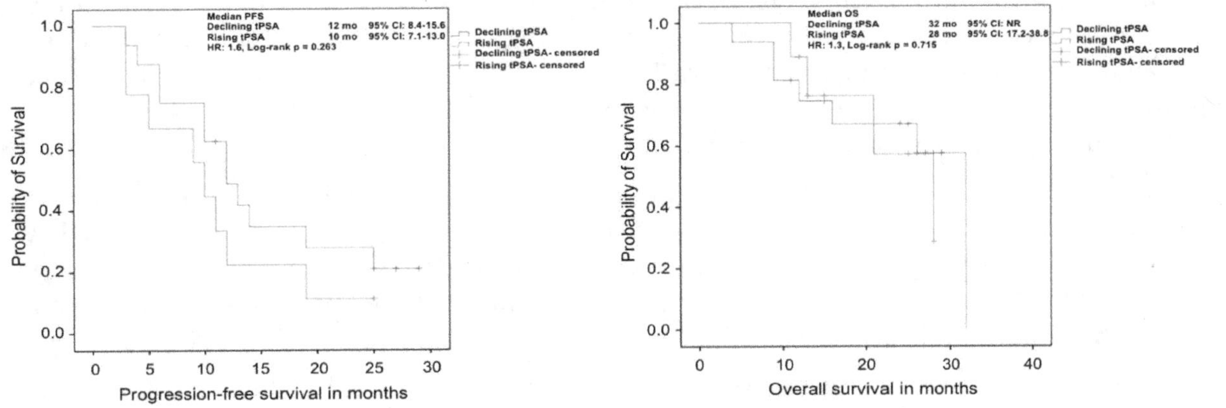

(a) (b)

Figure 4. Kaplan–Meier analyses of (**a**) progression free survival; and (**b**) overall survival of mCRPC patients treated with Abiraterone with rising or declining tPSA values after 8–12 weeks of therapy.

3. Discussion

To our knowledge, the relevance of fPSA and [−2]proPSA as well as PHI in patients with mCRPC under Abiraterone has not been investigated thus far. Standard monitoring of therapy is mainly based on the measurement of tPSA as well as radiological criteria and the general condition of the patients like the assessment of ECOG performance status [27].

Among the group of patients with mCRPC, a large proportion of up to 90% shows bone metastases [28]. During early imaging, especially in the first three to six months of therapy, an early "bone-flare" can occur in a relevant amount of patients, which can lead to incorrect classification as progressive disease (PD) [29,30].

The most common parameter being used for determination of treatment success under any therapy for mCRPC is tPSA. Here, comparable to the above-mentioned "bone-flare", a "PSA-flare" can occur under therapy with Abiraterone [10]. These common phenomena of everyday practice leave the burden to decide whether a therapy should be terminated or continued to the clinician. This dilemma holds especially true in asymptomatic or oligosymptomatic patients, since lack of clinical information can render decision making in some cases impossible. Therefore, in the case of biochemical progression only, current guidelines recommend continuing treatment until unequivocal information on progression is evident [31].

The data concerning monitoring of response or progression at an early stage of treatment are contradictory. PSA-flare has been reported to occur under other therapies than Abiraterone, like Docetaxel [32] and could be caused by a delayed response or rapid cell destruction with release of tPSA to the circulation [10]. Under treatment with Abiraterone, immediate or delayed tPSA-responses are common, but there are patients who will not show a tPSA-decline at all [10,33]. In our cohort, as well, a PSA-flare was seen in three patients, which is in line with the previously described 10% in other cohorts [10]. These three patients showed various duration of response to Abiraterone and stayed under treatment for nine, 26 and 38 months. Thus, the early differentiation between "PSA-flare" and true PD is difficult and remains mostly unresolved. This clinical dilemma can be even more complex if a possible "bone-flare" is suspected [29,30].

Although a significant tPSA decline of at least 50% from baseline was found in a large proportion of the patients treated within the registration trials for Abiraterone (COU-AA-301 and COU-AA-302), tPSA-changes were not found to be independent prognosticators for survival outcomes [1,2]. These non-straightforward findings are in line with our results. In our cohort, the median change of tPSA at 8–12 weeks of Abiraterone-therapy was a prognosticator for a PFS < 12 vs. ≥ 12 months ($p = 0.02$) with a decline resulting in a longer PFS, but the univariate cox-regression analysis showed no significant association (HR 1.6, $p = 0.29$); this may be due to our relatively small cohort. For this reason, no multivariate analysis was performed.

Some alternative biomarkers were recently evaluated. In contrast to tPSA, CTCs do not show a "flare" phenomenon and therefore could be ideal as a surrogate for OS [34]. In this context, several studies reported that the post-therapy CTC enumeration could be considered to be an independent prognostic parameter for OS [9,35]. However, due to costs, a relevant rate of falsely negative results and a lack of easily available assays the broad use of CTC enumeration remains limited [34].

Additionally, few retrospective studies report a trend for baseline LDH values above the range of normal limits being inversely associated with survival outcomes [12,35]. However, LDH is a very unspecific biomarker of cell necrosis in many tumor types including mCRPC and probably only reflects tumor burden as well as cell turnover as a marker of cancer aggressiveness [34].

Because of this lack of broadly available surrogate markers, we analyzed the potential of readily accessible biomarkers that are already being used in different settings within prostate cancer.

Until now, the role of fPSA is limited to the diagnosis of prostate cancer [19]. A lower proportion of %fPSA can be found in men with prostate cancer compared to patients with benign prostate enlargement [36]. Clinicians aim to avoid unnecessary biopsies by the measurement of fPSA, especially in cases with a mild tPSA elevation of 4–10 ng/mL. Additionally, a correlation between fPSA and the aggressiveness of the prostate cancers was shown [37].

More recent investigations demonstrated that this correlation with aggressiveness is even higher for the subform-proportion of %[−2]proPSA and PHI [23,24]. In addition, both parameters are currently considered to be the strongest predictors for presence of prostate cancer [21–23,38] with a higher specificity compared to fPSA and tPSA [22].

Due to the correlation between PSA subforms and the aggressiveness of the tumor we assumed that these parameters could play a role as surrogate biomarkers under therapy of mCRPC as well. Our results underline the non-straightforward data regarding early rising tPSA measurements with no validity concerning therapy outcomes. In contrast, we were able to show a trend towards rising [−2]proPSA, fPSA and, less importantly, PHI in patients with shorter OS and PFS at an early stage of treatment. Compared to tPSA, we need to consider that tPSA was taken into account for the definition of PD during treatment with Abiraterone. This might be an explanation for the less obvious separation of the curves during Kaplan–Meier analyses when comparing tPSA to fPSA and [−2]proPSA. However, our data suggest that fPSA and [−2]proPSA might be further studied as potential parameters for the prognostication of therapy response under early treatment with Abiraterone in case of non-straightforward development of PSA-values. The relative changes of both, median [−2]proPSA and fPSA values, were shown to be almost equal.

Our study is limited due to its relatively small cohort of only 25 patients recruited in a single center. Further larger studies are needed to explore the potential prognostic and predictive impact of fPSA and [−2]proPSA in mCRPC treated with Abiraterone.

4. Materials and Methods

4.1. Patients

Twenty-five patients with mCRPC presenting at the Prostate Center of the University Hospital Muenster (Münster, Germany), and receiving Abiraterone-therapy between March 2012 and July 2014, were reviewed. They had given written informed consent before participating and ethics committee-approval was granted for this study.

All patients presented with confirmed mCRPC, defined by prostate cancer working group 2 (PCWG2) criteria [31], in either pre- or post-chemotherapy setting (20 of them received Abiraterone in a pre- and 5 in a post-chemotherapy setting) suitable for Abiraterone-treatment. The pre-chemotherapy patients were asymptomatic or oligo-symptomatic, not requiring opiates and had a pain level of no more than 3 out of 10 on the numeric-rating-scale. Patients receiving Abiraterone in the post-chemotherapy setting had previously documented PD either on or after docetaxel chemotherapy. One of the 25 patients had received Enzalutamide previously. All patients in our study were either on a stable dose of an antiresorptive agent (i.e., Zoledronic acid or Denosumab) at least three months prior to the start of Abiraterone and during the whole treatment phase or did not receive antiresorptive medication at all. The patients were not systematically followed up with 12-weekly imaging when no PD was suspected, but when biochemical progression was evident, or when clinical progression occurred, even when there was no biochemical progression. CT-, MRI- or PSMA-PET-CT-scans of thorax, abdomen and pelvis were used for the evaluation of soft tissue metastases. Bone scans were done to acquire additional information on baseline bone metastases. PD was defined by RECIST 1.1 criteria [39] for cross-sectional imaging and by PCWG2 criteria for bone scans [31].

A physician with large expertise in the treatment of mCRPC assessed the current response status i.e., complete remission (CR), partial remission (PR), stable disease (SD) or PD at each visit. For defining PD, deterioration of general condition, worsening of pain or laboratory constellations (rising tPSA) and imaging were taken into account, according to PCWG2 criteria. Rising tPSA alone was not sufficient to define progression. The results of PSA-subform analysis, which was done in a retrospective setting, were not taken into consideration for therapeutic decisions.

All patients presented the day before the start of Abiraterone-therapy to have blood drawn for baseline analysis, two and four weeks after initiation of therapy and every four weeks thereafter.

4.2. Analysis of PSA Subforms

Blood samples were allowed to clot at room temperature and then centrifuged at $1600\times g$ for 15 min at 4 °C. Taking into account the stability issue of [−2]proPSA, serum samples were frozen at −80 °C within 3 h after blood draw [40]. After thawing of the frozen samples at room temperature, samples were processed immediately and used to determine tPSA, fPSA, [−2]proPSA on the Access II instrument, WHO-calibrated (Beckman Coulter, Krefeld, Germany) for the timepoints 'baseline', '8–12 weeks under therapy' and 'progression'. Furthermore, %fPSA, %[−2]proPSA and PHI were calculated.

We carried out the analyses according to the manufacturers' instructions on the AccessII-instrument (Beckman-Coulter, Krefeld, Germany)—batch numbers: tPSA (470206), fPSA (470202) and [−2]proPSA (434426). The results for PSA-subforms exceeded the measuring range of the instrument in many cases, with [−2]proPSA values up to 8000 pg/mL. Therefore, dilution was necessary. Due to a nonlinear response with serial dilution of the proPSA kit diluent, we used the LowCross-Buffer® (CANDOR Bioscience GmbH, Wangen, Germany, lot number 100A766f) as sample diluent in order to reduce nonspecific binding and cross-reactivities of the antibodies and matrix effects from blood serum. This procedure helped to minimize interferences in this assay and improves the reliability of the results. When dilution of serum samples was necessary due to very high [−2]proPSA values, all the other parameters were measured within the same diluted sample.

4.3. Statistical Methods

The descriptive statistics are reported as medians with IQR for continuous variables and as populations and frequencies for categorical variables. We performed the Mann–Whitney–Wilcoxon Test to determine the significance of the differences between categorical and continuous variables, respectively. We used the Kaplan–Meier-estimates for survival analyses. Univariate analysis of the different biomarkers was done with Cox-regression-models. Hazard ratios are given with 95% confidence intervals. All reported p-values are two-sided and statistical significance was assumed with a $p \leq 0.05$. SPSS-Statistics V.22 (IBM Inc., Armonk, NY, USA) was used for statistical assessment.

5. Conclusions

When added to tPSA information, which is traditionally used as therapy response indicator, changes of fPSA and [−2]proPSA at 8–12 weeks of Abiraterone-therapy may be a promising therapy control marker to help physicians make meaningful decisions on whether to stop or to continue Abiraterone-therapy in men with mCRPC but need to be further studied. Due to its better availability, the measurement of fPSA seems to be more feasible than [−2]proPSA.

Acknowledgments: The authors acknowledge the free-of-charge supply of PSA reagents by Beckman Coulter (Krefeld, Germany), and the assistance of Hilla Bürgel, Barbara Kloke and Beate Pepping-Schefers from the Prostate Center Muenster (Münster, Germany) in archiving and handling of the samples. We additionally thank Maria Eveslage of the Institute of Biostatistics and Clinical Research (Münster, Germany) for support regarding the statistical analysis.

Author Contributions: Katrin Schlack participated in the design of the study, helped in acquisition of data, in statistical analysis, and drafting of the manuscript; Laura-Maria Krabbe participated in statistical analysis and critical revision of the manuscript; Manfred Fobker participated in optimizing the assay for [−2]proPSA in very high levels and critical revision of the manuscript; Andres Jan Schrader participated in critical revision of the manuscript; Axel Semjonow participated in interpretation of serial dilution experiments, statistical analysis and critical revision of the manuscript; Martin Boegemann conceived of the study and participated in its design and coordination, performed part of the statistical analysis, and helped to draft the manuscript.

Abbreviations

mCRPC	metastatic Castration Resistant Prostate Cancer
ADT	Androgen-Deprivation Therapy
PSA	Prostate Specific Antigen
tPSA	total PSA
ECOG	Eastern Cooperative Oncology Group performance status
PFS	Progression Free Survival
CTC	Circulating Tumor Cells
LDH	Lactate Dehydrogenase
OS	Overall Survival
fPSA	free PSA
PHI	Prostate Health Index
IQR	Interquartile Range
HR	Hazard Ratio
CI	Confidence Interval
NR	Not Reached
PD	Progressive Disease
PCWG2	Prostate Cancer Working Group 2
CR	Complete Remission
PR	Partial Remission
SD	Stable Disease

References

1. Ryan, C.J.; Smith, M.R.; Fizazi, K.; Saad, F.; Mulders, P.F.; Sternberg, C.N.; Miller, K.; Logothetis, C.J.; Shore, N.D.; Small, E.J.; et al. Abiraterone acetate plus prednisone versus placebo plus prednisone in chemotherapy-naive men with metastatic castration-resistant prostate cancer (COU-AA-302): Final overall survival analysis of a randomised, double-blind, placebo-controlled phase 3 study. *Lancet Oncol.* **2015**, *16*, 152–160. [CrossRef]
2. Logothetis, C.J.; Basch, E.; Molina, A.; Fizazi, K.; North, S.A.; Chi, K.N.; Jones, R.J.; Goodman, O.B.; Mainwaring, P.N.; Sternberg, C.N.; et al. Effect of abiraterone acetate and prednisone compared with placebo and prednisone on pain control and skeletal-related events in patients with metastatic castration-resistant prostate cancer: Exploratory analysis of data from the COU-AA-301 randomised trial. *Lancet Oncol.* **2012**, *13*, 1210–1217. [PubMed]
3. Kantoff, P.W.; Higano, C.S.; Shore, N.D.; Berger, E.R.; Small, E.J.; Penson, D.F.; Redfern, C.H.; Ferrari, A.C.; Dreicer, R.; Sims, R.B.; et al. Sipuleucel-t immunotherapy for castration-resistant prostate cancer. *N. Engl. J. Med.* **2010**, *363*, 411–422. [CrossRef] [PubMed]
4. Loriot, Y.; Miller, K.; Sternberg, C.N.; Fizazi, K.; de Bono, J.S.; Chowdhury, S.; Higano, C.S.; Noonberg, S.; Holmstrom, S.; Mansbach, H.; et al. Effect of enzalutamide on health-related quality of life, pain, and skeletal-related events in asymptomatic and minimally symptomatic, chemotherapy-naive patients with metastatic castration-resistant prostate cancer (prevail): Results from a randomised, phase 3 trial. *Lancet Oncol.* **2015**, *16*, 509–521. [PubMed]

5. Fizazi, K.; Scher, H.I.; Miller, K.; Basch, E.; Sternberg, C.N.; Cella, D.; Forer, D.; Hirmand, M.; de Bono, J.S. Effect of enzalutamide on time to first skeletal-related event, pain, and quality of life in men with castration-resistant prostate cancer: Results from the randomised, phase 3 affirm trial. *Lancet Oncol.* **2014**, *15*, 1147–1156. [CrossRef]
6. Berthold, D.R.; Pond, G.R.; Soban, F.; de Wit, R.; Eisenberger, M.; Tannock, I.F. Docetaxel plus prednisone or mitoxantrone plus prednisone for advanced prostate cancer: Updated survival in the TAX 327 study. *J. Clin. Oncol.* **2008**, *26*, 242–245. [CrossRef] [PubMed]
7. Petrylak, D.P.; Tangen, C.M.; Hussain, M.H.; Lara, P.N., Jr.; Jones, J.A.; Taplin, M.E.; Burch, P.A.; Berry, D.; Moinpour, C.; Kohli, M.; et al. Docetaxel and estramustine compared with mitoxantrone and prednisone for advanced refractory prostate cancer. *N. Engl. J. Med.* **2004**, *351*, 1513–1520. [CrossRef] [PubMed]
8. Sartor, O.; Coleman, R.; Nilsson, S.; Heinrich, D.; Helle, S.I.; O'Sullivan, J.M.; Fossa, S.D.; Chodacki, A.; Wiechno, P.; Logue, J.; et al. Effect of radium-223 dichloride on symptomatic skeletal events in patients with castration-resistant prostate cancer and bone metastases: Results from a phase 3, double-blind, randomised trial. *Lancet Oncol.* **2014**, *15*, 738–746. [CrossRef]
9. De Bono, J.S.; Logothetis, C.J.; Molina, A.; Fizazi, K.; North, S.; Chu, L.; Chi, K.N.; Jones, R.J.; Goodman, O.B., Jr.; Saad, F.; et al. Abiraterone and increased survival in metastatic prostate cancer. *N. Engl. J. Med.* **2011**, *364*, 1995–2005. [CrossRef] [PubMed]
10. Burgio, S.L.; Conteduca, V.; Rudnas, B.; Carrozza, F.; Campadelli, E.; Bianchi, E.; Fabbri, P.; Montanari, M.; Carretta, E.; Menna, C.; et al. PSA flare with abiraterone in patients with metastatic castration-resistant prostate cancer. *Clin. Genitourin. Cancer* **2015**, *13*, 39–43. [CrossRef] [PubMed]
11. Danila, D.C.; Morris, M.J.; de Bono, J.S.; Ryan, C.J.; Denmeade, S.R.; Smith, M.R.; Taplin, M.E.; Bubley, G.J.; Kheoh, T.; Haqq, C.; et al. Phase II multicenter study of abiraterone acetate plus prednisone therapy in patients with docetaxel-treated castration-resistant prostate cancer. *J. Clin. Oncol.* **2010**, *28*, 1496–1501. [CrossRef] [PubMed]
12. Scher, H.I.; Heller, G.; Molina, A.; Attard, G.; Danila, D.C.; Jia, X.; Peng, W.; Sandhu, S.K.; Olmos, D.; Riisnaes, R.; et al. Circulating tumor cell biomarker panel as an individual-level surrogate for survival in metastatic castration-resistant prostate cancer. *J. Clin. Oncol.* **2015**, *33*, 1348–1355. [CrossRef] [PubMed]
13. Danila, D.C.; Heller, G.; Gignac, G.A.; Gonzalez-Espinoza, R.; Anand, A.; Tanaka, E.; Lilja, H.; Schwartz, L.; Larson, S.; Fleisher, M.; et al. Circulating tumor cell number and prognosis in progressive castration-resistant prostate cancer. *Clin. Cancer Res.* **2007**, *13*, 7053–7058. [CrossRef] [PubMed]
14. Danila, D.C.; Fleisher, M.; Scher, H.I. Circulating tumor cells as biomarkers in prostate cancer. *Clin. Cancer Res.* **2011**, *17*, 3903–3912. [CrossRef] [PubMed]
15. Lilja, H.; Christensson, A.; Dahlen, U.; Matikainen, M.T.; Nilsson, O.; Pettersson, K.; Lovgren, T. Prostate-specific antigen in serum occurs predominantly in complex with α 1-antichymotrypsin. *Clin. Chem.* **1991**, *37*, 1618–1625. [PubMed]
16. Lilja, H.; Stenman, U.H. Successful separation between benign prostatic hyperplasia and prostate cancer by measurement of free and complexed psa. *Cancer Treat. Res.* **1996**, *88*, 93–101. [PubMed]
17. Stenman, U.H.; Leinonen, J.; Alfthan, H.; Rannikko, S.; Tuhkanen, K.; Alfthan, O. A complex between prostate-specific antigen and alpha 1-antichymotrypsin is the major form of prostate-specific antigen in serum of patients with prostatic cancer: Assay of the complex improves clinical sensitivity for cancer. *Cancer Res.* **1991**, *51*, 222–226. [PubMed]
18. Mikolajczyk, S.D.; Rittenhouse, H.G. Pro psa: A more cancer specific form of prostate specific antigen for the early detection of prostate cancer. *Keio J. Med.* **2003**, *52*, 86–91. [CrossRef] [PubMed]
19. Tosoian, J.; Loeb, S. Psa and beyond: The past, present, and future of investigative biomarkers for prostate cancer. *Sci. World J.* **2010**, *10*, 1919–1931. [CrossRef] [PubMed]
20. Mikolajczyk, S.D.; Marks, L.S.; Partin, A.W.; Rittenhouse, H.G. Free prostate-specific antigen in serum is becoming more complex. *Urology* **2002**, *59*, 797–802. [CrossRef]
21. Lazzeri, M.; Briganti, A.; Scattoni, V.; Lughezzani, G.; Larcher, A.; Gadda, G.M.; Lista, G.; Cestari, A.; Buffi, N.; Bini, V.; et al. Serum index test %[−2]proPSA and prostate health index are more accurate than prostate specific antigen and %fPSA in predicting a positive repeat prostate biopsy. *J. Urol.* **2012**, *188*, 1137–1143. [CrossRef] [PubMed]

22. Catalona, W.J.; Partin, A.W.; Sanda, M.G.; Wei, J.T.; Klee, G.G.; Bangma, C.H.; Slawin, K.M.; Marks, L.S.; Loeb, S.; Broyles, D.L.; et al. A multicenter study of [−2]pro-prostate specific antigen combined with prostate specific antigen and free prostate specific antigen for prostate cancer detection in the 2.0 to 10.0 ng/mL prostate specific antigen range. *J. Urol.* **2011**, *185*, 1650–1655. [CrossRef] [PubMed]
23. Lazzeri, M.; Haese, A.; Abrate, A.; de la Taille, A.; Redorta, J.P.; McNicholas, T.; Lughezzani, G.; Lista, G.; Larcher, A.; Bini, V.; et al. Clinical performance of serum prostate-specific antigen isoform [−2]proPSA (p2PSA) and its derivatives, %p2PSA and the prostate health index (PHI), in men with a family history of prostate cancer: Results from a multicentre european study, the prometheus project. *BJU Int.* **2013**, *112*, 313–321. [PubMed]
24. Stephan, C.; Jung, K.; Semjonow, A.; Schulze-Forster, K.; Cammann, H.; Hu, X.; Meyer, H.A.; Bogemann, M.; Miller, K.; Friedersdorff, F. Comparative assessment of urinary prostate cancer antigen 3 and TMPRSS2: Erg gene fusion with the serum [−2]proprostate-specific antigen-based prostate health index for detection of prostate cancer. *Clin. Chem.* **2013**, *59*, 280–288. [CrossRef] [PubMed]
25. Fossati, N.; Buffi, N.M.; Haese, A.; Stephan, C.; Larcher, A.; McNicholas, T.; de la Taille, A.; Freschi, M.; Lughezzani, G.; Abrate, A.; et al. Preoperative prostate-specific antigen isoform p2PSA and its derivatives, %p2PSA and prostate health index, predict pathologic outcomes in patients undergoing radical prostatectomy for prostate cancer: Results from a multicentric european prospective study. *Eur. Urol.* **2015**, *68*, 132–138. [CrossRef] [PubMed]
26. Fossati, N.; Lazzeri, M.; Haese, A.; McNicholas, T.; de la Taille, A.; Buffi, N.M.; Lughezzani, G.; Gadda, G.M.; Lista, G.; Larcher, A.; et al. Clinical performance of serum isoform [−2]proPSA (p2PSA), and its derivatives %p2PSA and the prostate health index, in men aged <60 years: Results from a multicentric european study. *BJU Int.* **2015**, *115*, 913–920. [PubMed]
27. Woo, H.H.; Begbie, S.; Gogna, K.; Mainwaring, P.N.; Murphy, D.G.; Parnis, F.; Steer, C.; Davis, I.D. Multidisciplinary consensus: A practical guide for the integration of abiraterone into clinical practice. *Asia Pac. J. Clin. Oncol.* **2014**, *10*, 228–236. [CrossRef] [PubMed]
28. Roghmann, F.; Antczak, C.; McKay, R.R.; Choueiri, T.; Hu, J.C.; Kibel, A.S.; Kim, S.P.; Kowalczyk, K.J.; Menon, M.; Nguyen, P.L.; et al. The burden of skeletal-related events in patients with prostate cancer and bone metastasis. *Urol. Oncol.* **2015**, *33*, e9–e18. [CrossRef] [PubMed]
29. Ryan, C.J.; Shah, S.; Efstathiou, E.; Smith, M.R.; Taplin, M.E.; Bubley, G.J.; Logothetis, C.J.; Kheoh, T.; Kilian, C.; Haqq, C.M.; et al. Phase II study of abiraterone acetate in chemotherapy-naive metastatic castration-resistant prostate cancer displaying bone flare discordant with serologic response. *Clin. Cancer Res.* **2011**, *17*, 4854–4861. [CrossRef] [PubMed]
30. Johns, W.D.; Garnick, M.B.; Kaplan, W.D. Leuprolide therapy for prostate cancer: An association with scintigraphic "flare" on bone scan. *Clin. Nucl. Med.* **1990**, *15*, 485–487. [CrossRef] [PubMed]
31. Scher, H.I.; Halabi, S.; Tannock, I.; Morris, M.; Sternberg, C.N.; Carducci, M.A.; Eisenberger, M.A.; Higano, C.; Bubley, G.J.; Dreicer, R.; et al. Design and end points of clinical trials for patients with progressive prostate cancer and castrate levels of testosterone: Recommendations of the prostate cancer clinical trials working group. *J. Clin. Oncol.* **2008**, *26*, 1148–1159. [CrossRef] [PubMed]
32. Berthold, D.R.; Pond, G.R.; Roessner, M.; de Wit, R.; Eisenberger, M.; Tannock, A.I. TAX-327 investigators Treatment of hormone-refractory prostate cancer with docetaxel or mitoxantrone: Relationships between prostate-specific antigen, pain, and quality of life response and survival in the TAX-327 study. *Clin. Cancer Res.* **2008**, *14*, 2763–2767. [CrossRef] [PubMed]
33. Leibowitz-Amit, R.; Templeton, A.J.; Omlin, A.; Pezaro, C.; Atenafu, E.G.; Keizman, D.; Vera-Badillo, F.; Seah, J.A.; Attard, G.; Knox, J.J.; et al. Clinical variables associated with psa response to abiraterone acetate in patients with metastatic castration-resistant prostate cancer. *Ann. Oncol.* **2014**, *25*, 657–662. [CrossRef] [PubMed]
34. Armstrong, A.J.; Eisenberger, M.A.; Halabi, S.; Oudard, S.; Nanus, D.M.; Petrylak, D.P.; Sartor, A.O.; Scher, H.I. Biomarkers in the management and treatment of men with metastatic castration-resistant prostate cancer. *Eur. Urol.* **2012**, *61*, 549–559. [CrossRef] [PubMed]
35. Scher, H.I.; Jia, X.; de Bono, J.S.; Fleisher, M.; Pienta, K.J.; Raghavan, D.; Heller, G. Circulating tumour cells as prognostic markers in progressive, castration-resistant prostate cancer: A reanalysis of IMMC38 trial data. *Lancet Oncol.* **2009**, *10*, 233–239. [CrossRef]

36. De Angelis, G.; Rittenhouse, H.G.; Mikolajczyk, S.D.; Blair Shamel, L.; Semjonow, A. Twenty years of PSA: From prostate antigen to tumor marker. *Rev. Urol.* **2007**, *9*, 113–123. [PubMed]
37. Catalona, W.J.; Partin, A.W.; Slawin, K.M.; Brawer, M.K.; Flanigan, R.C.; Patel, A.; Richie, J.P.; deKernion, J.B.; Walsh, P.C.; Scardino, P.T.; et al. Use of the percentage of free prostate-specific antigen to enhance differentiation of prostate cancer from benign prostatic disease: A prospective multicenter clinical trial. *JAMA* **1998**, *279*, 1542–1547. [CrossRef] [PubMed]
38. Abrate, A.; Lughezzani, G.; Gadda, G.M.; Lista, G.; Kinzikeeva, E.; Fossati, N.; Larcher, A.; Dell'Oglio, P.; Mistretta, F.; Buffi, N.; et al. Clinical use of [−2]proPSA (p2PSA) and its derivatives (%p2PSA and prostate health index) for the detection of prostate cancer: A review of the literature. *Korean J. Urol.* **2014**, *55*, 436–445. [CrossRef] [PubMed]
39. Eisenhauer, E.A.; Therasse, P.; Bogaerts, J.; Schwartz, L.H.; Sargent, D.; Ford, R.; Dancey, J.; Arbuck, S.; Gwyther, S.; Mooney, M.; et al. New response evaluation criteria in solid tumours: Revised recist guideline (version 1.1). *Eur. J. Cancer* **2009**, *45*, 228–247. [CrossRef] [PubMed]
40. Semjonow, A.; Kopke, T.; Eltze, E.; Pepping-Schefers, B.; Burgel, H.; Darte, C. Pre-analytical in vitro stability of [−2]proPSA in blood and serum. *Clin. Biochem.* **2010**, *43*, 926–928. [CrossRef] [PubMed]

6

Prostate Cancer Detection and Prognosis: From Prostate Specific Antigen (PSA) to Exosomal Biomarkers

Xavier Filella * and Laura Foj

Department of Biochemistry and Molecular Genetics (CDB), Hospital Clínic, IDIBAPS, C/Villarroel, 170, 08036 Barcelona, Catalonia, Spain; lfoj@clinic.cat
* Correspondence: xfilella@clinic.cat

Academic Editor: Carsten Stephan

Abstract: Prostate specific antigen (PSA) remains the most used biomarker in the management of early prostate cancer (PCa), in spite of the problems related to false positive results and overdiagnosis. New biomarkers have been proposed in recent years with the aim of increasing specificity and distinguishing aggressive from non-aggressive PCa. The emerging role of the prostate health index and the 4Kscore is reviewed in this article. Both are blood-based tests related to the aggressiveness of the tumor, which provide the risk of suffering PCa and avoiding negative biopsies. Furthermore, the use of urine has emerged as a non-invasive way to identify new biomarkers in recent years, including the *PCA3* and *TMPRSS2:ERG* fusion gene. Available results about the PCA3 score showed its usefulness to decide the repetition of biopsy in patients with a previous negative result, although its relationship with the aggressiveness of the tumor is controversial. More recently, aberrant microRNA expression in PCa has been reported by different authors. Preliminary results suggest the utility of circulating and urinary microRNAs in the detection and prognosis of PCa. Although several of these new biomarkers have been recommended by different guidelines, large prospective and comparative studies are necessary to establish their value in PCa detection and prognosis.

Keywords: prostate cancer detection; biomarker; prostate specific antigen (PSA); prostate health index; 4Kscore; PCA3 score; miRNAs; exosomal biomarkers

---

1. Introduction

Prostate cancer (PCa) remains a medical challenge, since it is one of the most frequently diagnosed tumors and a common cause of cancer death among men in western countries [1]. The introduction of the measurement of prostate specific antigen (PSA) in the mid-eighties of last century represented a major innovation in the management of patients with PCa. PSA, or human kallicrein 3 (hK3), is a glandular kallikrein with abundant expression in the prostate encoded by the *KLK3* gene. The sequential measurement of PSA allows the monitoring of the response to treatment and the assessment of its effectiveness. PSA is also widely used in the detection of PCa, despite its low specificity, with false positive results in patients with benign prostatic hyperplasia (BPH). Biopsy is only positive in around 25% of patients with PSA in the range between 2 and 10 μg/L. Elevated levels of PSA are particularly found in patients with enlarged prostate volume [2]. Age-specific PSA reference ranges and PSA density have been proposed to avoid this effect, increasing the specificity of PSA. Moreover, prostate volume is a key element in multivariate PCa risk calculators [3].

More recently, several studies have shown that single nucleotide polymorphisms (SNPs) in the *KLK3* gene or other related genes can influence PSA serum levels. Gudmundsson et al. [4] detected a significant association between PSA serum levels and SNPs at six loci, finding the strongest association for SNPs located near or in the *KLK3* gene. Furthermore, some of these SNPs could be associated with predisposition to PCa and PCa aggressiveness [5]. Genetic effect on PSA expression advocates a genetic correction of PSA serum levels. Unnecessary biopsies could be avoided in genetically high PSA producers, while necessary biopsies could be performed in genetically low PSA producers. Helfand et al. [6] suggested a genetically personalized interpretation of PSA serum levels to obtain more accurate results. According to these authors, genetic correction of PSA serum levels could decrease the number of potentially unnecessary biopsies by approximately 18% to 22%, improving the use of PSA as a screening tool.

A major harm of PCa screening is overdiagnosis, defined as the diagnosis of patients whose cancer never surfaces clinically during lifetime. Active surveillance is now accepted as a valuable strategy in the management of low-risk PCa, decreasing the negative effects of overdiagnosis and overtreatment. The criteria for the selection of patients for active surveillance include several variables, such as a PSA lower than 10 μg/L, a Gleason score lower than 7 and a low number of cylinders affected by the tumor [7]. However, PCa characterization based on these findings is not ideal [8]. The availability of more accurate inclusion criteria would lead to an improvement in the management of patients with early PCa.

The introduction of a new biomarker in PCa should fulfil the dual purpose of providing increased specificity and—being related to the aggressiveness of the tumor—differentiating aggressive cancers from non-aggressive cancers. Several PSA derivatives have been proposed as PCa biomarkers with this aim. The percentage of free PSA to total PSA (%fPSA) was introduced three decades ago for the detection of PCa, but this test improves clinical information only when levels reach extreme values [9].

More recently, fPSA has been found to include the isoforms BPSA, proPSA and iPSA [10] (Figure 1), with usefulness in the detection of PCa. A commercial immunoassay for the measurement of [−2]proPSA, the most stable form of proPSA, has been developed. The Prostate Health Index has been proposed as a new index for PCa detection, combining serum concentrations of [−2]proPSA, fPSA and total PSA, according to the formula $([-2]\text{proPSA}/\text{fPSA})^{*} \sqrt{\text{total PSA}}$. In addition, an index based on the measurement of total PSA, fPSA, intact PSA (iPSA) and human kallicrein 2 (hK2) in combination with clinical and demographic data, called the 4Kscore, has been proposed for the detection of high-risk PCa.

Furthermore, the development of molecular biology has allowed the study of genes associated with PCa. Numerous studies have evaluated the utility of the *PCA3* gene and more recently the *TMPRSS2:ERG* fusion gene has also been investigated. On the other hand, the study of microRNAs (miRNAs) has opened an emerging field for the research of these biomarkers in the detection and prognosis of PCa.

Several sources for the study of these potential novel biomarkers for PCa are being analyzed, each one with its advantages and disadvantages. The measurement in plasma or serum has the advantage of being a consolidated media, for which commercial automated assays are available. However, the study of the *PCA3* gene in urine obtained after performing a prostate massage has opened a new way for the study of new biomarkers for PCa. Urine, due to the anatomic proximity of the prostate gland to the urethra, may allow the detection of biomarkers for PCa, particularly when the sample is enriched with prostate cells by performing a slight prostate massage. In addition, the protein content of the urine is lower than in serum and plasma, so that some interferences caused by excess of proteins can be reduced, thus facilitating the detection of new biomarkers. Finally, exosomal biomarkers obtained from blood or urine have been suggested as novel diagnostic and prognostic indicators for several cancers, e.g., PCa. Figure 2 shows a timeline for the identification of PCa biomarkers from the discovery of PSA till the current moment.

The aim of our article was to review the usefulness of blood and urine biomarkers in the detection and prognosis of PCa.

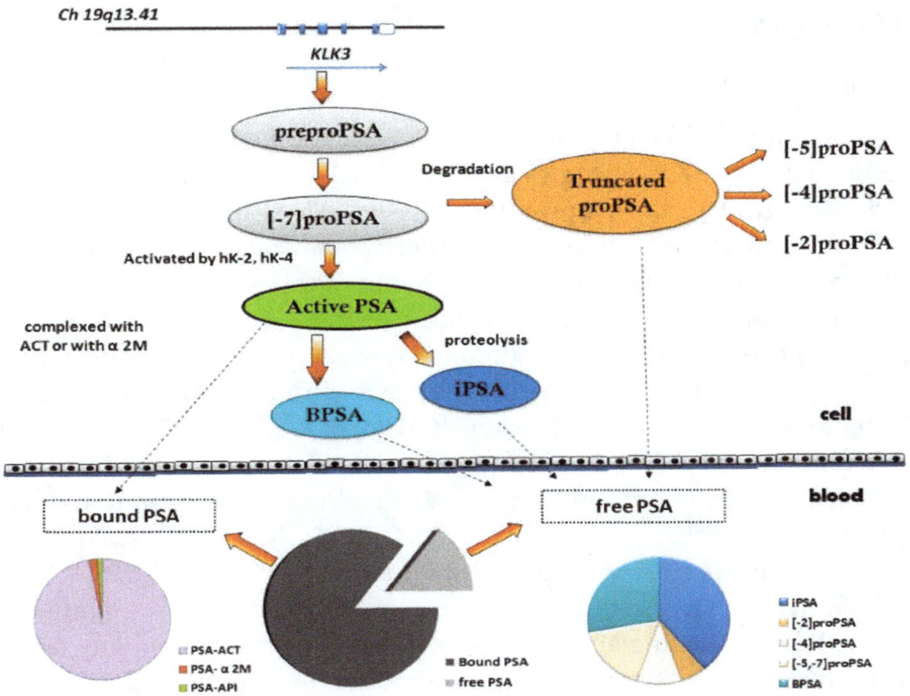

Figure 1. Molecular forms of PSA. The arrows with dashed line mean the forms of PSA that go from the cell to the blood. PSA: prostate specific antigen, BPSA: benign PSA, iPSA: intact PSA, PSA-ACT: Alpha 1-antichymotrypsin-PSA, PSA-API: alpha1-trypsin inhibitor PSA, PSA-A2M: alpha 2 macroglobulin, hK-2: human kallicrein 2, hk-4: human kallicrein 4.

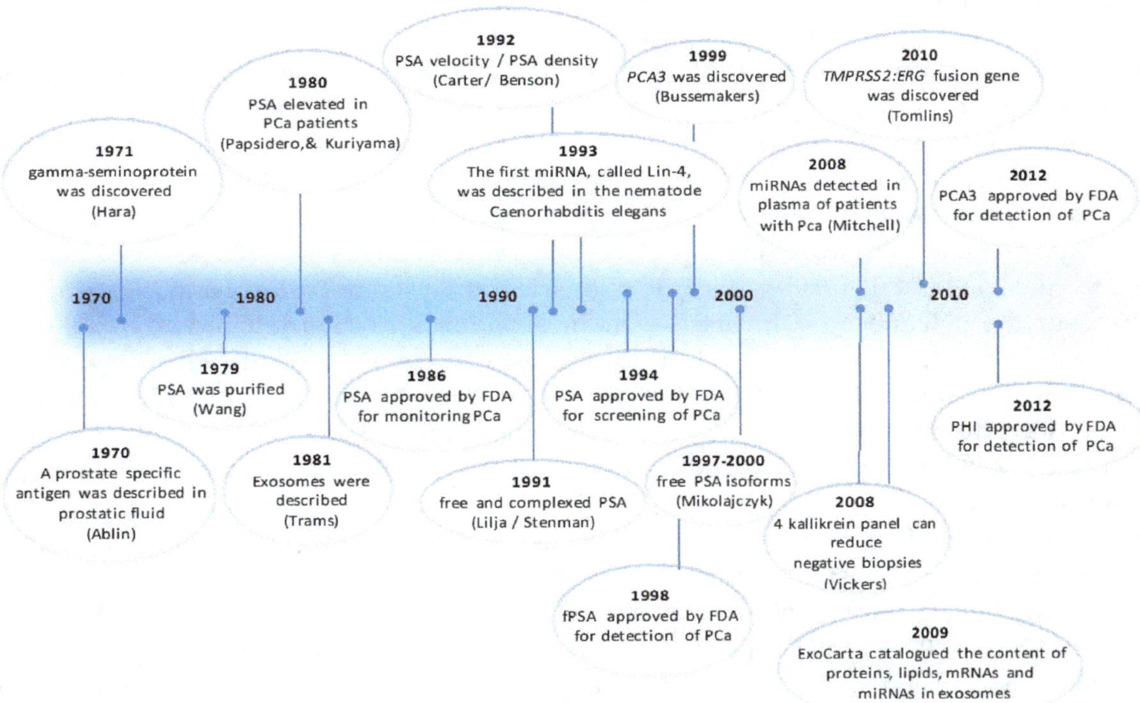

Figure 2. Timeline for the identification of PCa biomarkers. Most important events related to PCa markers from 1970 till the present. PSA: prostate specific antigen, miRNA: microRNA, PCa: prostate cancer, fPSA: free PSA, PHI: prostate health index.

2. Blood-Based PCa Biomarkers

2.1. Prostate Health Index (PHI)

The Prostate Health Index (PHI) was approved by the Food and Drug Administration (FDA) in June 2012 for the detection of PCa in men aged 50 or older, with a PSA between 4 and 10 μg/L and a non-suspicious digital rectal examination (DRE). Also, this test is recommended by the National Comprehensive Cancer Network for patients who have never undergone a biopsy or after a negative biopsy, considering that results higher than 35 are related to a high probability of PCa [11]. Several authors agree with the usefulness of the PHI and percentage of [−2]proPSA to fPSA (%[−2]proPSA) to predict the biopsy outcome. Two multicenter studies, including 1362 and 646 patients, highlight the value of these tests in patients with PSA values between 2 and 10 μg/L. Stephan et al. [12] reported an area under the curve (AUC) of 0.72 and 0.74 for %[−2]proPSA and the PHI, respectively, while Lazzeri et al. [13] reported an AUC of 0.67 for both biomarkers.

Two meta-analyses published in 2013 and 2014 corroborate these results, documenting AUCs from 0.635 to 0.78 for %[−2]proPSA and from 0.69 to 0.781 for the PHI [14,15]. Both meta-analyses underlined that these tests outperform the results obtained with PSA and %fPSA. This point has been confirmed by a subsequent meta-analysis comparing the PHI and %fPSA in patients with total PSA between 2 and 10 μg/L [16], showing an AUCs of 0.74 and 0.63, respectively for the PHI and %fPSA.

The three mentioned meta-analyses also agree regarding the relation of the PHI and %[−2]proPSA with the aggressiveness of the tumor. This fact has been documented by Loeb et al. [17] in a study that evaluated 658 male candidates to biopsy with PSA values between 4 and 10 μg/L. The authors noted that the AUC to identify a clinically significant PCa was 0.698 for the PHI, while it was only 0.654 for %fPSA. Also, Fossati et al. [18] indicated that both the PHI and %[−2]proPSA predicted a pathologic stage T3 and a Gleason score ≥7 in the surgical specimen after evaluating a series of 489 patients treated with radical prostatectomy.

Moreover, several studies have suggested that the addition of the PHI and %[−2]proPSA to multivariate models based on the combination of PSA and various clinical and demographic variables provides better clinical performance for the prediction of PCa. Stephan et al. [19] reported that the AUC increased from 0.69 to 0.75 when [−2]proPSA or the PHI were added to a multivariable model based on patient age, prostate volume, DRE, PSA and %fPSA. Similarly, Guazzoni et al. [20] showed an improvement in the AUC by including %[−2]proPSA (0.82) or the PHI (0.83) in a model based on the patient age, prostate volume, PSA and %fPSA (0.72). Finally, Filella et al. [21] showed that the AUC increased from 0.762 to 0.802 (using a logistic regression analysis) or 0.815 (using an artificial neural network) when the PHI and %[−2]proPSA were included in a multivariate model based on patient age, prostate volume, PSA and %fPSA. Moreover, this study showed a relationship between prostate volume and the PHI values, highlighting that prostate volume is a key factor in the interpretation of PHI results. According to these authors, the performance of the PHI changed in relation to prostate volume, finding AUCs of 0.818, 0.716 and 0.654 for patients with small, medium and large prostate volume, respectively.

Lughezzani et al. [22] developed a PHI based nomogram for predicting PCa evaluating 729 patients undergoing prostate biopsy. The PHI increased significantly the accuracy obtained using a multivariable logistic regression model based on patient age, prostate volume, DRE and biopsy history from 0.73 to 0.80. External validation of this model was provided by a multicenter European study based on 833 patients, showing an accuracy of 0.752 [23]. More recently, Roobol et al. [24] showed analogous results validating this nomogram on 1185 men from four European sites, obtaining an accuracy of 0.75 for all PCa and 0.69 for clinically relevant PCa (clinical stage > T2b and/or a biopsy Gleason score ≥ 7). Similar results were found in this study by adding the PHI to the European Randomized Study of Prostate Cancer (ERSPC) risk calculator, obtaining an accuracy of 0.72 for all PCa and 0.68 for clinically relevant PCa. Despite these positive results, the authors concluded that only limited reductions in the rate of unnecessary biopsies are possible when models are updated adding the PHI. More optimistic are the conclusions of a recent cost-effectiveness study of PCa detection using the PHI [25]. The authors used a micro simulation model based on the results of the ERSPC trial to compare the effects of screening using the PHI and those using only PSA. The model predicted a reduction of 23% in negative biopsies for men with PSA between 3 and 10 µg/L, concluding that PHI testing is 11% more cost-effective than screening only based on PSA.

2.2. Kallikrein Panel

The 4Kscore is a risk calculation for the detection of PCa on the biopsy based on the measurement of a 4-kallikrein panel combined with the patient age, DRE and biopsy history. The 4-kallikrein panel includes the measurement of total PSA, fPSA, iPSA and hK2, a kallikrein with high homology with PSA. The test provides information about the probability of having a high-risk PCa. Therefore, the aim is no longer to indicate a biopsy to detect PCa, but it is intended only to detect aggressive tumors with a Gleason score of 7 or higher. Although the 4Kscore does not have the approval of the FDA, in June 2015 the National Comprehensive Cancer Network recommended the use of this test for the detection of high-risk PCa for patients who have never undergone biopsy or after a negative biopsy [11].

The test was developed after studies performed by the group led by Lilja and Vickers, from Memorial Sloan-Kettering Cancer Center, who conducted an extensive research in collaboration with several European centers. The AUCs for the 4-kallikrein panel reported in all these studies for the detection of high-risk PCa were higher than those for a PSA based model [26–32]. The AUCs obtained for the 4-kallikrein panel ranged between 0.793 and 0.870, while the AUCs for the PSA based model ranged from 0.658 to 0.816. Similar differences were observed when the corresponding clinical models to predict high-risk PCa were compared. The AUCs for the model combining PSA, patient age and DRE ranged from 0.709 to 0.868, while the AUCs ranged from 0.798 to 0.903 when fPSA, iPSA and hK2 were also included.

Prostate volume is a crucial factor influencing PSA serum levels and it is usually included in PCa risk calculators. However, according to results published by Carlsson et al. [33], prostate volume is not affecting the performance of a 4-kallicrein panel in PCa detection. This group studied these biomarkers in two cohorts of 2914 and 740 patients with PSA $\geq$3 µg/L. In the first cohort, the AUC increased from 0.856 to 0.860 when the prostate volume was added to a model based on a 4-kallikrein panel, patient age and DRE, while in the second cohort the AUC was identical including or not prostate volume (0.802).

All results published about the 4Kscore before 2014 were obtained in retrospective European cohorts. In 2015, a prospective multicenter study developed in United States was published [34]. This evaluation, which included 1012 patients scheduled for prostate biopsy, confirmed the results shown in previous studies. The AUC obtained for the 4Kscore test in the detection of high-risk PCa was 0.82. The study documented that 58% of biopsies could be saved using a cut-off value of 15%, although 4.7% of high-risk PCa would not be detected. Using a cut-off value of 6%, the reduction in the number of biopsies was of 30%, but in contrast, only 1.3% of high-risk tumors were not detected.

On the other hand, a study based on a cohort collected in Sweden since 1986, in which samples of included subjects were collected at the age of 40, 50 and 60, showed the predictive value of the 4Kscore [35]. The result of this test assessed at 50 and 60 years old allowed the classification of the patients into two groups according to the probability of developing distant metastasis 20 years later. Patients with PSA $\geq$3 µg/L at 60 years old were classified using a cut-off for the 4Kscore of 7.5 in two groups with a significantly different risk of developing distant metastasis. Similarly, the 4Kscore was also predictive using a cut-off of 5 considering patients with PSA $\geq$2 µg/L at 50 years old.

3. Urine-Based PCa Biomarkers

3.1. PCA3

PCA3 (prostate cancer gene 3, previously referred as *DD3*) is a gene that transcribes a long non-coding mRNA that is overexpressed in PCa tissue (Figure 3). The PCA3 test is the score calculated measuring the concentration of *PCA3* mRNA in relation to PSA mRNA, which is used to normalize *PCA3* signals. Measurements are performed in the urine obtained after performing a prostate massage to enrich prostate cell content. This test, based on quantitative real time polymerase chain reaction (qRT-PCR) technology, obtained the European Conformity in November 2006 and was approved by the FDA in 2012 with the aim of deciding the repetition of a prostate biopsy in men more than 50 years old who have one or more previous negative biopsies and results of PCA3 score higher than 25. The 2015 clinical guide of the National Comprehensive Cancer Network for the early detection of PCa [11] considered PCA3 score as a useful test to decide the repetition of a biopsy in patients with a previous negative biopsy, suggesting the use of 35 as the discriminating value.

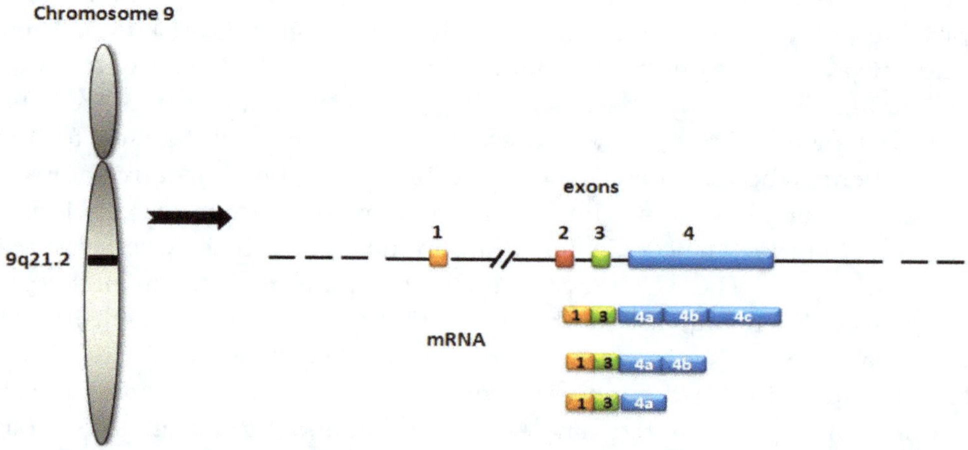

Figure 3. *PCA3* gene structure. The most frequent transcript contains exons 1, 3, 4a, and 4b.

The available results suggest that the PCA3 score can be useful in detecting PCa, especially in patients with a previous negative biopsy [36]. However, the definition of the best discriminating value is controversial. A multicenter study led by Haese [37] indicated that a score of 35 provides the optimal balance between sensitivity (47%) and specificity (72%). Similar results have been recently reported in a meta-analysis published by Hu et al. [38] including 16 studies that used 35 as the cut-off to decide when to perform a biopsy. These authors documented an overall sensitivity of 57% and an overall specificity of 71%, concluding that, although high quality further studies are missing, the PCA3 score is a useful test in the detection of PCa. However, a large group of tumors were not diagnosed when a biopsy was indicated in patients with a PCA3 score higher than 35. In the aforementioned study of Haese et al. [37], 67% of biopsies would have been saved using the discriminating value of 35, but 21% of high-grade PCa would not have been diagnosed. In the same study, using a discriminating value of 20, the saved biopsies were only from 44%, but 9% of high-grade PCa were not detected.

These data have been confirmed by Crawford et al. [39] in a multicenter study involving 1913 patients, 802 of which with PCa. These authors point out that the traditional score of 35 allowed a reduction of 77% in biopsies, but the number of false negatives was large, because PCa was detected in 413 of 1275 patients (32%) with a PCA3 score lower than 35, of which 195 had a Gleason score of 7 or higher. However, by lowering the discriminating value to 10, the number of undiagnosed tumors was reduced to 108, of which 52 had a Gleason score lower than 7. This study also points out that PCa was only detected in 86 of 114 patients with a PCA3 score $\geq$100. It is somewhat paradoxical because initial studies presented *PCA3* as an overexpressed gene in PCa tissue between 10- and 100-fold relative to non-neoplastic tissue [40]. In this way, Schröder et al. [41] showed a low positive predictive value (38.9%) for a PCA3 score $\geq$100, even when significant efforts to detect a PCa were performed.

Finally, the relationship between PCA3 score and the aggressiveness of the tumor is also controversial. Merola et al. [42], in a group of 114 patients with PCa, observed a significant association between the PCA3 score and Gleason score (p = 0.02). Moreover, Chevli et al. [43] in a study based on 3073 patients observed that the PCA3 score is related to the Gleason score, with mean values of 47.5 and 58.5 for patients with a Gleason score of 6 and 7 or higher, respectively. However, this study also shows that the AUC to predict high-grade PCa is lower than that obtained with PSA (0.679 vs. 0.682, respectively). Other authors do not find any correlation between the PCA3 score and Gleason score, without explanations for this divergence [44,45].

The accumulated data on the PCA3 score generate an important expectation. Nevertheless, the available evidence about its usefulness is not enough, as noted by a comparative analysis published by Bradley et al. [46] based on 34 observational studies. The majority of studies suggest that the diagnostic accuracy of the PCA3 score is clearly superior to that of PSA. In this regard, however, Roobol et al. [47] highlight the influence of the bias caused by the use of PSA in the selection of the population included in *PCA3* studies. In their report, the authors try to minimize this bias by not only performing the biopsy when PSA was greater than 3 μg/L, but also when the PCA3 score was lower than 10. The obtained data showed less difference in the AUCs than in other studies (0.581 and 0.635 for PSA and PCA3 score, respectively).

3.2. *TMPRSS2:ERG* Fusion Gene

The gene fusion involving *ERG* (v-ets erythroblastosis virus E26 oncogene homologs) and the androgen regulated gene *TMPRSS2* (transmembrane serine protease isoform 2) (Figure 4) was reported in 2005 by Tomlins et al. [48]. Aberrant fusion of the *TMPRSS2* gene with the *ERG* gene is observed in 15%–59% of PCa [49], but there are not unanimous results regarding its association with disease prognosis. Differences could be explained in relation to the exon involved in the fusion [50] or due to the presence of multiple copies of the fusion gene, showing a reduced prostate cancer-specific survival in those patients whose tumor had multiple copies of the fusion gene [51].

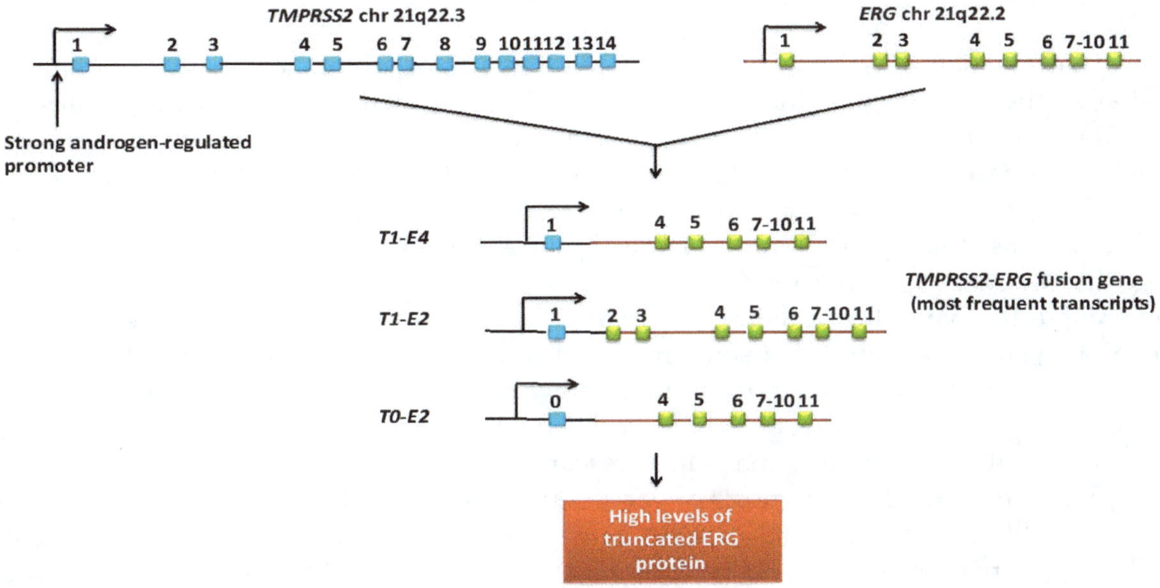

Figure 4. The *TMPRSS2:ERG* fusion gene and its most frequent transcripts. The most frequent transcripts of the *TMPRSS2:ERG* fusion gene consist in the fusion of exon 1 of *TMPRSS2* to either exon 2 or 4 of *ERG* (T1-E4 or T1-E2). These transcripts encode for N-terminal truncated ERG proteins. Exon 1 from *TPRSS2* is non-codifying. Transcription of the gene *TMPRSS2* can start not only from its first exon, exon 1, but also from an alternative first exon (exon 0).

The *TMPRSS2:ERG* gene rearrangements are studied in urine samples obtained after a prostate massage using qRT-PCR. A ratio with PSA mRNA is used to normalize *TMPRSS2:ERG* signals. The combination of the TMPRSS2:ERG score with the PCA3 score has been proposed as a way to improve the prediction of the presence of PCa on the biopsy. A multicenter study published by

Leyten et al. [52] prospectively evaluated the diagnostic utility of PCA3 and TMPRSS2:ERG scores in 443 patients who underwent a biopsy and found that both scores significantly increased the predictive value obtained with the risk calculator ERSPC, which includes PSA and several clinical variables. The AUC increased from 0.799 to 0.833 for the risk calculator ERSPC when PCA3 score was added, and to 0.842 when PCA3 and TMPRSS2:ERG scores were added. In addition, TMPRSS2-ERG, but not PCA3, was associated with the Gleason score and the tumor clinical stage.

More recently, Tomlins et al. [53] also proposed the combination of PCA3 and TMPRSS2:ERG scores with PSA serum levels as a useful tool for detecting PCa. The study, prospectively conducted in three centers and based on 1244 patients who underwent biopsy, showed the value of PCA3 and TMPRSS2:ERG scores when they were added to the PCPT (Prostate Cancer Prevention Trial) risk calculator, also based on PSA and several clinical variables. The AUC increased from 0.639 for the PCPT risk calculator to 0.739 and to 0.762 by adding the TMPRSS2:ERG score alone or the TMPRSS2:ERG score plus the PCA3 score, respectively. Both biomarkers were also evaluated to predict high-risk PCa, being the respective AUCs of 0.707 (for the PCPT risk calculator), 0.752 (plus *TMPRSS2:ERG*) and 0.779 (plus *TMPRSS2:ERG* and PCA3). The model that brings together the PCPT risk calculator, PCA3 and TMPRSS2:ERG scores, called My Prostate score (MiPS), would allow the avoidance of 36% of biopsies using a discriminating value of 15%, although it would cease to diagnose 1.6% of high-risk tumors.

The value of MiPS has been questioned by Stephan et al. [54] comparing PCA3, *TMPRSS2:ERG*, PSA and PHI in a series of 246 patients, including 110 patients with PCa. The authors obtained an AUC for MiPS of 0.748. The highest accuracy was found for a model including PCA3 and the PHI, with AUCs of 0.757 and 0.752, when an artificial neural network and the logistic regression analysis were used, respectively. The authors argued that the clinical potential of the TMPRSS2:ERG score is limited because of its low prevalence in PCa patients.

4. miRNAs

miRNAs are small (17–22 nucleotides) non-coding RNAs, which negatively regulate the gene expression at the posttranscriptional level by base-pairing to the complementary sites in their target mRNAs, resulting in a repression or degradation of the target. The number of identified miRNAs has progressively increased since 1993, when the first miRNA was described in the nematode *Caenorhabditis elegans*. Currently, the number of miRNAs described according to the database mirbase.org is 28,645 miRNAs (miRBase, release 21 June 2014) [55], 2588 of which are found in humans, targeting the vast majority of mRNAs.

Several studies have shown their participation in the development and progression of cancer. Calin et al. [56] showed in 2002 that some miRNAs were suppressed or downregulated in chronic lymphocytic leukemia. The number of studies that evaluate their usefulness as biomarkers has been increasing since 2008, when Lawrie et al. [57] proposed a profile of circulating miRNAs as a diagnostic tool in patients with B-cell lymphoma. Many research findings prove the usefulness of circulating miRNAs in the detection and prognosis of various tumors and in the prediction of the response to treatment, revealing robust signatures of miRNAs that distinguish healthy controls from patients with cancer. However, these results should be contextualized because of differences in the methodology used in the available studies. Witwer [58] underlines that limited overlap has been observed between the findings of similar studies in the same disease, probably due to methodological reasons. Indeed, although miRNAs are stable enough in plasma and serum, optimization and standardization of the methodology used for the miRNAs measurement is required to obtain high quality results. So far, there are still differences due to the type of sample (with differences between serum and plasma, and also related to plasma, among the different anticoagulants); the specific reagent used in the isolation of miRNA; the performance of a preamplification to obtain more Cdna; and the platform used for the qRT-PCR (AbiPrism, LightCycle, etc.), the use of endogenous (none of which behaves as ideal control) or exogenous controls (e.g., cel-miR-39) to normalize the results, and the calculation method used, of which probably $\Delta\Delta C_t$ is the most frequent (Figure 5).

The development of digital PCR could improve the performance of qRT-PCR and would remove the dependence for a reference miRNA for normalization. Besides, the introduction of digital count technologies, such as next-generation sequencing (NGS) and the NanoString nCounter System has supplied new tools for miRNA profiling [59]. As opposed to microarrays and qRT-PCR, NGS enables the discovery of new miRNAs in addition to the confirmation of known miRNAs. It beats the limitations of microarrays that have background signal and cross-hybridization problems. Another recent novelty for miRNA profiling is the NanoString nCounter system, a hybridization-based technology, which consists on direct digital detection of RNA molecules of interest using target-specific, colour-coded probe pairs without the requirement of reverse transcription or cDNA amplification.

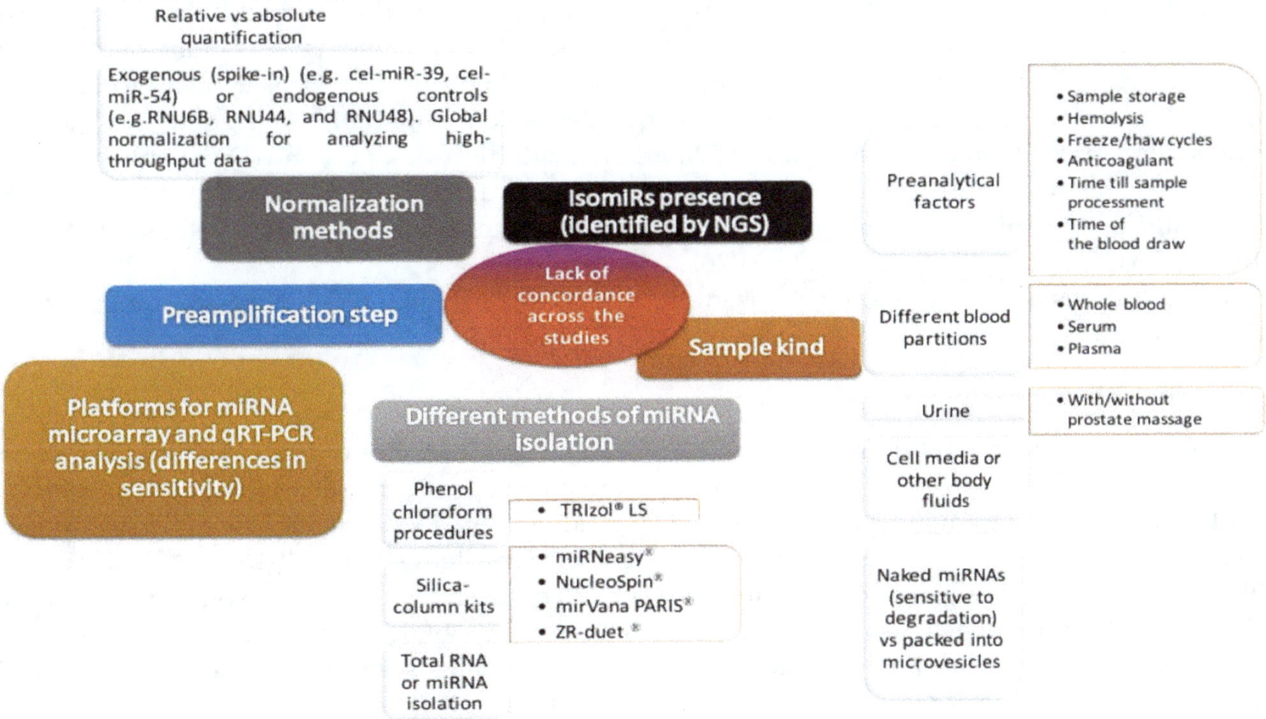

Figure 5. Sources of lack of concordance across the different studies. miRNA: microRNA, NGS: next generation sequencing.

The expression of aberrant miRNAs has been demonstrated in PCa, playing a critical role in tumor initiation, development and progression [60]. Mitchell et al. [61] were the first to show that miRNAs are present in the plasma of patients with PCa in a remarkably stable manner, noting that miR-141 is significantly elevated in patients with advanced PCa compared to healthy controls. Subsequently, several studies based on microarrays have identified several miRNAs signatures with utility in the diagnosis and prognosis of PCa. However, the differences among these panels are substantial and only miR-141, miR-375 and miR-21 repeatedly appear in various studies [62]. Prominently, Mihelich et al. [63] retrospectively studied the serum levels of 21 miRNAs in 100 PCa patients in stages T1–T2. The authors found a signature composed by 14 miRNAs (let-7a, miR-24, miR-26b, miR-30c, miR-93, miR-100, miR-103, miR-106a, miR-107, miR-130b, miR-146a, miR-223, miR-451, and miR-874) to distinguish accurately (negative predictive value of 0.939) high-grade PCa from low-grade PCa. Seven of these miRNAs (miR-451, miR-106a, miR-223, miR-107, miR-130b, let-7a and miR-26b) were also significantly lower in PCa patients with biochemical recurrence after radical prostatectomy compared with those without biochemical recurrence. Similarly, Chen et al. [64] identified, in plasma, a panel of five miRNAs (miR-622, miR-1285, let-7e, let-7c, and miR-30c) to discriminate CaP from BPH and healthy controls with high sensitivity and specificity. On the other hand, Moltzahn et al. [65] found AUCs from 0.812 to 0.928 for miR-106a, miR-1274, miR-93, miR-223, miR-874, miR-1207 and miR-24, showing a trend to correlate with the CAPRA score, a PCa risk assessment based on patient age, PSA serum levels, clinical tumor stage, the Gleason score and the percentage of positive biopsy cores. The authors reported the up-regulation of miR-30c, miR-93, miR-106a, miR-223 and miR-451 in patients with high-risk PCa compared with low-risk PCa. It should be noted that opposite results have been indicated by Mihelich et al. [63], showing that these miRNAs were highly expressed in BPH and low-risk PCa compared with high-risk PCa. These differences could be attributed to deficiencies in the standardization of the collection and measurement of miRNAs.

Although the clinical usefulness of miRNAs in urine has been investigated by several authors, no comprehensive evaluation has been reported till the present moment. Studies have been done in several urine fractions, including whole urine, urinary pellet and the cell-free urinary fraction. The enrichment with prostatic cells after a prostate massage has been also assayed. Preliminary results suggest that the measurement of urinary miRNAs may be valuable as biomarkers in the management of patients with early PCa, although conclusions of the available studies are based on a short series of patients [62]. Recently, Salido-Guadarrama et al. [66] identified a miR-100/200b signature in the urine obtained after prostate massage comparing 73 patients with high-risk PCa and 70 patients with BPH. The AUC for this signature (0.738) was higher than the obtained AUCs for total PSA (0.681) and %fPSA (0.710). Adding the miR-100/200b signature to a multivariate model based on age, DRE, total PSA and %fPSA the AUC increased from 0.816 to 0.876.

Contributions regarding the clinical usefulness of miRNAs in blood and urine are summarized in Table 1.

5. Exosomal Biomarkers

Exosomes are small (30–150 nm) double lipid membrane vesicles of endocytic origin secreted by most cell types, that contain proteins, lipids and nucleic acids. Information about the molecules identified in exosomes from multiple organisms is provided in the ExoCarta database (http://exocarta.org/). Currently, ExoCarta contains information on 41,860 protein entries, 4946 mRNA entries and 2838 miRNA entries that have been identified from 286 exosomal studies. Exosomes were initially described by Trams et al. [67] as exfoliated membrane vesicles, obtained from neoplasic cell cultures. Their presence has later been confirmed in serum and plasma as well as in other biological fluids, including urine, saliva, ascites, breast milk and amniotic fluid. The study of new biomarkers in exosomes is a promising field because they are remarkably stable in body fluids and their content is protected from enzymatic degradation by the exosomal lipid bilayer [68,69].

Cancer cells have been shown to release high levels of exosomes, which may influence tumor initiation, growth and progression as well as drug resistance. Actually, a significantly higher amount of exosomes has been found in serum from ovarian cancer patients in comparison with healthy subjects or patients with benign ovarian diseases. Also, the amount of exosomes has been correlated with the clinical stage in ovarian cancer, showing high levels in patients at an advanced stage [70]. Duijvesz et al. [71] showed that CD9 and CD63 exosomal biomarkers in urine collected after DRE were significantly higher in men with PCa. Analogous results have been found in other tumors, including lung cancer, colorectal cancer and chronic lymphocytic leukemia [72–74].

The emerging involvement of exosomes in intercellular communication focuses on their role in carcinogenesis. Tumor derived exosomes exchange information with other cancer cells and also with other cell types, including stroma and extracellular matrix cells, establishing favorable conditions for tumor growth and invasion. Exosomes can stimulate target cells through different ways, including the interaction with specific membrane receptors, endocitosis and the horizontal transfer of proteins and RNA species, such as mRNA, large non-coding RNA molecules and miRNAs [75]. Available evidence showed that exosomes derived from cancer cells actively contribute to the progression of disease [76]. Franzen et al. [77] reported that epithelial-to-mesenchymal transition in urothelial cells is induced by muscle invasive bladder cancer exosomes. Similar data have been shown in PCa. Abd Elmageed et al. [78] demonstrated that exosomes from PCa cells can induce the neoplastic transformation of adipose derived stem cells through the horizontal transfer of several oncogenic factors, including the oncomiRs miR-125b, miR-130b and miR-155. Besides, according to Hosseini-Beheshti et al. [79], exosomes derived from PCa cells could contribute to cancer progression, reducing apoptosis, increasing cancer cell proliferation, and inducing cell migration in LNCaP and RWPE-1 cells.

In spite of the growing interest in the role of exosomes in several diseases and their use for functional studies and biomarker discovery, no standard method is available to acquire highly pure and well-characterized exosomes. The most common method for exosomes isolation is differential ultracentrifugation, which consists of multiple centrifugation steps with increasing centrifugal strength to sequentially pellet cells (300 g), microvesicles (10,000 g) and exosomes (100,000 g) [80]. Many variations to these speeds are implemented in practice. Serial filtration through 0.45 and 0.2 mm filters is used optionally before exosome pelleting. Furthermore, density gradient based isolation, using sucrose or iodixanol (OptiPrep™, Sigma-Aldrich, St. Louis, MO, USA), can be used to obtain more pure exosome preparations. Commercial easy-to-use reagents have recently been developed, including precipitation solutions, such as ExoQuick™ or Total Exosome Isolation™ kits, and column-based assays, such as exoRNeasy Serum/Plasma. Transmission electron microscopy or immuno electron microscopy can be performed to check the presence of exosomes. Furthermore, Western blot and ELISA assays can be used to detect several exosomal markers (such as CD9, CD63 and CD81) in order to identify the isolated vesicles as exosomes (Figure 6).

Few studies have evaluated exosomal biomarkers in PCa detection and prognosis. Proteome of urinary exosomes has been analyzed using mass spectrometry to identify proteins by Øverbye et al. [81] in 15 healthy subjects and 16 PCa patients. This study showed that 246 proteins were significantly altered in urinary exosomes of PCa patients. The authors found that 17 proteins presented sensitivities above 60% at 100% specificity. The highest sensitivities were observed for transmembrane protein 256 (TM256) (94%), LAMTOR1 (81%) and ADIRF (81%). Furthermore, the authors reported an AUC of 0.87 for TM256, which increased to 0.94 by combining with LAMTOR1.

Comparison of *PCA3* and *TMPRSS2:ERG* between urinary sediment and exosomes has been reported by Dijkstra et al. [82], concluding that exosomes seem to be a more robust source of biomarkers, although a significant proportion of samples are not assessable because they do not reach the analytical detection limit. Exosomal *PCA3* and *TMPRSS2:ERG* levels were significantly higher when urine was collected after a prostate massage. More recently, published results by this group based on 29 men undergoing prostate biopsies showed that *PCA3* and *ERG* perform better in whole urine than in urinary sediment or exosomes [83]. No significant differences were found for both biomarkers in exosomes comparing PCa and non-PCa patients.

Opposite results have been reported by Donovan et al. [84] evaluating the combination of exosomal *PCA3* and *ERG* mRNA in the detection of high-grade PCa. The authors studied both biomarkers in first-catch urine samples obtained without prostate massage from 195 patients submitted for initial biopsy because of PSA serum levels within the gray zone. They showed that the EXO106 score (the sum of normalized exosomal *PCA3* and *ERG* mRNA levels) is related to the Gleason score, showing higher results in patients with a Gleason score $\geq$7. The authors proposed to combine the EXO106 score with PSA, age, race and PCa family history for the detection of high PCa, showing negative and positive predictive values of 97.5% and 34.5%, respectively (AUC: 0.803).

Several authors suggested that exosomes obtained from blood and urine are a consistent source of miRNA for disease biomarker detection [85–88], although some doubts have been presented by other researchers underlying that exosomes in standard preparations do not carry a biologically significant amount of miRNAs [89]. Moreover, according to Arroyo et al. [90], vesicle associated miRNAs only represent a minority, while around 90% of miRNAs in the circulation are present in a non-membrane-bound form. Instead, Gallo et al. [91] showed that the majority of miRNAs detectable in serum and saliva are concentrated in exosomes. Moreover, Cheng et al. [85] showed that in urine the highest proportion of miRNA was extracted from exosomes.

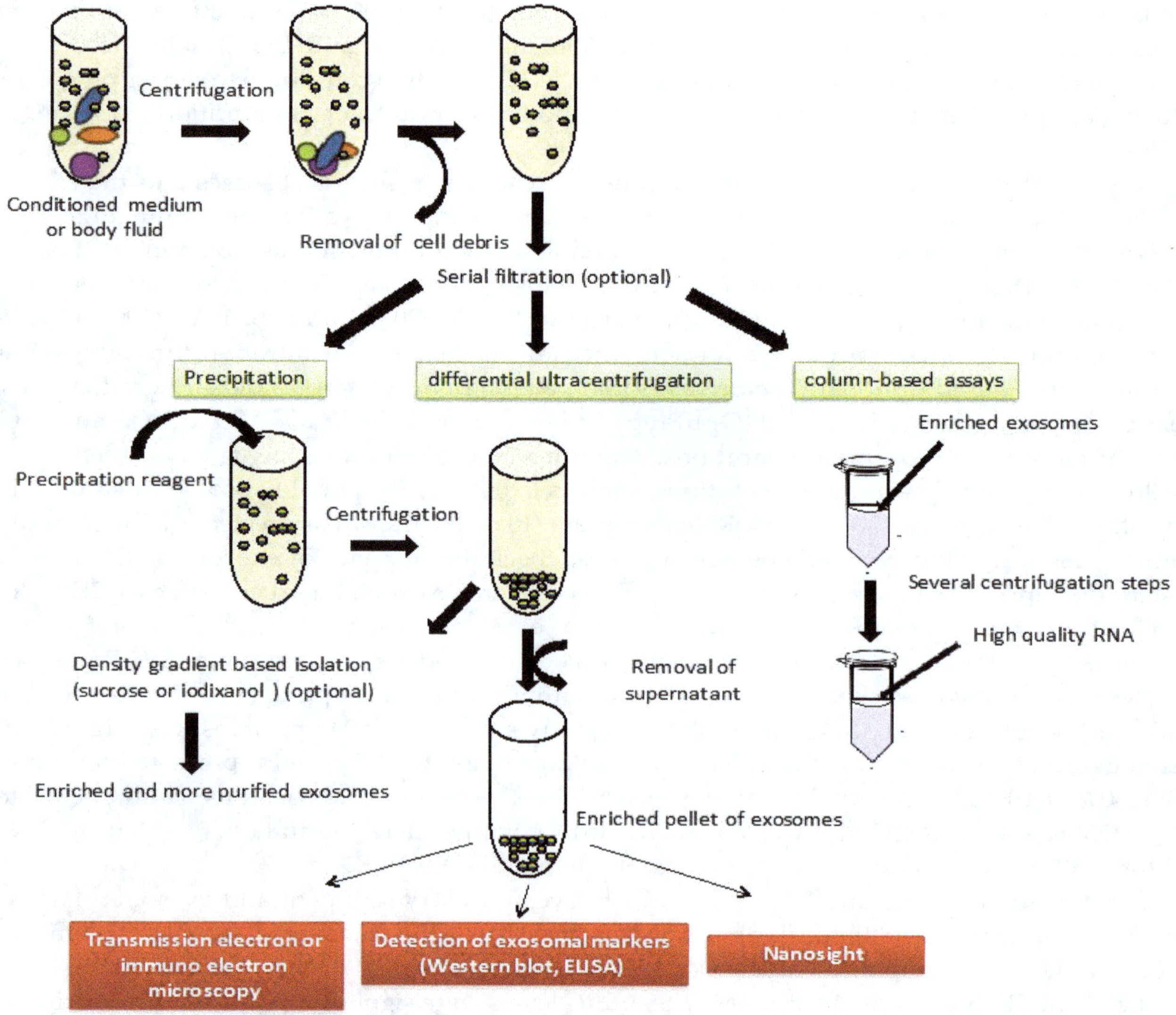

Figure 6. Exosome isolation procedures. The different size particles contained in body fluids or conditioned media are drawn as different color circles.

Actually, some studies have evaluated the usefulness of exosomes' miRNAs in PCa management (Table 1). Li et al. [92] showed that the level of the miR-141 was significantly higher in exosomes compared with the whole serum. Also, these authors reported that the level of serum exosomal miR-141 was significantly higher in PCa patients compared with BPH patients and healthy controls, finding the most elevated levels in patients with metastatic PCa. Moreover, Huang et al. [93] found that the levels of plasma exosomal miR-1290 and miR-375 were significantly associated with poor overall survival. The addition of these new biomarkers into a clinical prognostic model improved predictive performance with a time-dependent AUC increase from 0.66 to 0.73. On the other hand, Bryzgunova et al. [94] demonstrated promising results in the detection of PCa, analyzing miR-19b in urinary exosomes isolated by differential centrifugation. Finally, Samsonov et al. [95] indicated that miR-21, miR-141 and miR-574 were upregulated in PCa patients compared with healthy controls in urinary exosomes isolated by a lectin-based exosomes agglutination method. Nevertheless, only miR-141 was found to be significantly upregulated when urinary exosomes were isolated by differential centrifugation.

Table 1. microRNAs studies in PCa patients.

Reference	Body Fluid	miRNAs Analyzed	Methodology	Patients	Clinical Results
Mitchell et al. 2008 [61]	Serum	miR-100, -125b, -141, -143, -205, and -296	qRT-PCR	25 metastatic PCa and 25 matched healthy controls	AUC of 0.907 for miR-141 comparing PCa and healthy
Mihelich et al. 2015 [63]	Serum	21 miRNAs	qRT-PCR	100 no treated PCa (50 low-grade, 50 high-grade) and 50 BPH	A panel combining let-7a, miR-103, -451, -24, -26b, -30c, -93, -106a, -223, -874, -146a, -125b, -100, -107 and -130b distinguish high-grade PCa from low-grade PCa and BPH
Chen et al. 2012 [64]	Plasma	1146 miRNAs, 8 selected miRNAs for validation study	Illumina's Human miRNA microarray, qRT-PCR	Screening set: 17 BPH and 25 CaP. Validation set: 44 BPH, 54 healthy controls and 80 CaP	A panel combining miR-622, -1285, -30c, let-7e and let-7c discriminate CaP from BPH (AUC: 0.924) or healthy controls (AUC: 0.860)
Moltzahn et al. 2011 [65]	Serum	384 miRNAs, 12 miRs selected for validation study	multiplex qRT-PCR	12 low-risk PCa, 12 intermediate-risk PCa, 12 high-risk PCa and 12 healthy controls	AUCs: miR-106a, 0.928; miR-1274, 0.928; miR-93, 0.907; miR-223, 0.876; miR-874, 0.845; miR-1207, 0.812; miR-24: 0.778. miR-93, -106a and -24 differentiate healthy and metastatic groups
Salido-Guadarrama et al. 2016 [66]	urine obtained after prostate massage	364 miRNAs	MicroRNA TaqMan Low Density Array, qRT-PCR	73 patients with high-risk PCa and 70 patients with BPH	AUC for miR-100/200b signature was 0.738. Adding the miR-100/200b signature to a multivariate model based on age, DRE, total PSA and %fPSA the AUC increased from 0.816 to 0.876
Li et al. 2015 [92]	serum exosomes	miR-141	qRT-PCR	Serum vs. exosomes cohort: 20 PCa, 20 BPH, 20 healthy controls	Serum exosomal miR-141 was significantly higher in PCa patients compared with BPH patients and healthy controls
Huang et al. 2015 [93]	Plasma exosomes	let-7c, miR-30a/e, -99a, -1246, -1290, -16, -125a, and -375	Illumina HiSeq2000 platform, qRT-PCR	Screening cohort: 23 CRPC patients. Follow-up cohort: 100 CRPC patients	Plasma exosomal miR-1290 and miR-375 were significantly associated with poor overall survival
Bryzgunova et al. 2016 [94]	total extracellular vesicles and exosome-enriched fractions	miR-19b, -25, -125b, and -205	qRT-PCR	20 healthy controls and 14 untreated PCa patients	Detection of miR-19b versus miR-16 in total vesicles and exosome-enriched fractions achieved 100%/93% and 95%/79% specificity/sensitivity in distinguishing cancer patients from healthy individuals, respectively, demonstrating the diagnostic value of urine extracellular vesicles. miR-19b in total extracellular vesicles distinguishes cancer patients from healthy individuals with a sensitivity of 93% and a specificity of 100%
Samsonov et al. 2016 [95]	Urinary exosomes	miR-21, -107, -141, -221, -298, -326, -375, -432, -574, -2110, -625, -301a, -191	qRT-PCR	35 PCa patients and 35 healthy controls	miR-21, -141 and -574 were upregulated in PCa patients compared with healthy controls in urinary exosomes

AUC: area under the curve, BPH: benign prostatic hyperplasia, CRPC: castration resistant prostate cancer, PCa: prostate cancer.

More recently, NGS technologies revealed the presence of sequence variants of miRNAs, called isomiRs, showing their utility as biomarkers. They are generated from a single miRNA locus through the miRNA processing and maturation process. Koppers-Lalic et al. [96] identified that isomiRs of miR-21, miR-375 and miR-204 measured in urinary extracellular vesicles could distinguish control men from PCa patients. The authors found an AUC of 0.821 for these set of isomiRs, meanwhile the AUC corresponding to the mature miRNA was 0.661. The existence of isomiRs could explain disagreements about the usefulness of miRNAs in PCa detection.

Preliminary results about exosomal biomarkers are promising, although contradictory results have been published. New advances in standardization of isolation and characterization procedures together with larger clinical studies are required to assess the clinical usefulness of exosomes.

6. Conclusions

PCa is a very heterogeneous tumor, including patients with a low-risk of progression, in which cancer-specific survival rates exceeded 99% at a 15-year follow-up. The percentage of low-risk PCa has been estimated by Klotz [97] to be between 50% and 60% of new diagnosed cases. However, the survival rate decreases considerably for men with aggressive PCa. Specific gene-expression patterns have been identified for PCa subclasses. Recently, Rubin et al. [98] have reported specific genomic profiles related to the Gleason score, showing that few driver mutations and no polyploidy are associated with tumors with a Gleason score lower than 7. In this regard, to label those patients with a Gleason 6 or lower as having cancer has been put into question [99,100].

New biomarkers have been recently introduced for the management of early PCa, offering improvement in detection and some are useful in differentiating between aggressive and non-aggressive PCa. In this article, we have underlined recent advances in the discovery of PCa biomarkers related to aggressiveness. The 4kscore is defined to identify with high accuracy an individual patient's risk for aggressive PCa. Also, high values of PHI are associated with tumor aggressiveness. Besides, both tests outperform the specificity of tPSA and %fPSA. Furthermore, although the most appropriate cut-off for the PCA3 score still has to be established, it outperforms better than tPSA and %fPSA, although its relationship with the aggressiveness of the tumor is controversial. More results are necessary to identify more accurately the usefulness of emerging biomarkers based on molecular techniques, including the *TMPRSS2:ERG* fusion gene and exosomal and non-exosomal miRNAs. Furthermore, new efforts in the standardization of these methods are necessary to use these novel biomarkers routinely.

Available studies comparing PCa biomarkers showed non-conclusive results, although several studies have evaluated these biomarkers. Scattoni et al. [101] evaluated the PHI and PCA3 score in 211 patients undergoing initial (116) or repeat (95) prostate biopsy, finding that the PHI was significantly more accurate than the PCA3 score for predicting PCa (AUC 0.70 vs. 0.59). However, Stephan et al. [102] evaluated 246 patients, showing no significant differences in accuracy between the PCA3 score and the PHI (AUC 0.74 vs. 0.68), whereas the urinary *TMPRSS2:ERG* fusion gene failed to significantly improve the ability to detect PCa. On the other hand, only PSA and the PHI correlated with the Gleason score, whereas *PCA3*, %fPSA, and the *TMPRSS2:ERG* fusion gene did not. Instead, Tallon et al. [103] concluded that the PHI and urinary *PCA3* and *TMPRSS2:ERG* fusion gene are complementary predictors of cancer aggressiveness at radical prostatectomy. According to this group, the PCA3 score was related to tumor volume $\geq$0.5 mL and multifocality, while the PHI was related to tumor volume $\geq$0.5 mL, the Gleason score $\geq$7 and extracapsular extension. The *TMPRSS2:ERG* fusion gene was only related to the pathological T stage.

A comparison between the 4Kscore and the PHI was provided by Nordström et al. [104] evaluating the performance of these biomarkers in a series of 531 men with PSA levels between 3 and 15 μg/L. No significant differences were found between both tests in the detection of any-grade PCa as well as in the detection of high-grade PCa (AUCs: 0.69 and 0.718, respectively, for the 4Kscore; and 0.704 and 0.711, respectively, for the PHI). On the other hand, Vedder et al. [105] compared PCA3 and the 4Kscore in 708 patients in which biopsy was done when PSA was $\geq$3 μg/L or PCA3 score was $\geq$10.

The 4Kscore outperforms the PCA3 score (AUC 0.78 vs. 0.62) in men with elevated PSA, although the accuracy of the PCA3 score was higher in the global population (AUC 0.63 for PCA3 vs. 0.56 for the 4Kscore). Additionally, the authors showed that both tests increased the value of a base multivariate model (from 0.70 to 0.73 adding the PCA3 score and 0.71 adding the 4kscore), but significant differences were only found adding the PCA3 score ($p = 0.02$).

To summarize, in recent years, several new promising PCa biomarkers have been identified and found to be associated with tumor aggressiveness (Box 1). Multicenter prospective studies showed the utility of the PHI, the 4Kscore and the PCA3 score to reduce the number of unnecessary prostate biopsies in PSA tested men. Actually, these biomarkers have been recommended for different guidelines [11,106,107]. However, large prospective studies, avoiding bias due to preselection of patients according to PSA serum levels, are necessary to compare the value of these biomarkers. Also, new efforts are necessary to standardize the methodology for the measurement of exosomal and non-exosomal miRNAs to analyze accurately their usefulness in the management of patients with early PCa. Finally, the combined role of these biomarkers together with magnetic resonance imaging data would be elucidated [108–110]. Additionally, results obtained using blood and urinary biomarkers must be compared with promising data obtained with Prostate-specific membrane antigen (PSMA). PSMA is a transmembrane glycoprotein overexpressed in PCa cells. Results of PSMA serum levels in the detection of the PCa are inconclusive, but its expression is correlated with a higher Gleason score, PSA at diagnosis and advanced clinical stage. PSMA features enable this biomarker as an optimal target for developing imaging strategies for PCa. Recent results show that the use of PET probes targeting PSMA for imaging prostate cancer might improve detection of cancerous foci within the prostate, especially in patients with a previous negative prostate biopsy [111]. Further studies are necessary to better characterize new PCa biomarkers, but available publications show promising results to detect PCa and to distinguish patients with aggressive and non-aggressive PCa.

Box 1. Biomarkers in PCa detection and prognosis.

Prostate health index
Biomarkers measured: PSA, fPSA, [−2]proPSA
Sample: serum
Approved by the Food and Drug Administration (FDA)
Recommended by the National Comprehensive Cancer Network
Related to PCa aggressiveness

4Kscore
Biomarkers measured: PSA, fPSA, iPSA, hK2
Sample: serum
The test provides information about the probability of having a high-risk PCa
Recommended by the National Comprehensive Cancer Network
Related to PCa aggressiveness

PCA3 score
Biomarkers measured: mRNA *PCA3* in relation to mRNA *PSA*
Sample: urine obtained after prostate massage
Approved by the Food and Drug Administration (FDA)
Recommended by the National Comprehensive Cancer Network
Inconclusive results about its relationship with PCa aggressiveness

***TMPRSS2:ERG* fusion gene**
Biomarkers measured: mRNA *TMPRSS2:ERG* in relation to mRNA *PSA*
Sample: urine obtained after prostate massage
Preliminary results

miRNAs and other exosomal biomarkers
Sample: blood and urine
Directly related to development and progression of cancer
No standardized methodology
Preliminary results

References

1. Zhou, C.K.; Check, D.P.; Lortet-Tieulent, J.; Laversanne, M.; Jemal, A.; Ferlay, J.; Bray, F.; Cook, M.B.; Devesa, S.S. Prostate cancer incidence in 43 populations worldwide: An analysis of time trends overall and by age group. *Int. J. Cancer* **2016**, *138*, 1388–1400. [CrossRef] [PubMed]
2. Bohnen, A.M.; Groeneveld, F.P.; Bosch, J.L. Serum prostate-specific antigen as a predictor of prostate volume in the community: The Krimpen study. *Eur. Urol.* **2007**, *51*, 1645–1652. [CrossRef] [PubMed]
3. Roobol, M.J.; van Vugt, H.A.; Loeb, S.; Zhu, X.; Bul, M.; Bangma, C.H.; van Leenders, A.G.; Steyerberg, E.W.; Schröder, F.H. Prediction of prostate cancer risk: The role of prostate volume and digital rectal examination in the ERSPC risk calculators. *Eur. Urol.* **2012**, *61*, 577–583. [CrossRef] [PubMed]
4. Gudmundsson, J.; Besenbacher, S.; Sulem, P.; Gudbjartsson, D.F.; Olafsson, I.; Arinbjarnarson, S.; Agnarsson, B.A.; Benediktsdottir, K.R.; Isaksson, H.J.; Kostic, J.P.; et al. Genetic correction of PSA values using sequence variants associated with PSA levels. *Sci. Transl. Med.* **2010**, *2*, 62ra92. [CrossRef] [PubMed]
5. Helfand, B.; Roehl, K.A.; Cooper, P.R.; McGuire, B.B.; Fitzgerald, L.M.; Cancel-Tassin, G.; Cornu, J.N.; Bauer, S.; van Blarigan, E.L.; Chen, X.; et al. Associations of prostate cancer risk variants with disease aggressiveness: Results of the NCI-SPORE Genetics Working Group analysis of 18,343 cases. *Hum. Genet.* **2015**, *134*, 439–450. [CrossRef] [PubMed]
6. Helfand, B.T.; Loeb, S.; Hu, Q.; Cooper, P.R.; Roehl, K.A.; McGuire, B.B.; Baumann, N.A.; Catalona, W.J. Personalized prostate specific antigen testing using genetic variants may reduce unnecessary prostate biopsies. *J. Urol.* **2013**, *189*, 1697–1701. [CrossRef] [PubMed]
7. Heidenreich, A.; Bastian, P.J.; Bellmunt, J.; Bolla, M.; Joniau, S.; van der Kwast, T.; Mason, M.; Matveev, V.; Wiegel, T.; Zattoni, F.; et al. EAU guidelines on prostate cancer. Part 1: Screening; diagnosis; and local treatment with curative intent-update 2013. *Eur. Urol.* **2014**, *65*, 124–137. [CrossRef] [PubMed]
8. Palisaar, J.R.; Noldus, J.; Löppenberg, B.; von Bodman, C.; Sommerer, F.; Eggert, T. Comprehensive report on prostate cancer misclassification by 16 currently used low-risk and active surveillance criteria. *BJU Int.* **2012**, *110*, E172–E181. [CrossRef] [PubMed]
9. Lee, R.; Localio, A.R.; Armstrong, K.; Malkowicz, S.B.; Schwartz, J.S. A meta-analysis of the performance characteristics of the free prostate-specific antigen test. *Urology* **2006**, *67*, 762–768. [CrossRef] [PubMed]
10. Mikolajczyk, S.D.; Marks, L.S.; Partin, A.W.; Rittenhouse, H.G. Free prostate-specific antigen in serum is becoming more complex. *Urology* **2002**, *59*, 797–802. [CrossRef]
11. Prostate Cancer Early Detection. National Cancer Comprehensive Network Clinical Practice Guidelines in Oncology. Version 2. 2016. Available online: https://www.nccn.org/professionals/physician_gls/pdf/prostate_detection.pdf (accessed on 9 September 2016).
12. Stephan, C.; Vincendeau, S.; Houlgatte, A.; Cammann, H.; Jung, K.; Semjonow, A. Multicenter evaluation of [−2]proprostate-specific antigen and the prostate health index for detecting prostate cancer. *Clin. Chem.* **2013**, *59*, 306–314. [CrossRef] [PubMed]
13. Lazzeri, M.; Haese, A.; de la Taille, A.; Palou Redorta, J.; McNicholas, T.; Lughezzani, G.; Scattoni, V.; Bini, V.; Freschi, M.; Sussman, A.; et al. Serum isoform [−2]proPSA derivatives significantly improve prediction of prostate cancer at initial biopsy in a total PSA range of 2–10 ng/mL: A multicentric European study. *Eur. Urol.* **2013**, *63*, 986–994. [CrossRef] [PubMed]
14. Filella, X.; Giménez, N. Evaluation of [−2]proPSA and Prostate Health Index (phi) for the detection of prostate cancer: A systematic review and meta-analysis. *Clin. Chem. Lab. Med.* **2012**, *15*, 1–11. [CrossRef] [PubMed]
15. Wang, W.; Wang, M.; Wang, L.; Adams, T.S.; Tian, Y.; Xu, J. Diagnostic ability of %p2PSA and prostate health index for aggressive prostate cancer: A meta-analysis. *Sci. Rep.* **2014**, *4*, 5012. [CrossRef] [PubMed]
16. Bruzzese, D.; Mazzarella, C.; Ferro, M.; Perdonà, S.; Chiodini, P.; Perruolo, G.; Terracciano, D. Prostate health index vs. percent free prostate-specific antigen for prostate cancer detection in men with "gray" prostate-specific antigen levels at first biopsy: Systematic review and meta-analysis. *Transl. Res.* **2014**, *164*, 444–451. [PubMed]
17. Loeb, S.; Sanda, M.G.; Broyles, D.L.; Shin, S.S.; Bangma, C.H.; Wei, J.T.; Partin, A.W.; Klee, G.G.; Slawin, K.M.; Marks, L.S.; et al. The prostate health index selectively identifies clinically significant prostate cancer. *J. Urol.* **2015**, *193*, 1163–1169. [CrossRef] [PubMed]

18. Fossati, N.; Buffi, N.M.; Haese, A.; Stephan, C.; Larcher, A.; McNicholas, T.; de la Taille, A.; Freschi, M.; Lughezzani, G.; Abrate, A.; et al. Preoperative Prostate-specific Antigen isoform p2PSA and its derivatives; %p2PSA and Prostate Health Index; predict pathologic outcomes in patients undergoing radical prostatectomy for prostate cancer: Results from a multicentric European prospective study. *Eur. Urol.* **2015**, *68*, 132–138. [CrossRef] [PubMed]
19. Stephan, C.; Kahrs, A.M.; Cammann, H.; Lein, M.; Schrader, M.; Deger, S.; Miller, K.; Jung, K. A [−2]proPSA-based artificial neural network significantly improves differentiation between prostate cancer and benign prostatic diseases. *Prostate* **2009**, *69*, 198–207. [CrossRef] [PubMed]
20. Guazzoni, G.; Nava, L.; Lazzeri, M.; Scattoni, V.; Lughezzani, G.; Maccagnano, C.; Dorigatti, F.; Ceriotti, F.; Pontillo, M.; Bini, V.; et al. Prostate-specific antigen (PSA) isoform p2PSA significantly improves the prediction of prostate cancer at initial extended prostate biopsies in patients with total PSA between 2.0 and 10 ng/mL: Results of a prospective study in a clinical setting. *Eur. Urol.* **2011**, *60*, 214–222.
21. Filella, X.; Foj, L.; Alcover, J.; Augé, J.M.; Molina, R.; Jiménez, W. The influence of prostate volume in prostate health index performance in patients with total PSA lower than 10 μg/L. *Clin. Chim. Acta* **2014**, *436*, 303–307. [CrossRef] [PubMed]
22. Lughezzani, G.; Lazzeri, M.; Larcher, A.; Lista, G.; Scattoni, V.; Cestari, A.; Buffi, N.M.; Bini, V.; Guazzoni, G. Development and internal validation of a Prostate Health Index based nomogram for predicting prostate cancer at extended biopsy. *J. Urol.* **2012**, *188*, 1144–1150. [CrossRef] [PubMed]
23. Lughezzani, G.; Lazzeri, M.; Haese, A.; McNicholas, T.; de la Taille, A.; Buffi, N.M.; Fossati, N.; Lista, G.; Larcher, A.; Abrate, A.; et al. Multicenter European external validation of a prostate health index-based nomogram for predicting prostate cancer at extended biopsy. *Eur. Urol.* **2014**, *66*, 906–912. [CrossRef] [PubMed]
24. Roobol, M.J.; Moniek, M.; Vedder, M.M.; Nieboer, D.; Houlgatte, A.; Vincendeau, S.; Lazzeri, M.; Guazzoni, G.; Stephan, C.; Semjonow, A.; et al. Comparison of two prostate cancer risk calculators that include the Prostate Health Index. *Eur. Urol. Foucs* **2015**, *1*, 185–190.
25. Heijnsdijk, E.A.; Denham, D.; de Koning, H.J. The cost-efectiveness of prostate cancer detection with the use of Prostate Health Index. *Value Health* **2016**, *19*, 153–157. [CrossRef] [PubMed]
26. Vickers, A.J.; Cronin, A.M.; Aus, G.; Pihl, C.G.; Becker, C.; Pettersson, K.; Scardino, P.T.; Hugosson, J.; Lilja, H. A panel of kallikrein markers can reduce unnecessary biopsy for prostate cancer: Data from the European Randomized Study of Prostate Cancer Screening in Göteborg, Sweden. *BMC Med.* **2008**, *6*, 19. [CrossRef] [PubMed]
27. Vickers, A.; Cronin, A.; Roobol, M.; Savage, C.; Peltola, M.; Pettersson, K.; Scardino, P.T.; Schröder, F.; Lilja, H. Reducing unnecessary biopsy during prostate cancer screening using a four-kallikrein panel: An independent replication. *J. Clin. Oncol.* **2010**, *28*, 2493–2498. [CrossRef] [PubMed]
28. Vickers, A.J.; Cronin, A.M.; Roobol, M.J.; Savage, C.J.; Peltola, M.; Pettersson, K.; Scardino, P.T.; Schröder, F.H.; Lilja, H. A four-kallikrein panel predicts prostate cancer in men with recent screening: Data from the European Randomized Study of Screening for Prostate Cancer, Rotterdam. *Clin. Cancer Res.* **2010**, *16*, 3232–3239. [CrossRef] [PubMed]
29. Vickers, A.J.; Cronin, A.M.; Aus, G.; Pihl, C.G.; Becker, C.; Pettersson, K.; Scardino, P.T.; Hugosson, J.; Lilja, H. Impact of recent screening on predicting the outcome of prostate cancer biopsy in men with elevated prostate-specific antigen: Data from the European Randomized Study of Prostate Cancer Screening in Gothenburg, Sweden. *Cancer* **2010**, *116*, 2612–2620. [CrossRef] [PubMed]
30. Gupta, A.; Roobol, M.J.; Savage, C.J.; Peltola, M.; Pettersson, K.; Scardino, P.T.; Vickers, A.J.; Schröder, F.H.; Lilja, H. A four-kallikrein panel for the prediction of repeat prostate biopsy: Data from the European Randomized Study of Prostate Cancer screening in Rotterdam, Netherlands. *Br. J. Cancer* **2010**, *103*, 708–714. [CrossRef] [PubMed]
31. Benchikh, A.; Savage, C.; Cronin, A.; Salama, G.; Villers, A.; Lilja, H.; Vickers, A. A panel of kallikrein markers can predict outcome of prostate biopsy following clinical work-up: An independent validation study from the European Randomized Study of Prostate Cancer screening, France. *BMC Cancer* **2010**, *10*, 635. [CrossRef] [PubMed]
32. Vickers, A.J.; Gupta, A.; Savage, C.J.; Pettersson, K.; Dahlin, A.; Bjartell, A.; Manjer, J.; Scardino, P.T.; Ulmert, D.; Lilja, H. A panel of kallikrein marker predicts prostate cancer in a large; population-based cohort

followed for 15 years without screening. *Cancer Epidemiol. Biomark. Prev.* **2011**, *20*, 255–261. [CrossRef] [PubMed]

33. Carlsson, S.V.; Peltola, M.T.; Sjoberg, D.; Schröder, F.H.; Hugosson, J.; Pettersson, K.; Scardino, P.T.; Vickers, A.J.; Lilja, H.; Roobol, M.J. Can one blood draw replace transrectal ultrasonography-estimated prostate volume to predict prostate cancer risk? *BJU Int.* **2013**, *112*, 602–609. [CrossRef] [PubMed]
34. Parekh, D.J.; Punnen, S.; Sjoberg, D.D.; Asroff, S.W.; Bailen, J.L.; Cochran, J.S.; Concepcion, R.; David, R.D.; Deck, K.B.; Dumbadze, I.; et al. A Multi-institutional prospective trial in the USA confirms that the 4K score accurately identifies men with high-grade prostate cancer. *Eur. Urol.* **2015**, *68*, 464–470. [CrossRef] [PubMed]
35. Stattin, P.; Vickers, A.J.; Sjoberg, D.D.; Johansson, R.; Granfors, T.; Johansson, M.; Pettersson, K.; Scardino, P.T.; Hallmans, G.; Lilja, H. Improving the specificity of screening for lethal prostate cancer using Prostate-specific Antigen and a panel of kallikrein markers: A nested case-control study. *Eur. Urol.* **2015**, *68*, 207–213. [CrossRef] [PubMed]
36. Filella, X.; Foj, L.; Milà, M.; Augé, J.M.; Molina, R.; Jiménez, W. PCA3 in the detection and management of early prostate cancer. *Tumour Biol.* **2013**, *34*, 1337–1347. [CrossRef] [PubMed]
37. Haese, A.; de la Taille, A.; van Poppel, H.; Marberger, M.; Stenzl, A.; Mulders, P.F.; Huland, H.; Abbou, C.C.; Remzi, M.; Tinzl, M. Clinical utility of the PCA3 urine assay in European men scheduled for repeat biopsy. *Eur. Urol.* **2008**, *54*, 1081–1088. [CrossRef] [PubMed]
38. Hu, B.; Yang, H.; Yang, H. Diagnostic value of urine prostate cancer antigen 3 test using a cutoff value of 35 μg/L in patients with prostate cancer. *Tumour Biol.* **2014**, *35*, 8573–8580. [CrossRef] [PubMed]
39. Crawford, E.D.; Rove, K.O.; Trabulsi, E.J.; Qian, J.; Drewnowska, K.P.; Kaminetsky, J.C.; Huisman, T.K.; Bilowus, M.L.; Freedman, S.J.; Glover, W.L.; et al. Diagnostic performance of PCA3 to detect prostate cancer in men with increased prostate specific antigen: A prospective study of 1962 cases. *J. Urol.* **2012**, *188*, 1726–1731. [CrossRef] [PubMed]
40. Bussemakers, M.J.; van Bokhoven, A.; Verhaegh, G.W.; Smit, F.P.; Karthaus, H.F.; Schalken, J.A.; Debruyne, F.M.; Ru, N.; Isaacs, W.B. DD3: A new prostate-specific gene, highly overexpressed in prostate cancer. *Cancer Res.* **1999**, *59*, 5975–5979. [PubMed]
41. Schröder, F.H.; Venderbos, L.D.; van den Bergh, R.C.; Hessels, D.; van Leenders, G.J.; van Leeuwen, P.J.; Wolters, T.; Barentsz, J.; Roobol, M.J. Prostate cancer antigen 3: Diagnostic outcomes in men presenting with urinary prostate cancer antigen 3 scores ≥100. *Urology* **2014**, *83*, 613–616. [CrossRef] [PubMed]
42. Merola, R.; Tomao, L.; Antenucci, A.; Sperduti, I.; Sentinelli, S.; Masi, S.; Mandoj, C.; Orlandi, G.; Papalia, R.; Guaglianone, S.; et al. PCA3 in prostate cancer and tumor aggressiveness detection on 407 high-risk patients: A National Cancer Institute experience. *J. Exp. Clin. Cancer Res.* **2015**, *34*, 15. [CrossRef] [PubMed]
43. Chevli, K.K.; Duff, M.; Walter, P.; Yu, C.; Capuder, B.; Elshafei, A.; Malczewski, S.; Kattan, M.W.; Jones, J.S. Urinary PCA3 as a predictor for prostate cancer in a cohort of 3073 men undergoing initial prostate biopsy. *J. Urol.* **2014**, *191*, 1743–1748. [CrossRef] [PubMed]
44. Hessels, D.; van Gils, M.P.; van Hooij, O.; Jannink, S.A.; Witjes, J.A.; Verhaegh, G.W.; Schalken, J.A. Predictive value of PCA3 in urinary sediments in determining clinico-pathological characteristics of prostate cancer. *Prostate* **2010**, *70*, 10–16. [CrossRef] [PubMed]
45. Foj, L.; Milà, M.; Mengual, L.; Luque, P.; Alcaraz, A.; Jiménez, W.; Filella, X. Real-time PCR PCA3 assay is a useful test measured in urine to improve prostate cancer detection. *Clin. Chim. Acta* **2014**, *435*, 53–58. [CrossRef] [PubMed]
46. Bradley, L.A.; Palomaki, G.E.; Gutman, S.; Samson, D.; Aronson, N. Comparative effectiveness review: Prostate cancer antigen 3 testing for the diagnosis and management of prostate cancer. *J. Urol.* **2013**, *190*, 389–398. [CrossRef] [PubMed]
47. Roobol, M.J.; Schröder, F.H.; van Leeuwen, P.; Wolters, T.; van den Bergh, R.C.; van Leenders, G.J.; Hessels, D. Performance of the prostate cancer antigen 3 (*PCA3*) gene and prostate-specific antigen in prescreened men: Exploring the value of *PCA3* for a first-line diagnostic test. *Eur. Urol.* **2010**, *58*, 475–481. [CrossRef] [PubMed]
48. Tomlins, S.A.; Rhodes, D.R.; Perner, S.; Dhanasekaran, S.M.; Mehra, R.; Sun, X.W.; Varambally, S.; Cao, X.; Tchinda, J.; Kuefer, R.; et al. Recurrent fusion of TMPRSS2 and ETS transcription factor genes in prostate cancer. *Science* **2005**, *310*, 644–648. [CrossRef] [PubMed]
49. Boström, P.J.; Bjartell, A.S.; Catto, J.W.; Eggener, S.E.; Lilja, H.; Loeb, S.; Schalken, J.; Schlomm, T.; Cooperberg, M.R. Genomic predictors of outcome in prostate cancer. *Eur. Urol.* **2015**, *68*, 1033–1044. [CrossRef] [PubMed]

50. Boormans, J.L.; Porkka, K.; Visakorpi, T.; Trapman, J. Confirmation of the association of *TMPRSS2 (exon 0):ERG* expression and a favorable prognosis of primary prostate cancer. *Eur. Urol.* **2011**, *60*, 183–184. [CrossRef] [PubMed]
51. FitzGerald, L.M.; Agalliu, I.; Johnson, K.; Miller, M.A.; Kwon, E.M.; Hurtado-Coll, A.; Fazli, L.; Rajput, A.B.; Gleave, M.E.; Cox, M.E.; et al. Association of *TMPRSS2-ERG* gene fusion with clinical characteristics and outcomes: Results from a population-based study of prostate cancer. *BMC Cancer* **2008**, *8*, 230. [CrossRef] [PubMed]
52. Leyten, G.H.; Hessels, D.; Jannink, S.A.; Smit, F.P.; de Jong, H.; Cornel, E.B.; de Reijke, T.M.; Vergunst, H.; Kil, P.; Knipscheer, B.C.; et al. Prospective multicentre evaluation of *PCA3* and *TMPRSS2-ERG* gene fusions as diagnostic and prognostic urinary biomarkers for prostate cancer. *Eur. Urol.* **2014**, *65*, 534–542. [CrossRef] [PubMed]
53. Tomlins, S.A.; Day, J.R.; Lonigro, R.J.; Hovelson, D.H.; Siddiqui, J.; Kunju, L.P.; Dunn, R.L.; Meyer, S.; Hodge, P.; Groskopf, J.; et al. Urine *TMPRSS2:ERG* Plus PCA3 for individualized prostate cancer risk assessment. *Eur. Urol.* **2016**, *70*, 45–53. [CrossRef] [PubMed]
54. Stephan, C.; Cammann, H.; Jung, K. Urine *TMPRSS2:ERG* Plus PCA3 for individualized prostate cancer risk assessment. *Eur. Urol.* **2015**, *68*, e106–e107. [CrossRef] [PubMed]
55. Griffiths-Jones, S. miRBase: The microRNA sequence database. *Methods Mol. Biol. Clifton NJ* **2006**, *342*, 129–138.
56. Calin, G.A.; Dumitru, C.D.; Shimizu, M.; Bichi, R.; Zupo, S.; Noch, E.; Aldler, H.; Rattan, S.; Keating, M.; Rai, K.; et al. Frequent deletions and down-regulation of micro-RNA genes *miR15* and *miR16* at 13q14 in chronic lymphocytic leukemia. *Proc. Natl. Acad. Sci. USA* **2002**, *99*, 15524–15529. [CrossRef] [PubMed]
57. Lawrie, C.H.; Gal, S.; Dunlop, H.M.; Pushkaran, B.; Liggins, A.P.; Pulford, K.; Banham, A.H.; Pezzella, F.; Boultwood, J.; Wainscoat, J.S.; et al. Detection of elevated levels of tumour-associated microRNAs in serum of patients with diffuse large B-cell lymphoma. *Br. J. Haematol.* **2008**, *141*, 672–675. [CrossRef] [PubMed]
58. Witwer, K.W. Circulating microRNA biomarker studies: Pitfalls and potential solutions. *Clin. Chem.* **2015**, *61*, 56–63. [CrossRef] [PubMed]
59. Tam, S.; de Borja, R.; Tsao, M.S.; McPherson, J.D. Robust global microRNA expression profiling using next-generation sequencing technologies. *Lab. Investig.* **2014**, *94*, 350–358. [CrossRef] [PubMed]
60. ChunJiao, S.; Huan, C.; ChaoYang, X.; GuoMei, R. Uncovering the roles of miRNAs and their relationship with androgen receptor in prostate cancer. *IUBMB Life* **2014**, *66*, 379–386. [CrossRef] [PubMed]
61. Mitchell, P.S.; Parkin, R.K.; Kroh, E.M.; Fritz, B.R.; Wyman, S.K.; Pogosova-Agadjanyan, E.L.; Peterson, A.; Noteboom, J.; O'Briant, K.C.; Allen, A.; et al. Circulating microRNAs as stable blood-based markers for cancer detection. *Proc. Natl. Acad. Sci. USA* **2008**, *105*, 10513–10518. [CrossRef] [PubMed]
62. Filella, X.; Foj, L. miRNAs as novel biomarkers in the management of prostate cancer. *Clin. Chem. Lab. Med.* **2016**. [CrossRef] [PubMed]
63. Mihelich, B.L.; Maranville, J.C.; Nolley, R.; Peehl, D.M.; Nonn, L. Elevated serum microRNA levels associate with absence of high-grade prostate cancer in a retrospective cohort. *PLoS ONE* **2015**, *10*, e0124245. [CrossRef] [PubMed]
64. Chen, Z.H.; Zhang, G.L.; Li, H.R.; Luo, J.D.; Li, Z.X.; Chen, G.M.; Yang, J. A panel of five circulating microRNAs as potential biomarkers for prostate cancer. *Prostate* **2012**, *72*, 1443–1452. [CrossRef] [PubMed]
65. Moltzahn, F.; Olshen, A.B.; Baehner, L.; Peek, A.; Fong, L.; Stöppler, H.; Simko, J.; Hilton, J.F.; Carroll, P.; Blelloch, R.; et al. Microfluidic-based multiplex qRT-PCR identifies diagnostic and prognostic microRNA signatures in the sera of prostate cancer patients. *Cancer Res.* **2011**, *71*, 550–560. [CrossRef] [PubMed]
66. Salido-Guadarrama, A.I.; Morales-Montor, J.G.; Rangel-Escareño, C.; Langley, E.; Peralta-Zaragoza, O.; Cruz-Colin, J.L.; Rodriguez-Dorantes, M. Urinary microRNA-based signature improves accuracy of detection of clinically relevant prostate cancer within the prostate-specific antigen grey zone. *Mol. Med. Rep.* **2016**, *13*, 4549–4560. [CrossRef] [PubMed]
67. Trams, E.G.; Lauter, C.J.; Salem, N., Jr.; Heine, U. Exfoliation of membrane ecto-enzymes in the form of micro-vesicles. *Biochim. Biophys. Acta* **1981**, *645*, 63–70. [CrossRef]
68. Zhou, H.; Yuen, P.S.; Pisitkun, T.; Gonzales, P.A.; Yasuda, H.; Dear, J.W.; Gross, P.; Knepper, M.A.; Star, R.A. Collection; storage; preservation; and normalization of human urinary exosomes for biomarker discovery. *Kidney Int.* **2006**, *69*, 1471–1476. [CrossRef] [PubMed]

69. Ge, Q.; Zhou, Y.; Lu, J.; Bai, Y.; Xie, X.; Lu, Z. miRNA in plasma exosome is stable under different storage conditions. *Molecules* **2014**, *19*, 1568–1575. [CrossRef] [PubMed]
70. Taylor, D.D.; Gercel-Taylor, C. MicroRNA signatures of tumor-derived exosomes as diagnostic biomarkers of ovarian cancer. *Gynecol. Oncol.* **2008**, *110*, 13–21. [CrossRef] [PubMed]
71. Duijvesz, D.; Versluis, C.Y.; van der Fels, C.A.; Vredenbregt-van den Berg, M.S.; Leivo, J.; Peltola, M.T.; Bangma, C.H.; Pettersson, K.S.; Jenster, G. Immuno-based detection of extracellular vesicles in urine as diagnostic marker for prostate cancer. *Int. J. Cancer* **2015**, *137*, 2869–2878. [CrossRef] [PubMed]
72. Rabinowits, G.; Gercel-Taylor, C.; Day, J.M.; Taylor, D.D.; Kloecker, G.H. Exosomal microRNA: A diagnostic marker for lung cancer. *Clin. Lung Cancer* **2009**, *10*, 42–46. [CrossRef] [PubMed]
73. Silva, J.; Garcia, V.; Rodriguez, M.; Compte, M.; Cisneros, E.; Veguillas, P.; Garcia, J.M.; Dominguez, G.; Campos-Martin, Y.; Cuevas, J.; et al. Analysis of exosome release and its prognostic value in human colorectal cancer. *Genes Chromosomes Cancer* **2012**, *51*, 409–418. [CrossRef] [PubMed]
74. Yeh, Y.Y.; Ozer, H.G.; Lehman, A.M.; Maddocks, K.; Yu, L.; Johnson, A.J.; Byrd, J.C. Characterization of CLL exosomes reveals a distinct microRNA signature and enhanced secretion by activation of BCR signaling. *Blood* **2015**, *125*, 3297–3305. [CrossRef] [PubMed]
75. Ratajczak, M.Z.; Ratajczak, J. Horizontal transfer of RNA and proteins between cells by extracellular microvesicles: 14 years later. *Clin. Transl. Med.* **2016**, *5*, 7. [CrossRef] [PubMed]
76. O'Driscoll, L. Expanding on exosomes and ectosomes in cancer. *N. Engl. J. Med.* **2015**, *372*, 2359–2362. [CrossRef] [PubMed]
77. Franzen, C.A.; Blackwell, R.H.; Todorovic, V.; Greco, K.A.; Foreman, K.E.; Flanigan, R.C.; Kuo, P.C.; Gupta, G.N. Urothelial cells undergo epithelial-to-mesenchymal transition after exposure to muscle invasive bladder cancer exosomes. *Oncogenesis* **2015**, *4*, e163. [CrossRef] [PubMed]
78. Abd Elmageed, Z.Y.; Yang, Y.; Thomas, R.; Ranjan, M.; Mondal, D.; Moroz, K.; Fang, Z.; Rezk, B.M.; Moparty, K.; Sikka, S.C.; et al. Neoplastic reprogramming of patient-derived adipose stem cells by prostate cancer cell-associated exosomes. *Stem Cells* **2014**, *32*, 983–997. [CrossRef] [PubMed]
79. Hosseini-Beheshti, E.; Choi, W.; Weiswald, L.B.; Kharmate, G.; Ghaffari, M.; Roshan-Moniri, M.; Hassona, M.D.; Chan, L.; Chin, M.Y.; Tai, I.T.; et al. Exosomes confer pro-survival signals to alter the phenotype of prostate cells in their surrounding environment. *Oncotarget* **2016**. [CrossRef]
80. Thery, C.; Amigorena, S.; Raposo, G.; Clayton, A. Isolation and characterization of exosomes from cell culture supernatants and biological fluids. *Curr. Protoc. Cell Biol.* **2006**. [CrossRef]
81. Øverbye, A.; Skotland, T.; Koehler, C.J.; Thiede, B.; Seierstad, T.; Berge, V.; Sandvig, K.; Llorente, A. Identification of prostate cancer biomarkers in urinary exosomes. *Oncotarget* **2015**, *6*, 30357–30376. [PubMed]
82. Dijkstra, S.; Birker, I.L.; Smit, F.P.; Leyten, G.H.; de Reijke, T.M.; van Oort, I.M.; Mulders, P.F.; Jannink, S.A.; Schalken, J.A. Prostate cancer biomarker profiles in urinary sediments and exosomes. *J. Urol.* **2014**, *191*, 1132–1138. [CrossRef] [PubMed]
83. Hendriks, R.J.; Dijkstra, S.; Jannink, S.A.; Steffens, M.G.; van Oort, I.M.; Mulders, P.F.; Schalken, J.A. Comparative analysis of prostate cancer specific biomarkers PCA3 and ERG in whole urine; urinary sediments and exosomes. *Clin. Chem. Lab. Med.* **2016**, *54*, 483–492. [CrossRef] [PubMed]
84. Donovan, M.J.; Noerholm, M.; Bentink, S.; Belzer, S.; Skog, J.; O'Neill, V.; Cochran, J.S.; Brown, G.A. A molecular signature of PCA3 and ERG exosomal RNA from non-DRE urine is predictive of initial prostate biopsy result. *Prostate Cancer Prostatic Dis.* **2015**, *18*, 370–375. [CrossRef] [PubMed]
85. Cheng, L.; Sun, X.; Scicluna, B.J.; Coleman, B.M.; Hill, A.F. Characterization and deep sequencing analysis of exosomal and non-exosomal miRNA in human urine. *Kidney Int.* **2014**, *86*, 433–444. [CrossRef] [PubMed]
86. Cheng, L.; Sharples, R.A.; Scicluna, B.J.; Hill, A.F. Exosomes provide a protective and enriched source of miRNA for biomarker profiling compared to intracellular and cell-free blood. *J. Extracell. Vesicles* **2014**, *3*. [CrossRef] [PubMed]
87. Mall, C.; Rocke, D.M.; Durbin-Johnson, B.; Weiss, R.H. Stability of miRNA in human urine supports its biomarker potential. *Biomark. Med.* **2013**, *7*, 623–631. [CrossRef] [PubMed]
88. Hessvik, N.P.; Sandvigm, K.; Llorente, A. Exosomal miRNAs as Biomarkers for Prostate Cancer. *Front. Genet.* **2013**, *4*, 36. [CrossRef] [PubMed]
89. Chevillet, J.R.; Kang, Q.; Ruf, I.K.; Briggs, H.A.; Vojtech, L.N.; Hughes, S.M.; Cheng, H.H.; Arroyo, J.D.; Meredith, E.K.; Gallichotte, E.N.; et al. Quantitative and stoichiometric analysis of the microRNA content of exosomes. *Proc. Natl. Acad. Sci. USA* **2014**, *111*, 14888–14893. [CrossRef] [PubMed]

90. Arroyo, J.D.; Chevillet, J.R.; Kroh, E.M.; Ruf, I.K.; Pritchard, C.C.; Gibson, D.F.; Mitchell, P.S.; Bennett, C.F.; Pogosova-Agadjanyan, E.L.; Stirewalt, D.L.; et al. Argonaute2 complexes carry a population of circulating microRNAs independent of vesicles in human plasma. *Proc. Natl. Acad. Sci. USA* **2011**, *108*, 5003–5008. [CrossRef] [PubMed]
91. Gallo, A.; Tandon, M.; Alevizos, I.; Illei, G.G. The majority of microRNAs detectable in serum and saliva is concentrated in exosomes. *PLoS ONE* **2012**, *7*, e30679. [CrossRef] [PubMed]
92. Li, Z.; Ma, Y.Y.; Wang, J.; Zeng, X.F.; Li, R.; Kang, W.; Hao, X.K. Exosomal microRNA-141 is upregulated in the serum of prostate cancer patients. *Onco. Targets Ther.* **2015**, *9*, 139–148. [PubMed]
93. Huang, X.; Yuan, T.; Liang, M.; Du, M.; Xia, S.; Dittmar, R.; Wang, D.; See, W.; Costello, B.A.; Quevedo, F.; et al. Exosomal miR-1290 and miR-375 as prognostic markers in castration-resistant prostate cancer. *Eur. Urol.* **2015**, *67*, 33–41. [CrossRef] [PubMed]
94. Bryzgunova, O.E.; Zaripov, M.M.; Skvortsova, T.E.; Lekchnov, E.A.; Grigor'eva, A.E.; Zaporozhchenko, I.A.; Morozkin, E.S.; Ryabchikova, E.I.; Yurchenko, Y.B.; Voitsitskiy, V.E.; et al. Comparative Study of Extracellular Vesicles from the Urine of Healthy Individuals and Prostate Cancer Patients. *PLoS ONE* **2016**, *11*, e0157566. [CrossRef] [PubMed]
95. Samsonov, R.; Shtam, T.; Burdakov, V.; Glotov, A.; Tsyrlina, E.; Berstein, L.; Nosov, A.; Evtushenko, V.; Filatov, M.; Malek, A. Lectin-induced agglutination method of urinary exosomes isolation followed by mi-RNA analysis: Application for prostate cancer diagnostic. *Prostate* **2016**, *76*, 68–79. [CrossRef] [PubMed]
96. Koppers-Lalic, D.; Hackenberg, M.; Menezes, R.; Misovic, B.; Wachalska, M.; Geldof, A.; Zini, N.; Reijke, T.; Wurdinger, T.; Vis, A.; et al. Non-invasive prostate cancer detection by measuring miRNA variants (isomiRs) in urine extracellular vesicles. *Oncotarget* **2016**. [CrossRef]
97. Klotz, L. Low-risk prostate cancer can and should often be managed with active surveillance and selective delayed intervention. *Nat. Clin. Pract. Urol.* **2008**, *5*, 2–3. [CrossRef] [PubMed]
98. Rubin, M.A.; Girelli, G.; Demichelis, F. Genomic Correlates to the Newly Proposed Grading Prognostic Groups for Prostate Cancer. *Eur. Urol.* **2016**, *69*, 557–560. [CrossRef] [PubMed]
99. Carter, H.B.; Partin, A.W.; Walsh, P.C.; Trock, B.J.; Veltri, R.W.; Nelson, W.G.; Coffey, D.S.; Singer, E.A.; Epstein, J.I. Gleason score 6 adenocarcinoma: Should it be labeled as cancer? *J. Clin. Oncol.* **2012**, *30*, 4294–4296. [CrossRef] [PubMed]
100. Kulac, I.; Haffner, M.C.; Yegnasubramanian, S.; Epstein, J.I.; de Marzo, A.M. Should Gleason 6 be labeled as cancer? *Curr. Opin. Urol.* **2015**, *25*, 238–245. [CrossRef] [PubMed]
101. Scattoni, V.; Lazzeri, M.; Lughezzani, G.; de Luca, S.; Passera, R.; Bollito, E.; Randone, D.; Abdollah, F.; Capitanio, U.; Larcher, A.; et al. Head-to-head comparison of prostate health index and urinary PCA3 for predicting cancer at initial or repeat biopsy. *J. Urol.* **2013**, *190*, 496–501. [CrossRef] [PubMed]
102. Stephan, C.; Jung, K.; Semjonow, A.; Schulze-Forster, K.; Cammann, H.; Hu, X.; Meyer, H.A.; Bögemann, M.; Miller, K.; Friedersdorff, F. Comparative assessment of urinary prostate cancer antigen 3 and *TMPRSS2:ERG* gene fusion with the serum [−2]proprostate-specific antigen-based prostate health index for detection of prostate cancer. *Clin. Chem.* **2013**, *59*, 280–288. [CrossRef] [PubMed]
103. Tallon, L.; Luangphakdy, D.; Ruffion, A.; Colombel, M.; Devonec, M.; Champetier, D.; Paparel, P.; Decaussin-Petrucci, M.; Perrin, P.; Vlaeminck-Guillem, V. Comparative Evaluation of Urinary PCA3 and TMPRSS2:ERG Scores and Serum PHI in Predicting Prostate Cancer Aggressiveness. *Int. J. Mol. Sci.* **2014**, *15*, 13299–13316. [CrossRef] [PubMed]
104. Nordström, T.; Vickers, A.; Assel, M.; Lilja, H.; Grönberg, H.; Eklund, M. Comparison between the four-kallikrein panel and Prostate Health Index for predicting Prostate Cancer. *Eur. Urol.* **2015**, *68*, 139–146. [CrossRef] [PubMed]
105. Vedder, M.M.; de Bekker-Grob, E.W.; Lilja, H.G.; Vickers, A.J.; van Leenders, G.J.; Steyerberg, E.W.; Roobol, M.J. The added value of percentage of free to total Prostate-specific Antigen, PCA3, and a kallikrein panel to the ERSPC Risk Calculator for Prostate Cancer in prescreened Men. *Eur. Urol.* **2014**, *66*, 1109–1115. [CrossRef] [PubMed]
106. Mottet, N.; Bellmunt, J.; Briers, E.; Bolla, M.; Cornford, P.; de Santis, M.; Henry, A.; Joniau, S.; Lam, T.; Mason, M.D.; et al. EAU Guideliness Prostate Cancer. Available online: http://uroweb.org/guideline/prostate-cancer/ (accessed on 9 September 2016).

107. Vickers, A.J.; Eastham, J.A.; Scardino, P.T.; Lilja, H. The Memorial Sloan Kettering Cancer Center Recommendations for Prostate Cancer Screening. *Urology* **2016**, *91*, 12–18. [CrossRef] [PubMed]
108. De Visschere, P.J.; Briganti, A.; Fütterer, J.J.; Ghadjar, P.; Isbarn, H.; Massard, C.; Ost, P.; Sooriakumaran, P.; Surcel, C.I.; Valerio, M.; et al. Role of multiparametric magnetic resonance imaging in early detection of prostate cancer. *Insights Imaging* **2016**, *7*, 205–214. [CrossRef] [PubMed]
109. Porpiglia, F.; Cantiello, F.; de Luca, S.; Manfredi, M.; Veltri, A.; Russo, F.; Sottile, A.; Damiano, R. In-parallel comparative evaluation between multiparametric magnetic resonance imaging; prostate cancer antigen 3 and the prostate health index in predicting pathologically confirmed significant prostate cancer in men eligible for active surveillance. *BJU Int.* **2015**. [CrossRef] [PubMed]
110. Washino, S.; Okochi, T.; Saito, K.; Konishi, T.; Hirai, M.; Kobayashi, Y.; Miyagawa, T. Combination of PI-RADS score and PSA density predicts biopsy outcome in biopsy naïve patients. *BJU Int.* **2016**. [CrossRef] [PubMed]
111. Maurer, T.; Eiber, M.; Schwaiger, M.; Gschwend, J.E. Current use of PSMA-PET in prostate cancer management. *Nat. Rev. Urol.* **2016**, *13*, 226–235. [CrossRef] [PubMed]

7

Inherited Variants in Wnt Pathway Genes Influence Outcomes of Prostate Cancer Patients Receiving Androgen Deprivation Therapy

Jiun-Hung Geng [1,2], Victor C. Lin [3,4], Chia-Cheng Yu [5,6,7], Chao-Yuan Huang [8,9], Hsin-Ling Yin [10,11], Ta-Yuan Chang [12], Te-Ling Lu [13], Shu-Pin Huang [1,14,15,*] and Bo-Ying Bao [13,16,17,*]

1 Department of Urology, Kaohsiung Medical University Hospital, Kaohsiung 807, Taiwan; u9001090@hotmail.com
2 Department of Urology, Kaohsiung Municipal Hsiao-Kang Hospital, Kaohsiung 812, Taiwan
3 Department of Urology, E-Da Hospital, Kaohsiung 824, Taiwan; victorlin0098@yahoo.com.tw
4 School of Medicine for International Students, I-Shou University, Kaohsiung 840, Taiwan
5 Division of Urology, Department of Surgery, Kaohsiung Veterans General Hospital, Kaohsiung 813, Taiwan; ccyu@vghks.gov.tw
6 Department of Urology, School of Medicine, National Yang-Ming University, Taipei 112, Taiwan
7 Department of Pharmacy, Tajen University, Pingtung 907, Taiwan
8 Department of Urology, National Taiwan University Hospital, College of Medicine, National Taiwan University, Taipei 100, Taiwan; cyhuang0909@ntu.edu.tw
9 Department of Urology, National Taiwan University Hospital Hsin-Chu Branch, Hsinchu 300, Taiwan
10 Department of Pathology, Kaohsiung Medical University Hospital, Kaohsiung 807, Taiwan; schoolyin@gmail.com
11 Department of Pathology, Faculty of Medicine, College of Medicine, Kaohsiung Medical University, Kaohsiung 807, Taiwan
12 Department of Occupational Safety and Health, China Medical University, Taichung 404, Taiwan; tychang@mail.cmu.edu.tw
13 Department of Pharmacy, China Medical University, Taichung 404, Taiwan; lutl@mail.cmu.edu.tw
14 Department of Urology, Faculty of Medicine, College of Medicine, Kaohsiung Medical University, Kaohsiung 807, Taiwan
15 Graduate Institute of Medicine, College of Medicine, Kaohsiung Medical University, Kaohsiung 807, Taiwan
16 Sex Hormone Research Center, China Medical University Hospital, Taichung 404, Taiwan
17 Department of Nursing, Asia University, Taichung 413, Taiwan
* Correspondences: shpihu@yahoo.com.tw (S.-P.H.); bao@mail.cmu.edu.tw (B.-Y.B.)

Academic Editor: Carsten Stephan

Abstract: Aberrant Wnt signaling has been associated with many types of cancer. However, the association of inherited Wnt pathway variants with clinical outcomes in prostate cancer patients receiving androgen deprivation therapy (ADT) has not been determined. Here, we comprehensively studied the contribution of common single nucleotide polymorphisms (SNPs) in Wnt pathway genes to the clinical outcomes of 465 advanced prostate cancer patients treated with ADT. Two SNPs, *adenomatous polyposis coli* (*APC*) rs2707765 and rs497844, were significantly ($p \leq 0.009$ and $q \leq 0.043$) associated with both prostate cancer progression and all-cause mortality, even after multivariate analyses and multiple testing correction. Patients with a greater number of favorable alleles had a longer time to disease progression and better overall survival during ADT (p for trend ≤ 0.003). Additional, cDNA array and in silico analyses of prostate cancer tissue suggested that rs2707765 affects *APC* expression, which in turn is correlated with tumor aggressiveness and patient prognosis. This study identifies the influence of inherited variants in the Wnt pathway on the efficacy of ADT and highlights a preclinical rationale for using *APC* as a prognostic marker in advanced prostate cancer.

Keywords: prostate cancer; androgen deprivation therapy; outcomes; genetic variation; Wnt pathway

1. Introduction

Prostate cancer is the most common type of cancer in men worldwide, with 1.1 million cases and 307,000 related deaths in 2012. Most cases of prostate cancer are diagnosed and treated while the disease is localized. However, 10%–20% present with advanced-stage or metastatic prostate cancer, and others develop disseminated disease after definitive treatment [1]. Once an advanced-stage or metastatic prostate cancer is diagnosed, androgen deprivation therapy (ADT), which can be accomplished with either bilateral surgical or medical castration, is the standard systemic therapy [2,3]. Although the initial response rate of prostate cancer to ADT has been reported to be as high as 80%, ADT is not curative for prostate cancer, and many patients receiving ADT progress to castration-resistant prostate cancer (CRPC) within 18–30 months [4]. Once CRPC develops, a patient's life expectancy is approximately 16–18 months [5]. Several parameters, including the prostate-specific antigen (PSA) doubling time, PSA nadir, PSA level at ADT initiation, stage and Gleason score, have been reported as useful prognostic predictors of disease progression or survival in patients receiving ADT. However, the predictive ability of these parameters remains limited and might be improved by incorporating information on genetic variants, which may help to estimate disease progression and identify novel therapeutic targets.

The Wnt pathway is an evolutionarily-conserved signal transduction pathway that governs embryonic growth by directing processes, such as cell fate decisions, proliferation, neural patterning, polarity, migration and apoptosis [6,7]. The accumulated evidence has demonstrated that Wnt pathway aberrations are frequently associated with tumor development and the progression of many types of cancer, including colorectal cancer, hepatocellular cancer, breast cancer [8–15] and prostate cancer [16–20]. The best-known example, familial adenomatous polyposis, is an autosomal, dominantly inherited disease characterized by the development of polyps in the colon and rectum. It is most frequently caused by a mutation of the gene *adenomatous polyposis coli* (*APC*) [21,22]. In addition, mutations in β-catenin (*CTNNB1*) and *APC* have been identified in sporadic colorectal cancers and various other tumor types [15]. Although oncogenic mutations in Wnt pathway genes are rare in prostate cancer, increased expression levels of Wnt family proteins have been observed in clinical prostate cancer samples [18,23]. Additionally, the treatment of LNCaP human prostate cancer cells with conditioned medium containing the growth factor Wnt3a significantly enhanced cell growth in the absence of androgens, demonstrating that the Wnt pathway may represent a novel mechanism contributing to prostate cancer progression [24]. Therefore, it is reasonable to hypothesize that genetic variants in the Wnt signaling pathway could influence prostate cancer progression and might also contribute to the development of CRPC. In this study, we comprehensively evaluated the prognostic significance of 17 tagged single nucleotide polymorphisms (SNPs) in three key genes related to the Wnt pathway, *WNT1*, *APC* and *CTNNB1*, with regards to disease progression and all-cause mortality (ACM) in a cohort of prostate cancer patients treated with ADT.

2. Results

The demographic and clinicopathologic characteristics of the study participants are summarized in Table S1. With a median follow-up time of 92 months, 429 (92.3%) prostate cancer patients experienced disease progression after ADT. A total of 143 (30.8%) patients died at a median follow-up of 65 months. The clinical stage, Gleason score, PSA at ADT initiation, PSA nadir, time to PSA nadir and treatment modalities were associated with both disease progression and ACM ($p \leq 0.004$). The age at diagnosis was only correlated with the disease progression ($p < 0.001$).

Seventeen tagging SNPs in three core Wnt pathway genes, namely *CTNNB1*, *APC* and *WNT1*, were analyzed in this study. Details of the SNPs and their associations with disease progression and ACM during ADT are shown in Table S2. Seven *APC* SNPs were associated with disease progression or ACM with a nominal $p < 0.05$, according to a multivariate Cox model adjusted for age, clinical stage, Gleason score, PSA at ADT initiation, PSA nadir, time to PSA nadir and treatment modality. After adjusting for the false discovery rate (FDR) at the <0.05 level, four SNPs, namely *APC* rs3846716, rs2707765, rs41115 and rs497844, remained significantly associated with time to progression ($q \leq 0.012$; Table 1). Intriguingly, *APC* rs2707765 and rs497844 correlated significantly with a decreased risk of both disease progression and ACM ($q \leq 0.043$; Table 2). A gene-dosage effect on disease progression and ACM was found when two genetic loci of interest were analyzed in combination, with the hazards ratio decreasing as the number of protective alleles increased (p for trend ≤ 0.003; Table 3 and Figure 1).

Table 1. Association between htSNPs in *APC* and disease progression in prostate cancer patients treated with ADT.

SNP	Location	Allele	Event [a]	No Event [a]	Best Model	HR (95% CI) [b]	p [b]	q
rs3846716	5′ upstream	G>A	295/117/12	22/11/2	Dominant	0.67 (0.53–0.84)	<0.001	**0.009**
rs2289485	Intron	T>G	371/54/2	30/5/1	Additive	0.74 (0.56–0.99)	0.040	0.093
rs2707765	Intron	G>C	210/176/38	16/15/4	Additive	0.78 (0.67–0.91)	0.002	**0.009**
rs2431238	Intron	C>T	343/76/2	30/4/1	Additive	0.77 (0.60–0.99)	0.044	0.093
rs41115	Thr1493Thr	T>C	300/114/14	25/9/2	Dominant	0.71 (0.57–0.89)	0.003	**0.012**
rs497844	3′ downstream	C>T	301/107/15	24/10/1	Dominant	0.68 (0.54–0.85)	0.001	**0.009**

Abbreviations: htSNP, haplotype tagging single nucleotide polymorphism; *APC*, *adenomatous polyposis coli*; ADT, androgen deprivation therapy; HR, hazards ratio; CI, confidence interval; p, p-value; q, q-value. [a] The number represents major allele homozygotes, heterozygotes and minor allele homozygotes, respectively; [b] Multivariate Cox models adjusted for age, clinical stage, Gleason score, prostate-specific antigen (PSA) at ADT initiation, PSA nadir, time to PSA nadir and treatment modality. The major allele homozygotes were considered as the reference group, with a fixed HR = 1.00. $p < 0.05$ is in boldface.

Table 2. Association between htSNPs in *APC* and ACM in prostate cancer patients treated with ADT.

SNP	Location	Allele	Event [a]	No Event [a]	Best Model	HR (95% CI) [b]	p [b]	q
rs3846716	5′ upstream	G>A	106/32/2	211/96/12	Additive	0.65 (0.44–0.95)	0.026	0.055
rs2289485	Intron	T>G	129/12/0	272/47/3	Additive	0.46 (0.25–0.86)	0.014	0.054
rs2707765	Intron	G>C	77/54/9	149/137/33	Additive	0.68 (0.51–0.91)	0.009	**0.043**
rs17134945	Intron	A>G	130/12/0	276/43/3	Additive	0.52 (0.28–0.95)	0.033	0.057
rs41115	Thr1493Thr	T>C	108/31/3	217/92/13	Dominant	0.62 (0.41–0.95)	0.026	0.055
rs497844	3′ downstream	C>T	110/27/3	215/90/13	Dominant	0.51 (0.33–0.80)	0.003	**0.043**

Abbreviations: ACM, all-cause mortality. [a] The number represents major allele homozygotes, heterozygotes and minor allele homozygotes, respectively; [b] Multivariate Cox models adjusted for age, clinical stage, Gleason score, PSA at ADT initiation, PSA nadir, time to PSA nadir and treatment modality. The major allele homozygotes were considered as the reference group, with a fixed HR = 1.00. $p < 0.05$ is in boldface.

As a preliminary assessment of the putative functional roles of these SNPs, we investigated whether rs2707765 and rs497844 were associated with the differential expression of *APC*. The Genotype-Tissue Expression (GTEx) database revealed a significant trend toward increased *APC* mRNA expression in the prostate tissues of rs2707765 protective allele (C) carriers ($p = 0.018$; Figure 2, left) and rs497844 protective allele (T) carriers ($p = 0.21$; Figure 2, right). We used HaploReg to annotate these risk-associated SNPs and discover their potential causal link with the disease. rs2707765, rs497844 and several SNPs in strong linkage disequilibrium with them ($r^2 > 0.8$) (e.g., rs2431514 and rs2464803 for rs2707765 and rs712671 and rs455469 for rs497844) are situated within a locus showing promoter and enhancer histone marks, DNase hypersensitivity peaks and transcription factor binding in several cell lines (Tables S3 and S4). Together, rs2707765 and rs497844 might affect transcription factor binding, increase *APC* mRNA expression and reduce the aggressiveness of prostate cancer.

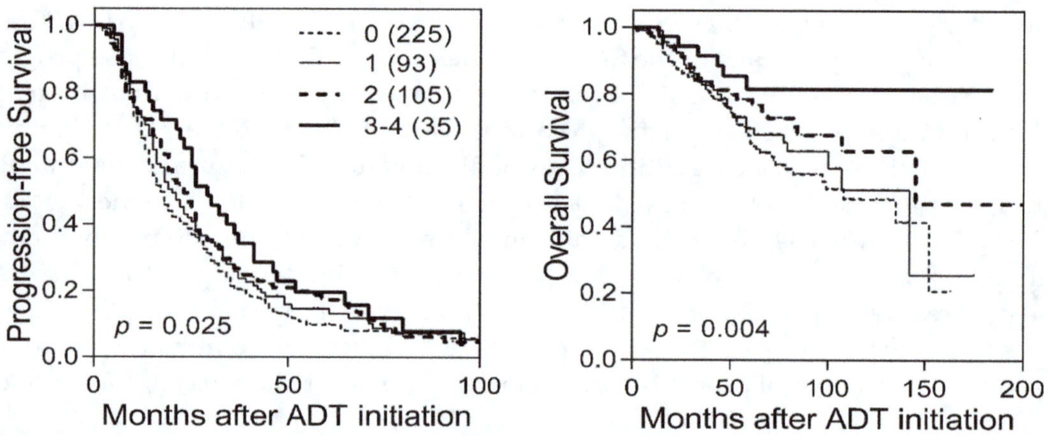

Figure 1. Kaplan-Meier curves of time to progression (**left** panel) and all-cause mortality (ACM) (**right** panel) during androgen deprivation therapy (ADT) for patients with 0, 1, 2 or 3–4 protective alleles at *APC* rs2707765 and rs497844. The protective alleles refer to C in rs2707765 and T in rs497844. The more protective alleles a prostate cancer patient carries, the longer their time to progression and ACM. Numbers in parentheses indicate the number of patients.

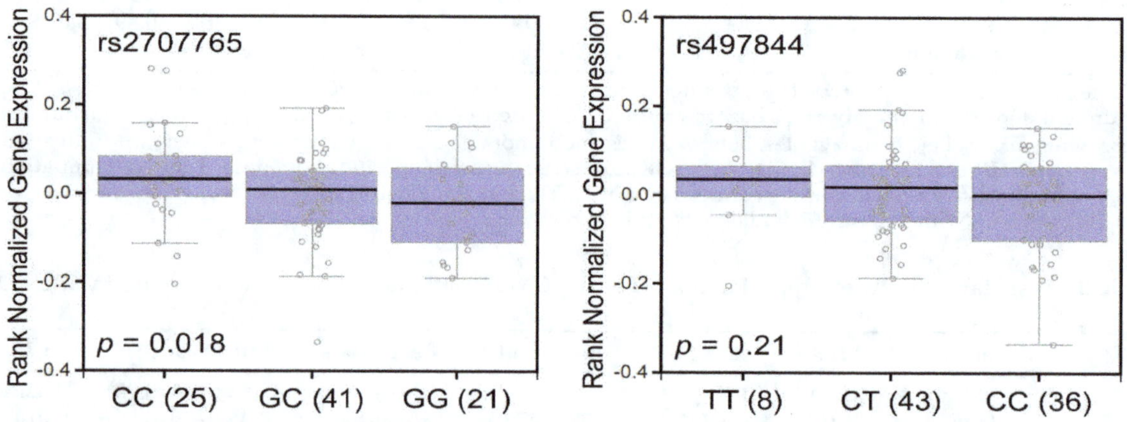

Figure 2. Correlation of rs2707765 and rs497844 genotypes and *APC* gene expression in prostate tissues. Boxplots represent *APC* mRNA expression according to the rs2707765 (**left** panel) and rs497844 (**right** panel) genotypes in 87 human prostate tissues (Genotype-Tissue Expression (GTEx) dataset). There is a trend toward increased *APC* mRNA expression in the prostate tissues of rs2707765 protective allele C carriers and rs497844 protective allele T carriers. The numbers in parentheses indicate the number of cases.

To determine whether *APC* expression is linked to prostate cancer progression, we performed a quantitative real-time polymerase chain reaction (qRT-PCR) analysis of *APC* transcripts using a prostate cancer complementary DNA (cDNA) array containing 48 tissue samples. A significant downregulation of *APC* expression was observed in cancer and more advanced stage cancer samples ($p \leq 0.048$; Figure 3A). To further confirm the relationship between *APC* expression and prostate cancer aggressiveness, we performed an in silico evaluation using publicly-available Memorial Sloan-Kettering Cancer Center Prostate Oncogenome datasets [25]. Our analysis revealed that more clinically-advanced prostate cancers, such as those with metastasis, had significantly lower levels of *APC* expression ($p < 0.001$; Figure 3B). Follow-up of this cohort established that *APC* homozygous deletion, mutation and mRNA downregulation were strongly associated with a worse recurrence-free survival ($p < 0.001$, Figure 3B).

Table 3. Cumulative effect of predictive markers on disease progression and ACM in prostate cancer patients treated with ADT.

No. of Protective Alleles [a]	Overall Patients, *n*	Disease Progression				ACM			
		Events, *n*	Median, *mo*	HR (95% CI) [b]	*p* [b]	Events, *n*	Median, *mo*	HR (95% CI) [b]	*p* [b]
0	225	109	17	1.00	-	77	108	1.00	-
1	93	86	20	0.91 (0.70–1.18)	0.467	30	142	0.76 (0.48–1.20)	0.240
2	105	96	23	0.72 (0.55–0.93)	**0.012**	27	145	0.60 (0.37–0.97)	**0.037**
3–4	35	32	29	0.56 (0.38–0.83)	**0.004**	6	NR [c]	0.36 (0.16–0.84)	**0.018**
Trend	-	-	-	0.84 (0.76–0.93)	**<0.001**	-	-	0.75 (0.62–0.90)	**0.003**

Abbreviations: mo, month. [a] Protective alleles refer to C in rs2707765 and T in rs497844; [b] Multivariate Cox models adjusted for age, clinical stage, Gleason score, PSA at ADT initiation, PSA nadir, time to PSA nadir and treatment modality; [c] NR means the median time-to-event has not been reached. $p < 0.05$ is in boldface.

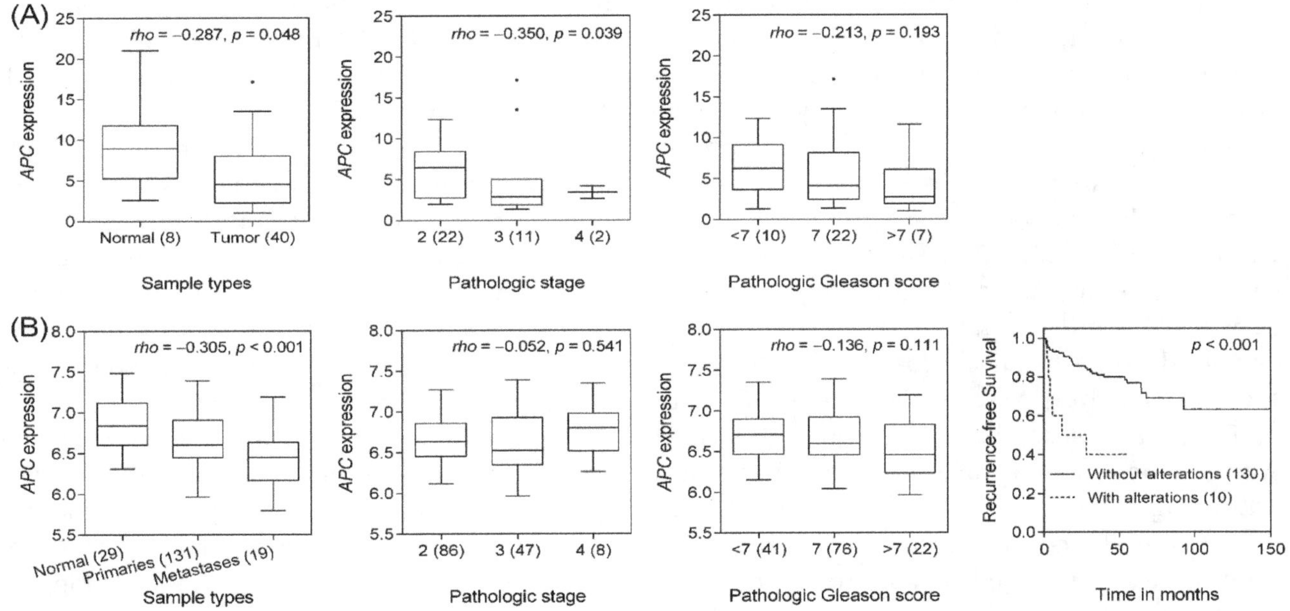

Figure 3. Correlation of *APC* mRNA expression with prostate cancer progression. (**A**) *APC* mRNA expression in 40 prostate cancers and eight normal human prostate tissue specimens, as determined by qRT-PCR, indicates that *APC* is downregulated in the cancer tissues, especially in those from patients with more advanced stages of cancer; (**B**) The associations between *APC* expression and prostate cancer aggressiveness were analyzed using an independent set of Memorial Sloan-Kettering Cancer Center Prostate Oncogenome data. Primary and metastatic prostate cancers display significantly lower *APC* mRNA expression. *rho*, Spearman's rank correlation coefficient. Data points beyond the quartiles are outliers. Kaplan-Meier curves of recurrence-free survival according to the alterations in *APC* are shown. Patients were dichotomized with or without *APC* homozygous deletion, mutation and mRNA downregulation. Numbers in parentheses indicate the number of patients.

3. Discussion

In this hypothesis-driven association study, we identified two SNPs in *APC*, namely rs2707765 and rs497844, as being associated with the efficacy of ADT. Notably, the relationships of these SNPs with disease progression and ACM persisted despite controlling for known prognostic factors and multiple comparison testing. This suggests that the patient genotype adds information beyond conventional factors. Moreover, rs2707765 affects *APC* expression, and a lower *APC* expression correlated with more aggressive cancer and a worse clinical outcome. These results support the connection between the Wnt pathway and prostate cancer progression.

APC is a multifunctional protein involved in a variety of cellular processes. Its best-known role is as a negative regulator of the Wnt pathway, but recent evidence also suggests that it has a role in regulating microtubule dynamics in mitosis. APC was found to associate with the plus-ends of microtubules that interact with kinetochores and to be required for the spindle checkpoint to prevent chromosome missegregation [26]. Many tumors exhibit chromosomal instability, which is probably caused by chromosome missegregation [27]. *APC* mutant mouse embryonic stem cells were reported to have multipolar spindles, indicating that *APC* mutations could lead to chromosomal instability through defective mitosis [28,29]. Therefore, it was postulated that mutations in *APC* lead to chromosomal instability and induce aberrant Wnt signaling, thus contributing to tumor progression. While *APC* is highly relevant with respect to chromosomal aberrations in human colorectal cancers [21,22], mutations in *APC* are rare in human prostate cancer [30]. Many studies have focused on *APC* hypermethylation, which might cause *APC* downregulation [31,32] and has been associated with clinicopathological features of tumor aggressiveness. In a systematic review and meta-analysis of studies on tissue samples, *APC* promoter hypermethylation was found to correlate with more advanced stages of prostate cancer [33]. Functional annotations derived from the Encyclopedia of DNA Elements (ENCODE) and Roadmap Epigenomics data indicate that rs2707765 and rs497844, as well as their linked SNPs, coincide with open chromatin regions that likely correspond to promoters or enhancers of *APC* (Tables S3 and S4). In addition, rs2707765 and rs497844 are predicted to influence the binding of several transcription factors, such as fetal Alz-50 reactive clone 1 (FAC1), activating transcription factor 3 (ATF3) and the E2 factor (E2F) family of transcription factors. These data were consistent with our findings that the protective alleles, rs2707765 C and rs497844 T, tend to have a higher expression of *APC* and a better response to therapy. Interestingly, our previous study also demonstrated a potential prognostic role of *APC* rs3846716 (although it did not reach the predefined significance threshold of $q < 0.05$ in ACM) with regards to post-radical prostatectomy recurrence for localized prostate cancer [34]. Taken together, these results highlight the importance of *APC* throughout all stages of cancer treatment.

The present study has several strengths. This is the first study to have assessed whether genetic variants in the Wnt pathway influence clinical outcomes for advanced prostate cancer patients receiving ADT. Using a cDNA array and after validation with a published dataset, we have also presented additional evidence for a role of *APC* in prostate cancer, namely that downregulated APC gene expression was associated with more aggressive cancer and a poor prognosis. The haplotype-tagging SNP approach ensured the exhaustive and detailed coverage of susceptibility alleles across the whole *APC* gene region. Moreover, complete clinical information and follow-up data allowed us to control for potential confounding factors. However, our study population comprised homogeneous Han Chinese individuals, and therefore, the findings might be less applicable to other ethnic groups. There are many important Wnt pathway genes that have not been investigated in the present study. Thus, further validation in larger interethnic cohorts and additional functional studies will be necessary to elucidate the underlying biological mechanisms.

4. Materials and Methods

4.1. Patient Selection and Data Collection

Our study population included prostate cancer patients treated from 1995–2009 at three medical centers in Taiwan: Kaohsiung Medical University Hospital (Kaohsiung, Taiwan), Kaohsiung Veterans General Hospital (Kaohsiung, Taiwan) and National Taiwan University Hospital (Taipei, Taiwan), as described previously [35]. The clinical characteristics at diagnosis were compiled from medical records, and patients were followed-up prospectively to evaluate whether the tested genetic variations could represent prognostic factors of clinical outcomes during ADT. After excluding patients with inadequate clinicopathological characteristics or follow-up periods, 465 patients remained in the cohort. Written informed consent was obtained from all participants, and the study was approved by the Institutional Review Board of Kaohsiung Medical University Hospital (#KMUHIRB-2013132; 21 January 2014; Kaohsiung, Taiwan).

Treatment outcomes, disease progression and ACM were measured and updated recently during a prospective follow-up in 2014. The PSA nadir was defined as the lowest PSA value achieved at any time during ADT treatment [36,37]. The time to PSA nadir was defined as the duration from the initiation of ADT to the PSA nadir [38]. Disease progression was defined as the presence of at least two consecutive increases in the PSA value more than one week apart that exceeded the PSA nadir [39]. The use of secondary hormone treatment for increasing PSA was also considered to be a progression event. The time to progression was defined as the duration from the start of ADT until disease progression. In this study, patients underwent regular monthly follow-up evaluations and PSA testing at three-month intervals. Causes of death were determined from the official cause of death registry provided by the Department of Health, Executive Yuan, Taipei, Taiwan. ACM was defined as the interval from ADT initiation to death from any cause.

4.2. Single Nucleotide Polymorphism (SNP) Selection and Genotyping

We used a tagging SNP approach to select genetic variants for the investigation of the genetic variability in three core genes of the Wnt pathway, namely *WNT1*, *APC* and *CTNNB1*. Eighteen tagged SNPs were selected from Han Chinese in Beijing HapMap data using Tagger with $r^2 \geq 0.8$ and a minor-allele frequency ≥ 0.2 [40,41]. Genomic DNA was extracted from the peripheral blood using QIAamp DNA Blood Mini Kit (Qiagen, Venlo, The Netherlands) following the manufacturer's instruction, and stored at -80 °C. Genotyping was performed using iPLEX® matrix-assisted laser desorption/ionization time-of-flight mass-spectrometry technology (Agena Bioscience, Hamburg, Germany) at the National Center for Genome Medicine, Academia Sinica, Taipei, Taiwan, as described previously [42]. The average genotype call rate for genotyped SNPs was 99.7%, and the average concordance rate was 100% among five duplicated control samples. One SNP, rs1798802, significantly deviated from the Hardy-Weinberg equilibrium ($p < 0.05$) and was removed, leaving 17 SNPs for further statistical analysis.

4.3. Human Tissue cDNA Array and TaqMan® qRT-PCR Analysis

The expression levels of *APC* and *β-actin* (*ACTB*) were measured using the TissueScan™ human prostate cancer cDNA array II, including 8 normal and 40 prostate cancer samples (OriGene Technologies, Rockville, MD, USA). qRT-PCR was performed using prevalidated TaqMan® gene expression assays (Applied Biosystems, Foster City, CA, USA) for *APC* (Hs01568269_m1) and *ACTB* (Hs01060665_g1), on a 7500 real-time PCR system (Applied Biosystems, Foster City, CA, USA) according to the manufacturer's instructions. The quantification of each sample was normalized using the house-keeping gene *ACTB*.

4.4. Statistical Analysis

The clinical characteristics of the study population were summarized as numbers and percentages of patients or median values with interquartile ranges. Associations of clinical characteristics with disease progression and ACM were estimated using the log-rank test or Cox regression analysis. The median follow-up time and 95% confidence intervals of disease progression and ACM were assessed using the reverse Kaplan-Meier method. Associations of genotyped SNPs with the time to progression and ACM were assessed using multivariate Cox models adjusted for known prognostic factors, including age, clinical stage, Gleason score, PSA at ADT initiation, PSA nadir, time to PSA nadir and treatment modality. For each SNP, three genetic models (dominant, recessive and additive) of inheritance were assessed. The model with the strongest likelihood was considered to be the best model for each SNP. Only additive and dominant models were assessed if the variant homozygotes were observed in <0.05 of the study population. While testing the selected 17 SNPs, the FDR was calculated to determine the degree to which the tests for association were prone to yielding false positive results, using the q-values method [43]. q-Values and two-sided p-values < 0.05 were considered to be statistically significant. SPSS software, Version 22.0.0 (IBM, Armonk, NY, USA), was used for the statistical analyses.

4.5. Bioinformatics Analysis

HaploReg Version 4.1 [44] was used to assess the evidence of regulatory potential for the associated SNPs. We used the GTEx data to examine the correlations between SNPs and gene expression levels in human prostate tissues [45]. To further validate our findings, the association between *APC* expression and prostate cancer aggressiveness was analyzed using data from the Memorial Sloan-Kettering Cancer Center Prostate Oncogenome [25].

5. Conclusions

We comprehensively evaluated haplotype-tagging SNPs in core genes of the Wnt pathway and provided the first evidence of an association between *APC* gene variants and outcomes in advanced prostate cancer patients. Our findings might influence personalized prostate cancer management by identifying patients who would not benefit from ADT.

Acknowledgments: This work was supported by the Ministry of Science and Technology of Taiwan (Grant Numbers 102-2628-B-039-005-MY3, 103-2314-B-037-060, 104-2314-B-650-006, 104-2314-B-037-052-MY3 and 105-2314-B-650-003-MY3), the Kaohsiung Medical University Hospital (Grant Number KMUH103-3R43), the E-Da Hospital (Grant Numbers EDPJ104059 and EDPJ105054) and the China Medical University (Grant Number CMU105-S-42). The funders had no role in study design, data collection and analysis, decision to publish nor the preparation of the manuscript. We thank Chao-Shih Chen for data analysis and the National Center for Genome Medicine, Ministry of Science and Technology of Taiwan, for technical support. The results published here are based in part on data generated by the GTEx, HaploReg, ENCODE and Roadmap Epigenomics projects.

Author Contributions: Jiun-Hung Geng, Victor C. Lin, Chia-Cheng Yu, Chao-Yuan Huang, Shu-Pin Huang and Bo-Ying Bao conceived of and designed the experiments. Hsin-Ling Yin, Ta-Yuan Chang and Te-Ling Lu performed the experiments and analyzed the data. All authors wrote, reviewed and approved the submission of the paper.

References

1. Djulbegovic, M.; Beyth, R.J.; Neuberger, M.M.; Stoffs, T.L.; Vieweg, J.; Djulbegovic, B.; Dahm, P. Screening for prostate cancer: Systematic review and meta-analysis of randomised controlled trials. *BMJ* **2010**, *341*, c4543. [CrossRef] [PubMed]
2. Harris, W.P.; Mostaghel, E.A.; Nelson, P.S.; Montgomery, B. Androgen deprivation therapy: Progress in understanding mechanisms of resistance and optimizing androgen depletion. *Nat. Clin. Pract. Urol.* **2009**, *6*, 76–85. [CrossRef] [PubMed]
3. Horwitz, E.M. Prostate cancer: Optimizing the duration of androgen deprivation therapy. *Nat. Rev. Urol.* **2009**, *6*, 527–529. [CrossRef] [PubMed]
4. Walczak, J.R.; Carducci, M.A. Prostate cancer: A practical approach to current management of recurrent disease. *Mayo Clin. Proc.* **2007**, *82*, 243–249. [CrossRef]
5. Pienta, K.J.; Bradley, D. Mechanisms underlying the development of androgen-independent prostate cancer. *Clin. Cancer Res.* **2006**, *12*, 1665–1671. [CrossRef] [PubMed]
6. Moon, R.T.; Miller, J.R. The APC tumor suppressor protein in development and cancer. *Trends Genet.* **1997**, *13*, 256–258. [CrossRef]
7. Spink, K.E.; Polakis, P.; Weis, W.I. Structural basis of the axin-adenomatous polyposis coli interaction. *EMBO J.* **2000**, *19*, 2270–2279. [CrossRef] [PubMed]
8. Logan, C.Y.; Nusse, R. The Wnt signaling pathway in development and disease. *Annu. Rev. Cell Dev. Biol.* **2004**, *20*, 781–810. [CrossRef] [PubMed]

9. Katoh, M. Wnt/pcp signaling pathway and human cancer (review). *Oncol. Rep.* **2005**, *14*, 1583–1588. [CrossRef] [PubMed]
10. Brennan, K.R.; Brown, A.M. Wnt proteins in mammary development and cancer. *J. Mammary Gland Biol. Neoplasia* **2004**, *9*, 119–131. [CrossRef] [PubMed]
11. Brown, A.M. Wnt signaling in breast cancer: Have we come full circle? *Breast Cancer Res.* **2001**, *3*, 351–355. [CrossRef] [PubMed]
12. Howe, L.R.; Brown, A.M. Wnt signaling and breast cancer. *Cancer Biol. Ther.* **2004**, *3*, 36–41. [CrossRef] [PubMed]
13. Park, J.Y.; Park, W.S.; Nam, S.W.; Kim, S.Y.; Lee, S.H.; Yoo, N.J.; Lee, J.Y.; Park, C.K. Mutations of β-catenin and AXIN I genes are a late event in human hepatocellular carcinogenesis. *Liver Int.* **2005**, *25*, 70–76. [CrossRef] [PubMed]
14. Takahashi, M.; Wakabayashi, K. Gene mutations and altered gene expression in azoxymethane-induced colon carcinogenesis in rodents. *Cancer Sci.* **2004**, *95*, 475–480. [CrossRef] [PubMed]
15. Clevers, H. Wnt breakers in colon cancer. *Cancer Cell* **2004**, *5*, 5–6. [CrossRef]
16. Mulholland, D.J.; Read, J.T.; Rennie, P.S.; Cox, M.E.; Nelson, C.C. Functional localization and competition between the androgen receptor and T-cell factor for nuclear β-catenin: A means for inhibition of the Tcf signaling axis. *Oncogene* **2003**, *22*, 5602–5613. [CrossRef] [PubMed]
17. Yardy, G.W.; Brewster, S.F. Wnt signalling and prostate cancer. *Prostate Cancer Prostatic Dis.* **2005**, *8*, 119–126. [CrossRef] [PubMed]
18. Verras, M.; Sun, Z. Roles and regulation of wnt signaling and β-catenin in prostate cancer. *Cancer Lett.* **2006**, *237*, 22–32. [CrossRef] [PubMed]
19. Bierie, B.; Nozawa, M.; Renou, J.P.; Shillingford, J.M.; Morgan, F.; Oka, T.; Taketo, M.M.; Cardiff, R.D.; Miyoshi, K.; Wagner, K.U.; et al. Activation of β-catenin in prostate epithelium induces hyperplasias and squamous transdifferentiation. *Oncogene* **2003**, *22*, 3875–3887. [CrossRef] [PubMed]
20. Chesire, D.R.; Isaacs, W.B. β-catenin signaling in prostate cancer: An early perspective. *Endocr. Relat. Cancer* **2003**, *10*, 537–560. [CrossRef] [PubMed]
21. Kinzler, K.W.; Nilbert, M.C.; Su, L.K.; Vogelstein, B.; Bryan, T.M.; Levy, D.B.; Smith, K.J.; Preisinger, A.C.; Hedge, P.; McKechnie, D.; et al. Identification of fap locus genes from chromosome 5q21. *Science* **1991**, *253*, 661–665. [CrossRef] [PubMed]
22. Nishisho, I.; Nakamura, Y.; Miyoshi, Y.; Miki, Y.; Ando, H.; Horii, A.; Koyama, K.; Utsunomiya, J.; Baba, S.; Hedge, P.; et al. Mutations of chromosome 5q21 genes in fap and colorectal cancer patients. *Science* **1991**, *253*, 665–669. [CrossRef] [PubMed]
23. Chen, G.; Shukeir, N.; Potti, A.; Sircar, K.; Aprikian, A.; Goltzman, D.; Rabbani, S.A. Up-regulation of Wnt-1 and β-catenin production in patients with advanced metastatic prostate carcinoma: Potential pathogenetic and prognostic implications. *Cancer* **2004**, *101*, 1345–1356. [CrossRef] [PubMed]
24. Verras, M.; Brown, J.; Li, X.; Nusse, R.; Sun, Z. Wnt3a growth factor induces androgen receptor-mediated transcription and enhances cell growth in human prostate cancer cells. *Cancer Res.* **2004**, *64*, 8860–8866. [CrossRef] [PubMed]
25. Hieronymus, H.; Schultz, N.; Gopalan, A.; Carver, B.S.; Chang, M.T.; Xiao, Y.; Heguy, A.; Huberman, K.; Bernstein, M.; Assel, M.; et al. Copy number alteration burden predicts prostate cancer relapse. *Proc. Natl. Acad. Sci. USA* **2014**, *111*, 11139–11144. [CrossRef] [PubMed]
26. Nathke, I.S. The adenomatous polyposis coli protein: The achilles heel of the gut epithelium. *Annu. Rev. Cell Dev. Biol.* **2004**, *20*, 337–366. [CrossRef] [PubMed]
27. Lengauer, C.; Kinzler, K.W.; Vogelstein, B. Genetic instabilities in human cancers. *Nature* **1998**, *396*, 643–649. [CrossRef] [PubMed]
28. Fodde, R.; Kuipers, J.; Rosenberg, C.; Smits, R.; Kielman, M.; Gaspar, C.; van Es, J.H.; Breukel, C.; Wiegant, J.; Giles, R.H.; et al. Mutations in the APC tumour suppressor gene cause chromosomal instability. *Nat. Cell Biol.* **2001**, *3*, 433–438. [CrossRef] [PubMed]
29. Kaplan, K.B.; Burds, A.A.; Swedlow, J.R.; Bekir, S.S.; Sorger, P.K.; Nathke, I.S. A role for the adenomatous polyposis coli protein in chromosome segregation. *Nat. Cell Biol.* **2001**, *3*, 429–432. [CrossRef] [PubMed]
30. Kypta, R.M.; Waxman, J. Wnt/β-catenin signalling in prostate cancer. *Nat. Rev. Urol.* **2012**, *9*, 418–428. [CrossRef] [PubMed]

31. Cho, N.Y.; Kim, J.H.; Moon, K.C.; Kang, G.H. Genomic hypomethylation and cpg island hypermethylation in prostatic intraepithelial neoplasm. *Virchows Arch.* **2009**, *454*, 17–23. [CrossRef] [PubMed]
32. Costa, V.L.; Henrique, R.; Jeronimo, C. Epigenetic markers for molecular detection of prostate cancer. *Dis. Markers* **2007**, *23*, 31–41. [CrossRef] [PubMed]
33. Chen, Y.; Li, J.; Yu, X.; Li, S.; Zhang, X.; Mo, Z.; Hu, Y. APC gene hypermethylation and prostate cancer: A systematic review and meta-analysis. *Eur. J. Hum. Genet.* **2013**, *21*, 929–935. [CrossRef] [PubMed]
34. Huang, S.P.; Ting, W.C.; Chen, L.M.; Huang, L.C.; Liu, C.C.; Chen, C.W.; Hsieh, C.J.; Yang, W.H.; Chang, T.Y.; Lee, H.Z.; et al. Association analysis of Wnt pathway genes on prostate-specific antigen recurrence after radical prostatectomy. *Ann. Surg. Oncol.* **2010**, *17*, 312–322. [CrossRef] [PubMed]
35. Bao, B.Y.; Pao, J.B.; Huang, C.N.; Pu, Y.S.; Chang, T.Y.; Lan, Y.H.; Lu, T.L.; Lee, H.Z.; Juang, S.H.; Chen, L.M.; et al. Polymorphisms inside micrornas and microrna target sites predict clinical outcomes in prostate cancer patients receiving androgen-deprivation therapy. *Clin. Cancer Res.* **2011**, *17*, 928–936. [CrossRef] [PubMed]
36. Stewart, A.J.; Scher, H.I.; Chen, M.H.; McLeod, D.G.; Carroll, P.R.; Moul, J.W.; D'Amico, A.V. Prostate-specific antigen nadir and cancer-specific mortality following hormonal therapy for prostate-specific antigen failure. *J. Clin. Oncol.* **2005**, *23*, 6556–6560. [CrossRef] [PubMed]
37. Kwak, C.; Jeong, S.J.; Park, M.S.; Lee, E.; Lee, S.E. Prognostic significance of the nadir prostate specific antigen level after hormone therapy for prostate cancer. *J. Urol.* **2002**, *168*, 995–1000. [CrossRef]
38. Choueiri, T.K.; Xie, W.; D'Amico, A.V.; Ross, R.W.; Hu, J.C.; Pomerantz, M.; Regan, M.M.; Taplin, M.E.; Kantoff, P.W.; Sartor, O.; et al. Time to prostate-specific antigen nadir independently predicts overall survival in patients who have metastatic hormone-sensitive prostate cancer treated with androgen-deprivation therapy. *Cancer* **2009**, *115*, 981–987. [CrossRef] [PubMed]
39. Ross, R.W.; Oh, W.K.; Xie, W.; Pomerantz, M.; Nakabayashi, M.; Sartor, O.; Taplin, M.E.; Regan, M.M.; Kantoff, P.W.; Freedman, M. Inherited variation in the androgen pathway is associated with the efficacy of androgen-deprivation therapy in men with prostate cancer. *J. Clin. Oncol.* **2008**, *26*, 842–847. [CrossRef] [PubMed]
40. De Bakker, P.I.; Yelensky, R.; Pe'er, I.; Gabriel, S.B.; Daly, M.J.; Altshuler, D. Efficiency and power in genetic association studies. *Nat. Genet.* **2005**, *37*, 1217–1223. [CrossRef] [PubMed]
41. Frazer, K.A.; Ballinger, D.G.; Cox, D.R.; Hinds, D.A.; Stuve, L.L.; Gibbs, R.A.; Belmont, J.W.; Boudreau, A.; Hardenbol, P.; Leal, S.M.; et al. A second generation human haplotype map of over 3.1 million SNPs. *Nature* **2007**, *449*, 851–861. [CrossRef] [PubMed]
42. Huang, S.P.; Huang, L.C.; Ting, W.C.; Chen, L.M.; Chang, T.Y.; Lu, T.L.; Lan, Y.H.; Liu, C.C.; Yang, W.H.; Lee, H.Z.; et al. Prognostic significance of prostate cancer susceptibility variants on prostate-specific antigen recurrence after radical prostatectomy. *Cancer Epidemiol. Biomark. Prev.* **2009**, *18*, 3068–3074. [CrossRef] [PubMed]
43. Storey, J.D.; Tibshirani, R. Statistical significance for genomewide studies. *Proc. Natl. Acad. Sci. USA* **2003**, *100*, 9440–9445. [CrossRef] [PubMed]
44. Ward, L.D.; Kellis, M. Haploreg: A resource for exploring chromatin states, conservation, and regulatory motif alterations within sets of genetically linked variants. *Nucleic Acids Res.* **2012**, *40*, D930–D934. [CrossRef] [PubMed]
45. Lonsdale, J.; Thomas, J.; Salvatore, M.; Phillips, R.; Lo, E.; Shad, S.; Hasz, R.; Walters, G.; Garcia, F.; Young, N.; et al. The genotype-tissue expression (GTEx) project. *Nat. Genet.* **2013**, *45*, 580–585. [CrossRef] [PubMed]

8

The Prostate Cancer Cells Resistant to Docetaxel as In Vitro Model for Discovering MicroRNAs Predictive of the Onset of Docetaxel Resistance

Lorenzo Bascetta [1,†], Arianna Oliviero [1,†], Romina D'Aurizio [2], Monica Evangelista [1], Alberto Mercatanti [1], Marco Pellegrini [2], Francesca Marrocolo [3], Sergio Bracarda [3,4] and Milena Rizzo [1,4,*]

1 Non-Coding RNA Laboratory, Institute of Clinical Physiology (IFC), National Research Council (CNR), via G. Moruzzi 1, 56124 Pisa, Italy; lorenzobascetta@hotmail.it (L.B.); arianna90oli@hotmail.it (A.O.); m.evangelista@ifc.cnr.it (M.E.); alberto.mercatanti@ifc.cnr.it (A.M.)

2 Laboratory for Integrative System Medicine (LISM), Institute of Informatics and Telematics (IIT), National Research Council (CNR), via G. Moruzzi 1, 56124 Pisa, Italy; romina.daurizio@gmail.com (R.D.); marco.pellegrini@iit.cnr.it (M.P.)

3 Department of Oncology, San Donato Hospital, Azienda USL Toscana Sud-Est, via P. Nenni 20, 52100 Arezzo, Italy; francesca.marrocolo@uslsudest.toscana.it (F.M.); sergio.bracarda@uslsudest.toscana.it (S.B.)

4 Istituto Toscano Tumori (ITT), via T. Alderotti 26/N, 50139 Firenze, Italy

* Correspondence: milena.rizzo@ifc.cnr.it

† These authors contributed equally to this work.

Abstract: On the grounds that miRNAs present in the blood of prostate cancer (PCa) patients are released in the growth medium by PCa cells, it is conceivable that PCa cells resistant to docetaxel (DCT) (DCT^R) will release miRNAs that may be found in PCa patients under DCT therapy if resistant PCa cells appear. We isolated DCT^R clones respectively from 22Rv1 and DU-145 PCa cell lines and performed through next-generation sequencing (NGS) the miRNAs profiles of the released miRNAs. The analysis of the NGS data identified 105 and 1 miRNAs which were differentially released in the growth medium of the 22Rv1/DCT^R and DU-145/DCT^R clones, respectively. Using additional filters, we selected 12 and 1 miRNA more released by all 22Rv1/DCT^R and DU-145/DCT^R clones, respectively. Moreover, we showed that 6 of them were more represented in the growth medium of the DCT^R cells than the ones of DCT-treated cells. We speculated that they have the pre-requisite to be tested as predictive biomarkers of the DCT resistance in PCa patients under DCT therapy. We propose the utilization of clones resistant to a given drug as in vitro model to identify the differentially released miRNAs, which in perspective could be tested as predictive biomarkers of drug resistance in tumor patients under therapy.

Keywords: prostate cancer cell lines; docetaxel resistance; circulating miRNAs; predictive biomarkers

---

1. Introduction

Prostate cancer (PCa) evolves into a condition known as castration-resistant prostate cancer (CRPC) when the androgen deprivation therapy fails. At this stage, docetaxel (DCT) represents the gold standard treatment [1]. Unfortunately, most patients develop resistance to the drug within a year from the beginning of the therapy, and the disease progresses [2]. The identification of biomarkers capable to predict in advance the onset of the DCT resistance could facilitate the shift towards alternative effective therapies, thus increasing the life expectancy of the patients.

MicroRNAs (miRNAs), and more recently circulating miRNAs (c-miRNA), have been proposed as molecules with a diagnostic and prognostic value for PCa [3,4] but only few studies explored c-miRNAs as predictive biomarker of DCT resistance [5,6].

We have already reported that PCa cells in vitro specifically released in the growth medium the same miRNAs found in the peripheral blood of PCa patients [7]. Therefore, it is conceivable that PCa cells resistant to DCT will release in the growth medium miRNAs that, if detected in the blood of PCa patients, could reveal the presence of DCT-resistant cells. To approach the problem, we isolated PCa cells resistant to DCT and used the next-generation sequencing (NGS) technology and bioinformatics tools to identify miRNAs differentially released in the growth medium by DCT-resistant cells (DCT^R-miRNAs). We also discussed that DCT^R-miRNAs may represent potential predictive biomarkers of the DCT resistance suitable to be tested in PCa patients under DCT therapy.

2. Results

2.1. Isolation of DCT^R Clones from 22Rv1 and DU-145 Prostate Cancer Cell Lines

We exposed for three days either 22Rv1 or DU-145 PCa cells to increasing concentrations of DCT and observed a dose-dependent inhibition of cell proliferation which reached a plateau phase at 4 nM concentration and 3 nM, respectively (Figure 1A,C). We then grew continuously 22Rv1 cells and DU-145 cells respectively in 4 nM and 3 nM DCT-containing medium until we observed colonies presumably resistant to DCT. We isolated and expanded as clones 6 independent colonies from both 22Rv1 cells (22Rv1/DCT^R clones) and DU-145 cells (DU-145/DCT^R clones). Afterwards, we tested them for the DCT resistance. We treated cells with increasing DCT concentration and showed that 22Rv1/DCT^R and DU-145/DCT^R clones were more resistant to DCT with respect to parental cell lines (Figure 1B,D).

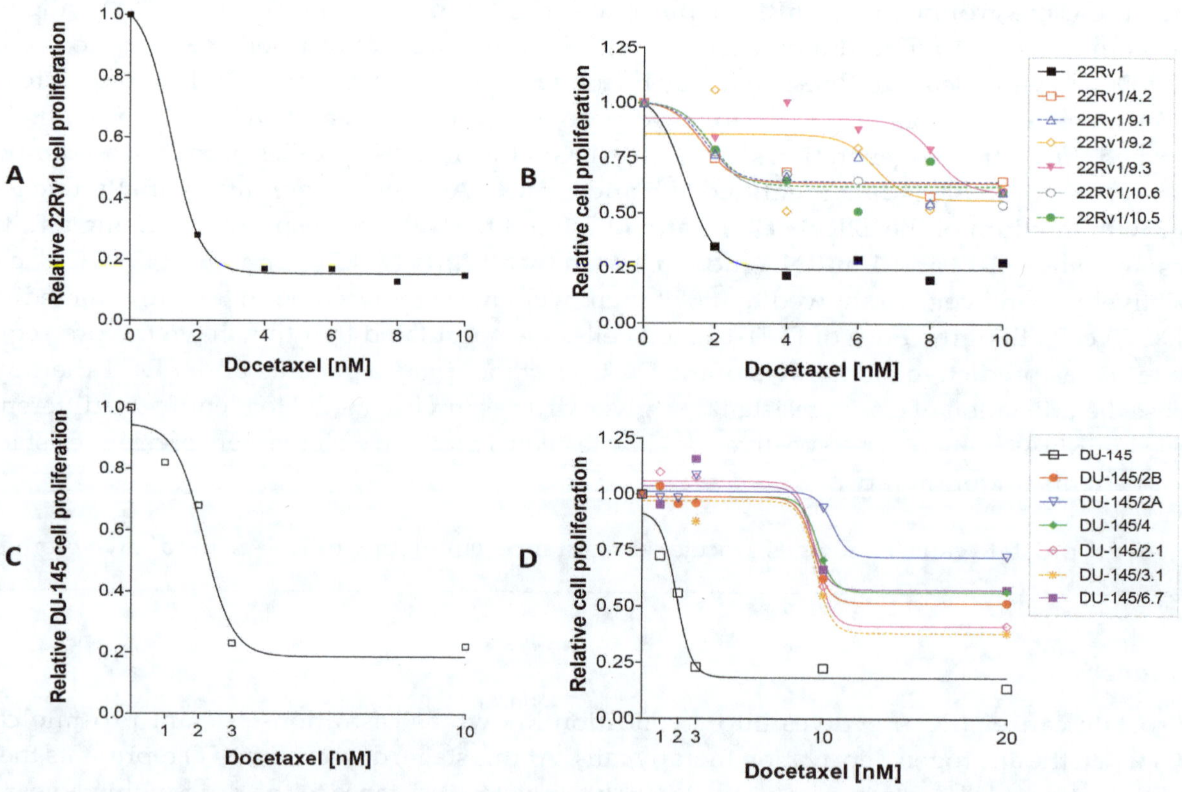

Figure 1. Effect of docetaxel (DCT) on DU-145 cell proliferation. Relative cell proliferation of 22Rv1 cells (**A**), 22Rv1/DCT^R clones (**B**), DU-145 cells (**C**) and DU-145/DCT^R clones (**D**) exposed to increasing concentrations of docetaxel for 72 h.

In addition, we showed that 22Rv1/DCT^R as well as DU-145/DCT^R clones presented expanded generation times (Figure 2A,B) and an acquired capability to extrude Rhodamine 123 (Figure 2C,D). These results, together with the upregulation of *MDR1* gene (Figure 2E,F), indicated that the drug export increase through the ABC transporters was at the basis of the DCT resistance in all clones. We tested also the expression of *BCL2* and *βIII tubulin* genes, whose upregulation is involved in the DCT resistance in PCa [8,9].

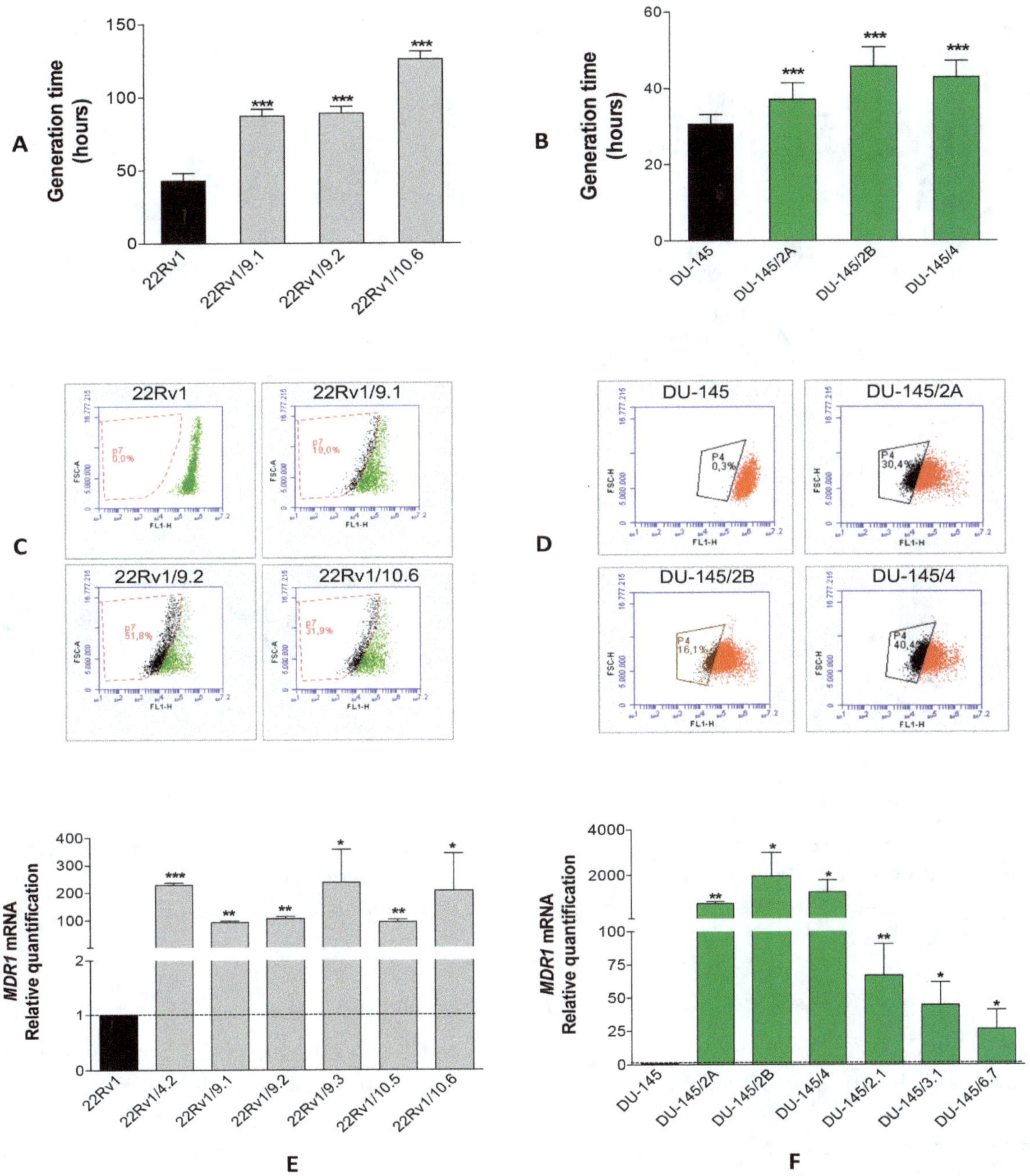

Figure 2. Characterization of DCT^R clones. Generation times (calculated dividing the hours in culture by the number of cell doublings) (**A**,**B**), percentage of cells which extruded Rh123 (**C**,**D**), *MDR1* mRNA relative quantification with qRT-PCR (**E**,**F**) in 22Rv1/DCT^R or DU-145/DCT^R clones with respect to parental cells (dotted line). Data were shown as mean ± SD from three independent experiments (* $p < 0.05$, ** $p < 0.01$, *** $p < 0.001$, unpaired t-test).

It is worth noting that while in 22Rv1/DCT^R clones the expression level of both *BCL2* (Figure 3A) and *βIII tubulin* (Figure 3B) genes did not change, these genes showed slight but significant variations in DU-145/DCT^R clones. In particular, *BCL2* was upregulated in DU-145/2B and DU-145/4 clones and downregulated in DU-145/2.1 and DU-145/6.7 clones (Figure 3B). In addition, *βIII tubulin* gene was upregulated in DU-145/2A clones and downregulated in DU-145/3.1 clones (Figure 3D).

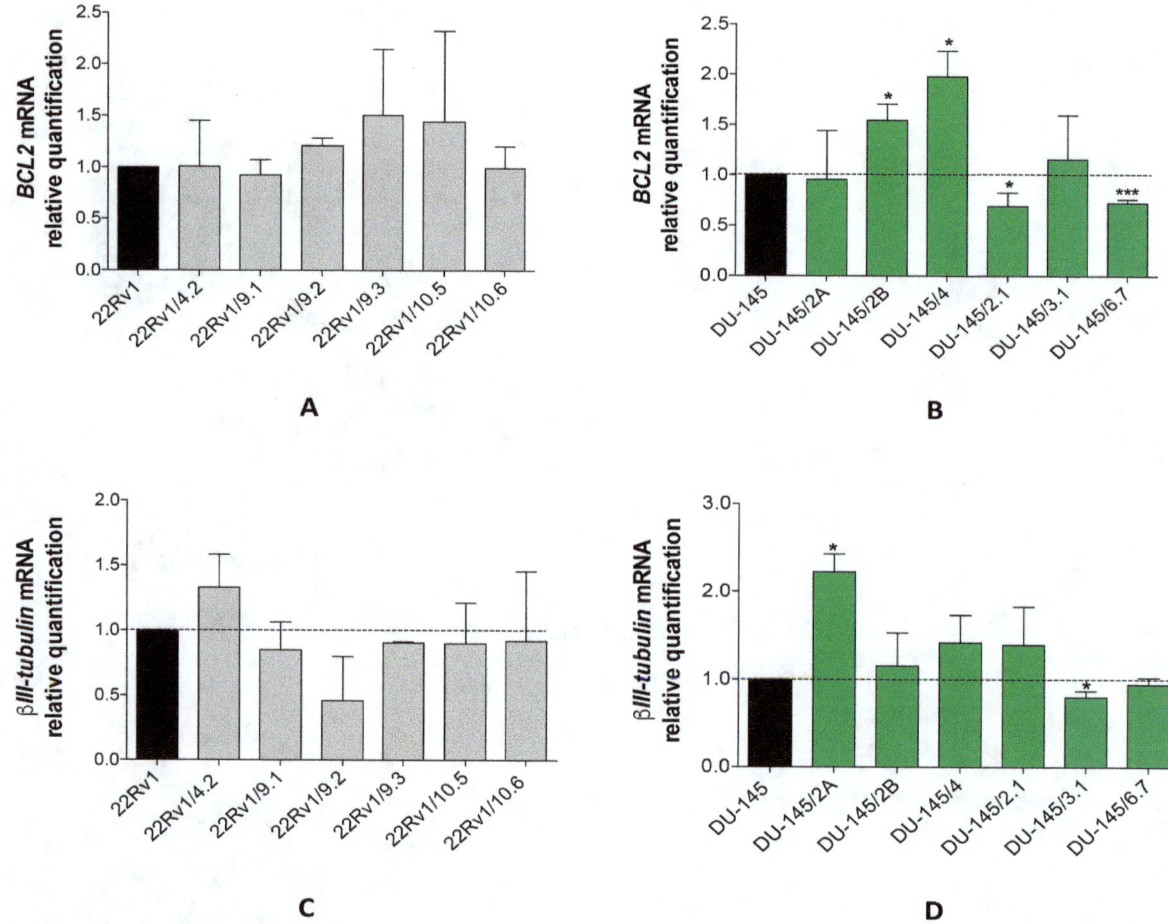

Figure 3. Characterization of DCT^R clones. *BCL2* (**A**,**B**) and *βIII tubulin* (**C**,**D**) mRNA relative quantification with qRT-PCR in 22Rv1/DCT^R or DU-145/DCT^R clones with respect to parental cells (dotted line). Data were shown as mean ± SD from three independent experiments (* $p < 0.05$, *** $p < 0.001$, unpaired t-test).

2.2. *Identification of miRNAs Differentially Released by DCT^R Clones*

We collected the growth medium of each 22Rv1/DCT^R and DU-145/DCT^R clone as well as the one of parental cells and performed the miRNAs expression profile using next-generation sequencing (small RNA-seq). We conducted the differential analysis to identify, for each PCa cell line, the miRNAs that were differentially released with a statistical significance from all DCT^R clones with respect to the corresponding parental cells. The analysis was performed using two different methods, i.e., DESeq2 and edgeR. For DU-145/DCT^R clones, the small RNA-seq experiment was conducted in two different runs. To test whether the experiment could suffer a batch effect on distribution of detected miRNAs, we performed a principal component analysis and observed a significant bias (Figure S1). Therefore, for DU-145/DCT^R clones, we use an additive model formula in the design formula of DESeq2 and edgeR. We identified 134 (with DESeq2) and 127 (with edgeR) miRNAs differentially released (FDR $\leq$ 0.01) by 22Rv1/DCT^R clones (Table S1) and 1 (with DESeq2) and 3 (with edgeR) miRNAs differentially released (FDR $\leq$ 0.01) by DU-145/DCT^R clones (Table S2). We then considered only the miRNAs identified by both algorithms which were 105 miRNAs for 22Rv1/DCT^R clones (44 more released miRNAs, 61 retained/less released miRNAs) and 1 more released miRNA for DU-145/DCT^R clones (Figure 4A). We then focused on miRNAs more released (red in Figure 4A) and we selected those whose average number of normalized reads (NR) in all 22Rv1/DCT^R (or DU-145/DCT^R) clones or in the corresponding parental cells was greater than 100 (Figure 4A, box i). Among them, we selected those with a difference greater than 10 NR ($\Delta > 10$) between the clone with the lowest value and the biological replicate of the parental cells with the highest value (Figure 4A, box ii). Thus, we identified 12 miRNAs for 22Rv1/DCT^R clones (Figure 4B) and 1 miRNA (miR-146a-5p) for DU-145/DCT^R clones (Figure 4C and Figure S2).

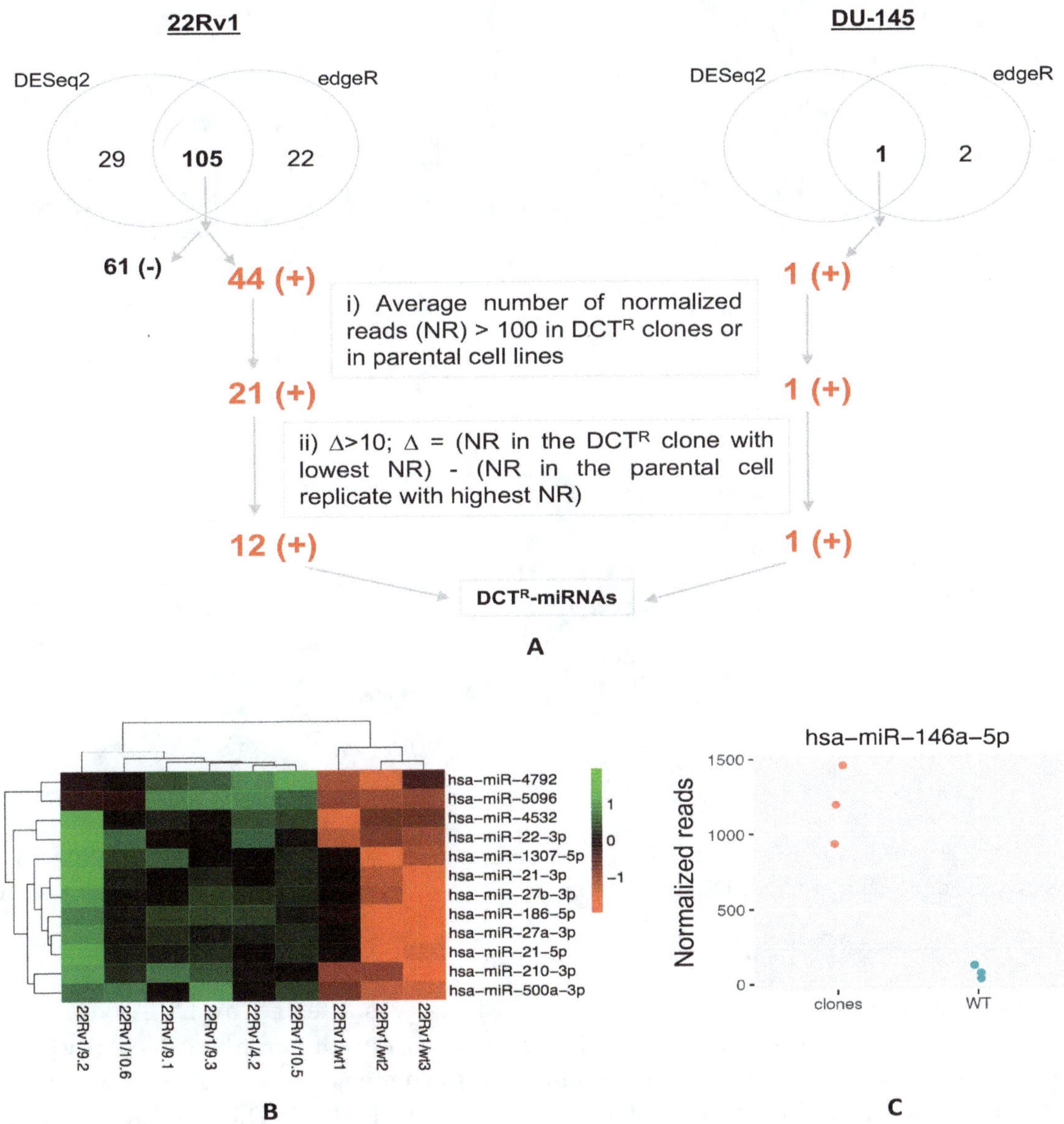

Figure 4. Extracellular miRNA profile of DCT^R clones. (**A**) Schematic representation of the selective criteria used to identify DCT^R-miRNAs in both 22Rv1/DCT^R and DU-145/DCT^R clones (+, more released; −, retained/less released); (**B**) Heatmap representing the result of DCT^R-miRNAs in 22Rv1/DCT^R clones and parental cells biological replicates (22Rv1WT1-3); (**C**) Normalized reads of miR-146a-5p in DU-145/DCT^R clones (red spots) and parental cells biological replicates (blue spots) of DU-145/2A, /2B and /4 clones (see Figure S2 for DU-145/2.1, /3.1 and /6.7 clones).

Finally, we validated the expression of these miRNAs (DCT^R-miRNAs) in the growth medium of both 22Rv1/DCT^R and DU-145/DCT^R clones by qRT-PCR. With the exception of miR-1307-5p (whose level showed a slight change), the levels of all DCT^R-miRNAs were higher in the growth medium of the DCT^R clones (Figure 5A,B) thus confirming the NGS data.

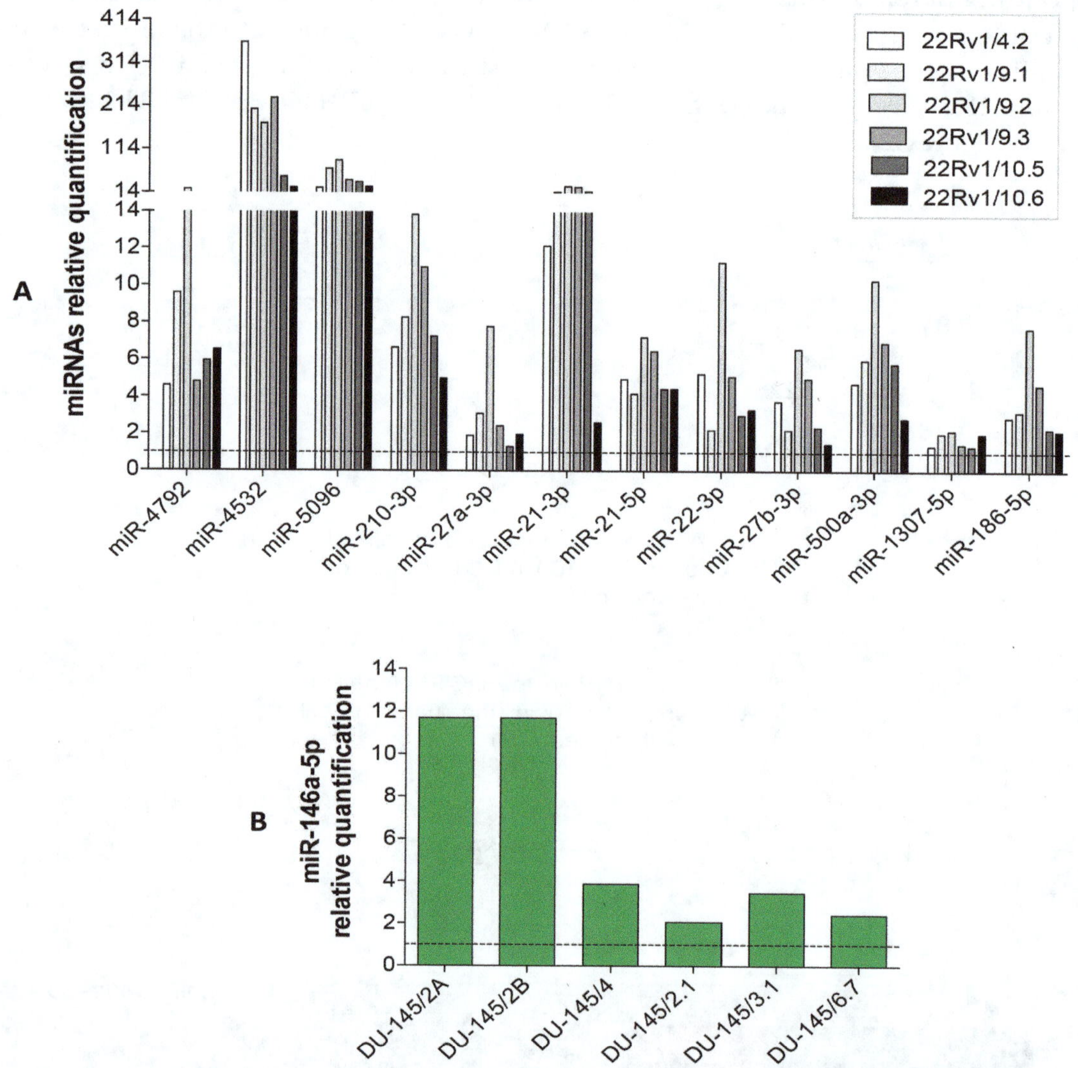

Figure 5. DCT^R-miRNAs validation. Relative quantification with qRT-PCR of DCT^R-miRNAs in the growth medium of 22Rv1/ (**A**) or DU-145/ (**B**) DCT^R clones with respect to parental cells (dotted line).

2.3. *DCT^R-miRNAs as Possible Biomarkers of DCT Resistance*

To evaluate whether the level of the DCT^R-miRNAs was affected by DCT, we measured by qRT-PCR the level of the 12 DCT^R-miRNAs in the growth medium of parental cells (22Rv1 or DU-145) treated for three days with DCT and we calculated the fold change of these miRNAs in comparison to that found in the growth medium of untreated cells (column B, Table 1). Then, we evaluated the mean fold change of the DCT^R-miRNAs (measured by qRT-PCR) in the growth medium of 22Rv1/DCT^R or DU-145/DCT^R clones with respect to that of the corresponding parental cells line (column A, Table 1). Finally, for each DCT^R-miRNAs, we calculate the ratio between the fold change value of DCT-treated versus untreated cells and the mean fold change of DCT^R-miRNA in 22Rv1/DCT^R or DU-145/DCT^R clones versus parental cells (column A/column B, Table 1). We observed that the level of 6 DCT^R-miRNAs was similar in cells either resistant to or treated with DCT, whereas the level of the remaining 6 DCT^R-miRNAs was higher (more than 2-fold) in cells resistant to DCT versus cells treated with DCT (Table 1, miRNAs underlined and in bold), suggesting that their differential release was specific of the DCT-resistant phenotype.

Table 1. DCT^R-miRNAs level in the growth medium of DCT^R clones or DCT-treated cells.

DCT^R/miRNAs	Column A *. DCT^R-miRNAs Level in DCT^R Clones Versus Parental Cells Growth Medium	Column B **. DCT^R-miRNAs Level in DCT-Treated Versus Untreated Cells Growth Medium	Column A/ Column B	Unpaired *t*-Test Pvalue (A Versus B)
miR-4792 ***	**8.94 ± 2.75**	**1.69 ± 0.11**	**5.27**	**$p < 0.05$**
miR-4532	**175.20 ± 50.66**	**2.10 ± 0.48**	**83.42**	**$p < 0.01$**
miR-5096	**48.61 ± 10.00**	**1.28 ± 0.03**	**37.97**	**$p < 0.001$**
miR-210-3p	**8.80 ± 1.13**	**2.28 ± 0.19**	**3.86**	**$p < 0.001$**
miR-27a-3p	3.48 ± 0.85	2.13 ± 0.2	1.63	NS
miR-21-3p	**17.7 ± 4.12**	**3.9 ± 0.49**	**4.53**	**$p < 0.01$**
miR-21-5p	**5.18 ± 0.43**	**2.49 ± 0.39**	**2.07**	**$p < 0.001$**
miR-22-3p	5.22 ± 1.21	3.86 ± 0.32	1.35	NS
miR-27b-3p	3.52 ± 0.77	4.29 ± 0.25	0.82	NS
miR-500a-3p	6.11 ± 1.01	3.78 ± 0.03	1.61	$p < 0.05$
miR-186-5p	3.82 ± 0.86	3.64 ± 0.43	1.05	NS
miR-146a-5p ****	5.87 ± 1.86	10.21 ± 1.46	0.57	NS

* Each value represents the mean ± SD of the DCT^R/miRNAs level in the DCT^R clones. ** Each value represents the mean ± SD of the DCT^R/miRNAs level in six biological replicates. *** DCT^R-miRNAs whose column A/column B value was higher than 2 are underlined and in bold. **** miR-146a-5p was the only miRNA selected from DU-145/DCT^R clones. NS, not significant.

2.4. Expression Level of Selected DCT^R-miRNAs in DCT^R Clones

To gain more insight into the differential release of the DCT^R-miRNAs by the DCT^R clones we measured the intracellular level of the DCT^R-miRNAs specifically associated with DCT-resistant phenotype (Table 1, underlined and in bold) in 22Rv1/DCT^R clones with respect to parental cell lines (Figure 6). We found that DCT^R-miRNAs were upregulated in 22Rv1/DCT^R clones (particularly miR-4532, miR-5096 and miR-210-3p) except for miR-21-3p and miR-21-5p whose level did not change significantly, suggesting that the release of DCT^R-miRNAs by DCT^R PCa cells could be mediated by both active or passive mechanisms.

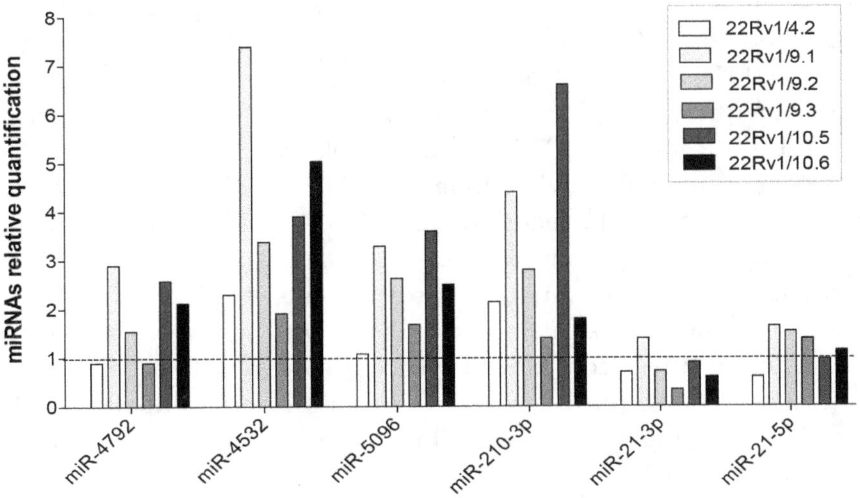

Figure 6. Intracellular level of selected DCT^R-miRNAs in 22Rv1/DCT^R clones. Relative quantification by qRT-PCR of DCT^R-miRNAs in the growth medium of 22Rv1/DCT^R clones with respect to parental cells (dotted line).

3. Discussion

Docetaxel (DCT) is the first line chemotherapy for patients who become insensitive to androgen deprivation therapy (castration-resistant prostate cancer, CRPC). Unfortunately, the DCT therapy frequently favors the development of DCT resistance in metastatic CRPC patients [2]. Hence, the discovery of biomarkers that indicate in advance the onset of DCT resistance could allow the early switch to other effective treatment options such as abiraterone acetate and enzalutamide [10,11]. While the detection of circulating miRNAs (c-miRNAs) in tumor patients is widely applied in clinical research [12–14], the detection of c-miRNAs in cancer patients under medical treatment is under-investigated, especially in PCa patients as confirmed by the poor availability of published data. So far, the change of miR-21 [5] and miR-210 [6] levels in the blood of PCa patients under DCT treatment have been associated with the clinical outcome. In addition, miR-141 [15,16], miR-146b-3p and miR-194 [16] have been shown to predict PCa clinical progression after therapies. Finally, in a recent work Lin et al. [17,18] demonstrated that miR-200a, miR-200b, miR-200c, miR-132, miR-375, miR-429 were associated with overall survival after DCT treatment.

In this work, we detected the miRNAs released by clones of 22Rv1 and DU-145 PCa cells resistant to DCT with the aim to identify those preferentially released by the DCT-resistant cells. The decision to isolate DCT^R clones from the androgen-dependent (22Rv1) and androgen-independent (DU-145) cell lines was due to the fact that DCT-based chemotherapy has become a therapeutic option not only for CRPC patients but also for those who have not yet reached the full androgen-independence [19]. In line with other data [20,21], we showed that the main molecular mechanism at the basis of the resistance of the DCT^R clones was the increase in the activity of the ABC membrane transporters, a family of ATP-dependent membrane-bound drug efflux pump that protects the tumor cells by cytotoxic drugs. In addition, we showed that both 22Rv1/DCT^R and DU-145/DCT^R clones had a generation time longer than those of the parental cell line. These data were in line with those obtained by Corcoran et al. [22]. We cannot exclude that the reduced growth rate of the DCT^R clones may contribute to the DCT-resistant phenotype.

Once the DCT^R clones were obtained, we detected miRNAs differentially released in the growth medium and selected those that passed several filters. First, we considered the miRNAs differentially released by all DCT^R clones derived from each cell line and this increased the probability that they could be those really released by DCT-resistant cells. Second, we focused on miRNAs that were more released and on these miRNAs we imposed a cut-off on normalized reads (NR > 100) as we believe that this level was adequate for an easier detection. Third, we selected miRNAs whose level were significantly different between DCT^R clones and parental cells by selecting not only the miRNAs more released by a $|\log2FC| > 1$, but also the miRNAs whose level between the DCT^R clone with the lower NR and the parental line replicate with the highest NR was greater than 10 ($\Delta > 10$). At the end, we selected 12 DCT^R-miRNAs and 1 DCT^R-miRNA released by 22Rv1/DCT^R and DU-145/DCT^R clones respectively. In our opinion, the low abundance of DU-145/DCT^R-miRNAs in comparison with 22Rv1/DCT^R-miRNAs depends on the fact that DU-145/DCT^R clones are more heterogeneous than 22Rv1/DCT^R clones as suggested by the molecular data (*BLC2* and *βIII tubulin* expression levels) and the different levels of *MDR1* activation. Another observation is that 22Rv1/DCT^R and DU-145/DCT^R clones did not release the same miRNAs. This finding is not completely surprising given that DCT^R clones derived from different tumor contexts and therefore the resistant phenotype may be different. As DCT resistance in PCa patients may arise from different tumor context as well, this observation underlines the importance of using more PCa cell lines to have a higher chance of identifying miRNAs which could potentially predict DCT resistance.

We then examined whether DCT^R-miRNAs could be potential biomarkers of DCT resistance. In particular, we evaluated whether the release of the DCT^R-miRNAs was affected also by the DCT treatment. We obtained promising results from the comparison of the DCT^R-miRNAs released in the growth medium by DCT^R clones and by parental cells treated with DCT for 3 days. We showed that the release of miR-4792, miR-4532, miR-5096, miR-210-3p, miR-21-3p and miR-21-5p were higher in the growth medium of DCT^R clones than in DCT-treated cells thus rendering these miRNAs specific of DCT-resistant cells and then promising putative biomarkers of DCT resistance.

To be a good biomarker, a miRNA should be highly released before the onset of the DCT resistance. So far, many c-miRNAs diagnostic/prognostic of PCa have been identified, but it is still unclear if these c-miRNAs are useful in the management of PCa patients under DCT therapy. At the moment, only two c-miRNAs (miR-21, miR-210) have been associated to the outcome of DCT therapy [5,6] and, as such, have characteristics of predicting the DCT resistance of PCa patients. It has been shown that miR-21 level was elevated in CRPC patients, especially in those who developed resistance after DCT chemotherapy [5]. In the same way, it was demonstrated that the serum levels of miR-210 was higher in patients whose disease was resistant to DCT treatment as assessed by change in prostate specific antigen (PSA) [6]. It is worth noticing that both miR-21 and miR-210 belong to the 6 DCT^R-miRNAs that were highly released only by cells resistant to DCT, suggesting that our approach to isolate DCT^R PCa cells and to select the differentially released miRNAs not affected by DCT treatment could represent a manner to discover miRNAs to be tested as predictive biomarkers of the DCT resistance. As a consequence, the other DCT^R-miRNAs specifically released by DCT^R cells (miR-4792, miR-4532, miR-5096), and not yet tested in PCa patients, represent promising candidates to be tested as DCT predictive biomarkers in PCa patients.

Finally, we considered the intracellular level of the 6 DCT^R-miRNAs in DCT^R clones to gain more insight on the miRNA release mechanism. We found that not all DCT^R-miRNAs were upregulated in all 22Rv1/DCT^R clones suggesting that the release of these miRNAs by DCT-resistant PCa cells may be also mediated by an active mechanism. There are several reports in favor of either a specific or non-specific secretion of miRNAs by the cells (for review see [23,24]).

Among the miRNAs that were more upregulated (i.e., miR-210-3p, miR-4532 and miR-5096), miR-210 has been found to be transcriptionally activated by the hypoxia-inducible factor 1 α (HIF-1α) [25]. In particular, Cheng et al. [6] demonstrated that the treatment of PCa cells with hypoxic conditions determined the upregulation and the release of miR-210 in the growth medium. In addition, they demonstrated that high miR-210 serum level is associated with therapy (hormone therapy in combination with chemotherapy) resistance in CRPC patients. Given that it is known that tumor hypoxia is associated with therapy resistance [26], the author suggested that an increased hypoxia response signaling is present in a subset of CRPC patients, leading to increased miR-210 level and therapy resistance. So, the upregulation/release of miR-210-3p by 22Rv1/DCT^R clones is in line with these data: we can only speculate that an increased hypoxia signaling could be associated with DCT resistance mechanism of 22Rv1/DCT^R clones. However, miR-210 has a central role in promoting cancer-associated fibroblast (CAF) formation in PCa [27], hence in cancer progression, suggesting that it may act as a signal molecule in tumor microenvironment. Regarding miR-5096 and miR-4532, since they have been recently discovered, there are no reports on their biological functions. However, there are two studies that demonstrated that the transfer of miR-5096 through the gap junctions from glioma cells to astrocyte [28] or to human microvascular endothelial cells [29] promotes the glioma invasion with an unknown mechanism suggesting an oncogenic role of this miRNA, in line with its upregulation in 22Rv1/DCT^R clones.

In conclusion, we showed that DCT resistant PCa cells release in the growth medium miRNAs whose level change in PCa patients resistant to DCT therapy, suggesting that clones resistant to DCT represent a good in vitro model to identify potential DCT predictive miRNAs to be tested as c-miRNA in PCa patients during DCT treatment. In addition, we showed that not all miRNA specifically released by DCT^R clones were upregulated, suggesting that the miRNAs release may be mediated also by an active mechanism. In perspective, this in vitro approach for discovering miRNAs predictive of the onset of drug resistance may be applied to other tumor types as well as other anticancer drugs.

4. Materials and Methods

4.1. Cells and Culture Conditions

DU-145 and 22Rv1 cell lines were grown in RPMI 1640 medium added of 10% fetal bovine serum, 1% penicillin/streptomycin 2 mM and 1% L-glutammine 2 mM (Euroclone, Milan, Italy). Cells were incubated at 37 °C in a humidified atmosphere containing 6% CO_2. For DCT treatment, cells were grown for 24 h and treated with DCT (Taxotere, 20 mg/mL, Sanofi Aventis, Milan, Italy) for 3 days.

4.2. Dose Response Curves

2×10^5 cells were seeded per well (6 wells multiplate) and exposed to increasing concentration of DCT (Taxotere, 20 mg/mL, Sanofi Aventis). At specified time points, cells were fixed in 2% paraformaldehyde in PBS (Oxoid, Altrincham, Cheshire, UK), and subsequently stained with 0.1% crystal violet (SIGMA, St. Louis, MO, USA) dissolved in 20% methanol (SIGMA) and let dry at room temperature. Cells were then lysed with 10% acetic acid and the optical density (OD 590 nm) of the solution, detected with ChroMate Microtetraplate Reader apparatus (Awareness Technology, Westport, CT, USA), was used to measure cell proliferation.

4.3. Isolation and Characterization of DCT-Resistant (DCT^R) Clones

To obtain DCT^R clones, 5×10^5 cells/100 mm diameter dish were grown in presence of DCT of either 3 nM (22Rv1) or 4 nM (DU-145). Each 3–4 days, the medium was removed and replaced with fresh selective medium until colonies formation (30–50 days). Thereafter, independent colonies were isolated and expanded to clonal populations. To verify whether clones were still resistant to DCT, cells were seeded at density of 2×10^4 cells/cm^2 and 24 h later exposed at increasing concentrations of DCT (range 1–20 nM). After 72 h exposure, cell proliferation was determined as reported above. The generation times were calculated dividing the hours in culture by the number of cell doublings calculated as [$\lg_2$ (final cell number/initial cell number)/$\lg_2$ 2].

4.4. Rhodamine 123 Exclusion Assay

The assay was performed as previously described [30] with some modifications. Briefly, for each sample of DU-145 or 22Rv1 cells and DCT^R clones, 2 aliquots of 4×10^4 cells/mL were incubated at 37 °C with 1 μL of Rhodamine 123 (Rh123) (1 mM, SIGMA) and with or without 1 μL of Verapamil (50 mM, SIGMA). After 30 min, cells were harvested and centrifuged and each aliquot was split into two aliquots and analyzed with FACScalibur cytofluorimeter (BD Biosciences, San Jose, CA, USA) immediately (aliquot 1) and after 1 h (aliquot 2). Rh123 green was recorded on FL1 channel and the gate was set to exclude fluorescence of both aliquot 1 samples and verapamil minus aliquot 2 sample. The Rh123 extrusion was detected in the verapamil plus aliquot 2 sample and expressed as percentage of cells with a fluorescence different from the one excluded from the gate.

4.5. Total RNA Isolation

Intracellular total RNA was extracted with miRNeasy mini kit (Qiagen, Hilden, Germany) following the manufacturer's instructions. For NGS experiment, extracellular total RNA was isolated from 2 mL growth medium with QIAamp circulating nucleic acid kit (Qiagen), following the manufacturer's instructions. For qRT-PCR analysis, extracellular total RNA extraction was performed as previously described [7].

4.6. miRNAs and mRNA Quantification

miRNAs and mRNAs quantification were performed as previously described [7]. Transcripts values were normalized to those obtained from the amplification of the internal control (GAPDH,

HPRT1, β-actin for mRNAs and U6, sno-44, sno-55, sno-110 for intracellular miRNA and cel-miR-39 for extracellular miRNAs).

4.7. *miRNA Profiling with Next-Generation Sequencing (NGS) Technology (Small RNA-Seq)*

The small RNA libraries were constructed using TruSeq Small RNA kit (Illumina, San Diego, CA, USA) according to the manufacturer's suggestions. cDNA libraries were loaded at six-plex level of multiplexing (~4 million reads per samples) into a flow cell V3, and sequenced in a single-reads mode (50 bp) on a MiSeq sequencer (Illumina). Raw reads were analyzed as described in Barsanti et al. [31]. Briefly, raw sequences were de-multiplexed using the Illumina pipline CASAVA v.1.8.2. software (Illumina). FastQC was used for quality check and primary reads were trimmed of adapters sequence using Cutadapt v1.2.1 [32]. Remaining reads, with a minimum length of 17 bzp and maximum 35 bp after trimming, were clustered for unique hits and mapped to pre-miRNA sequences present into the miRBase (rel. 21) employing miRExpress tool v 2.1.3 [33].

4.8. *Statistical Analysis*

Data are expressed as mean ± SD of at least three independent experiments, and analyzed with Student's *t*-test.

The differential analysis was performed using two different statistical methods implemented in the two packages, edgeR [34] and DESeq2 [35] of the R Bioconductor repository. Exact *p*-values were adjusted for multiple testing according to Benjamini–Hochberg procedure. In order to control the batch effect of the two sequencing runs of the DU-145/DCT^R clones experiment, the analysis was corrected for baseline differences between the batches using an additive model in the design formula of both edgeR and DESeq2 approaches.

The hierarchical clustering was performed using the mean centered Log2 normalized reads, the Euclidean distance and complete agglomerative method.

Acknowledgments: We would like to thank Stefania Biagini (Fondazione Toscana Gabriele Monasterio, FTGM, Pisa) for giving us taxotere and Giuseppe Rainaldi for critical reading of the manuscript. This work was supported by the Istituto Toscano Tumori (grant 2010-Giuseppe Rainaldi; grant 2013-Milena Rizzo).

Author Contributions: Milena Rizzo conceived and designed the experiments. Lorenzo Bascetta, Monica Evangelista, Arianna Oliviero and Milena Rizzo performed the experiments. Milena Rizzo, Lorenzo Bascetta, Arianna Oliviero analyzed the data. Romina D'Aurizio and Alberto Mercatanti analyzed the NGS data. Milena Rizzo wrote the paper. Sergio Bracarda, Marco Pellegrini, Francesca Marrocolo revised the manuscript.

References

1. Schurko, B.; Oh, W.K. Docetaxel chemotherapy remains the standard of care in castration-resistant prostate cancer. *Nat. Clin. Pract. Oncol.* **2008**, *5*, 506–507. [CrossRef] [PubMed]
2. Petrylak, D.P.; Tangen, C.M.; Hussain, M.H.; Lara, P.N., Jr.; Jones, J.A.; Taplin, M.E.; Burch, P.A.; Berry, D.; Moinpour, C.; Kohli, M.; et al. Docetaxel and estramustine compared with mitoxantrone and prednisone for advanced refractory prostate cancer. *N. Engl. J. Med.* **2004**, *351*, 1513–1520. [CrossRef] [PubMed]
3. Endzelins, E.; Melne, V.; Kalnina, Z.; Lietuvietis, V.; Riekstina, U.; Llorente, A.; Line, A. Diagnostic, prognostic and predictive value of cell-free miRNAs in prostate cancer: A systematic review. *Mol. Cancer* **2016**, *15*, 41. [CrossRef] [PubMed]
4. Filella, X.; Foj, L. miRNAs as novel biomarkers in the management of prostate cancer. *Clin. Chem. Lab. Med.* **2017**, *55*, 715–736. [CrossRef] [PubMed]
5. Zhang, H.L.; Yang, L.F.; Zhu, Y.; Yao, X.D.; Zhang, S.L.; Dai, B.; Zhu, Y.P.; Shen, Y.J.; Shi, G.H.; Ye, D.W. Serum miRNA-21: Elevated levels in patients with metastatic hormone-refractory prostate cancer and potential predictive factor for the efficacy of docetaxel-based chemotherapy. *Prostate* **2011**, *71*, 326–331. [CrossRef] [PubMed]

6. Cheng, H.H.; Mitchell, P.S.; Kroh, E.M.; Dowell, A.E.; Chery, L.; Siddiqui, J.; Nelson, P.S.; Vessella, R.L.; Knudsen, B.S.; Chinnaiyan, A.M.; et al. Circulating microRNA profiling identifies a subset of metastatic prostate cancer patients with evidence of cancer-associated hypoxia. *PLoS ONE* **2013**, *8*, e69239. [CrossRef] [PubMed]
7. Lucotti, S.; Rainaldi, G.; Evangelista, M.; Rizzo, M. Fludarabine treatment favors the retention of miR-485-3p by prostate cancer cells: Implications for survival. *Mol. Cancer* **2013**, *12*, 52. [CrossRef] [PubMed]
8. Yamanaka, K.; Rocchi, P.; Miyake, H.; Fazli, L.; So, A.; Zangemeister-Wittke, U.; Gleave, M.E. Induction of apoptosis and enhancement of chemosensitivity in human prostate cancer LNCaP cells using bispecific antisense oligonucleotide targeting *Bcl-2* and *Bcl-xL* genes. *BJU Int.* **2006**, *97*, 1300–1308. [CrossRef] [PubMed]
9. Terry, S.; Ploussard, G.; Allory, Y.; Nicolaiew, N.; Boissiere-Michot, F.; Maille, P.; Kheuang, L.; Coppolani, E.; Ali, A.; Bibeau, F.; et al. Increased expression of class III beta-tubulin in castration-resistant human prostate cancer. *Br. J. Cancer* **2009**, *101*, 951–956. [CrossRef] [PubMed]
10. Sartor, O.; Gillessen, S. Treatment sequencing in metastatic castrate-resistant prostate cancer. *Asian J. Androl.* **2014**, *16*, 426–431. [CrossRef] [PubMed]
11. Hathaway, A.R.; Baker, M.K.; Sonpavde, G. Emerging agents for the therapy of advanced prostate cancer. *Future Oncol.* **2015**, *11*, 2775–2787. [CrossRef] [PubMed]
12. Cheng, G. Circulating miRNAs: Roles in cancer diagnosis, prognosis and therapy. *Adv. Drug Deliv. Rev.* **2015**, *81*, 75–93. [CrossRef] [PubMed]
13. Larrea, E.; Sole, C.; Manterola, L.; Goicoechea, I.; Armesto, M.; Arestin, M.; Caffarel, M.M.; Araujo, A.M.; Araiz, M.; Fernandez-Mercado, M.; et al. New concepts in cancer biomarkers: Circulating miRNAs in liquid biopsies. *Int. J. Mol. Sci.* **2016**, *17*, 627. [CrossRef] [PubMed]
14. Armand-Labit, V.; Pradines, A. Circulating cell-free microRNAs as clinical cancer biomarkers. *Biomol. Concepts* **2017**, *8*, 61–81. [CrossRef] [PubMed]
15. Gonzales, J.C.; Fink, L.M.; Goodman, O.B., Jr.; Symanowski, J.T.; Vogelzang, N.J.; Ward, D.C. Comparison of circulating MicroRNA 141 to circulating tumor cells, lactate dehydrogenase, and prostate-specific antigen for determining treatment response in patients with metastatic prostate cancer. *Clin. Genitourin. Cancer* **2011**, *9*, 39–45. [CrossRef] [PubMed]
16. Selth, L.A.; Townley, S.L.; Bert, A.G.; Stricker, P.D.; Sutherland, P.D.; Horvath, L.G.; Goodall, G.J.; Butler, L.M.; Tilley, W.D. Circulating microRNAs predict biochemical recurrence in prostate cancer patients. *Br. J. Cancer* **2013**, *109*, 641–650. [CrossRef] [PubMed]
17. Lin, H.M.; Castillo, L.; Mahon, K.L.; Chiam, K.; Lee, B.Y.; Nguyen, Q.; Boyer, M.J.; Stockler, M.R.; Pavlakis, N.; Marx, G.; et al. Circulating microRNAs are associated with docetaxel chemotherapy outcome in castration-resistant prostate cancer. *Br. J. Cancer* **2014**, *110*, 2462–2471. [CrossRef] [PubMed]
18. Lin, H.M.; Mahon, K.L.; Spielman, C.; Gurney, H.; Mallesara, G.; Stockler, M.R.; Bastick, P.; Briscoe, K.; Marx, G.; Swarbrick, A.; et al. Phase 2 study of circulating microRNA biomarkers in castration-resistant prostate cancer. *Br. J. Cancer* **2017**, *116*, 1002–1011. [CrossRef] [PubMed]
19. James, N.D.; Sydes, M.R.; Clarke, N.W.; Mason, M.D.; Dearnaley, D.P.; Spears, M.R.; Ritchie, A.W.; Parker, C.C.; Russell, J.M.; Attard, G.; et al. Addition of docetaxel, zoledronic acid, or both to first-line long-term hormone therapy in prostate cancer (STAMPEDE): Survival results from an adaptive, multiarm, multistage, platform randomised controlled trial. *Lancet* **2016**, *387*, 1163–1177. [CrossRef]
20. O'Neill, A.J.; Prencipe, M.; Dowling, C.; Fan, Y.; Mulrane, L.; Gallagher, W.M.; O'Connor, D.; O'Connor, R.; Devery, A.; Corcoran, C.; et al. Characterisation and manipulation of docetaxel resistant prostate cancer cell lines. *Mol. Cancer* **2011**, *10*, 126. [CrossRef] [PubMed]
21. Zhu, Y.; Liu, C.; Nadiminty, N.; Lou, W.; Tummala, R.; Evans, C.P.; Gao, A.C. Inhibition of ABCB1 expression overcomes acquired docetaxel resistance in prostate cancer. *Mol. Cancer Ther.* **2013**, *12*, 1829–1836. [CrossRef] [PubMed]
22. Corcoran, C.; Rani, S.; O'Brien, K.; O'Neill, A.; Prencipe, M.; Sheikh, R.; Webb, G.; McDermott, R.; Watson, W.; Crown, J.; et al. Docetaxel-resistance in prostate cancer: Evaluating associated phenotypic changes and potential for resistance transfer via exosomes. *PLoS ONE* **2012**, *7*, e50999. [CrossRef] [PubMed]
23. Makarova, J.A.; Shkurnikov, M.U.; Wicklein, D.; Lange, T.; Samatov, T.R.; Turchinovich, A.A.; Tonevitsky, A.G. Intracellular and extracellular microRNA: An update on localization and biological role. *Prog. Histochem. Cytochem.* **2016**, *51*, 33–49. [CrossRef] [PubMed]

24. Turchinovich, A.; Tonevitsky, A.G.; Burwinkel, B. Extracellular miRNA: A collision of two paradigms. *Trends Biochem. Sci.* **2016**, *41*, 883–892. [CrossRef] [PubMed]
25. Huang, X.; Le, Q.T.; Giaccia, A.J. MiR-210-micromanager of the hypoxia pathway. *Trends Mol. Med.* **2010**, *16*, 230–237. [CrossRef] [PubMed]
26. Bertout, J.A.; Patel, S.A.; Simon, M.C. The impact of O_2 availability on human cancer. *Nat. Rev. Cancer* **2008**, *8*, 967–975. [CrossRef] [PubMed]
27. Taddei, M.L.; Cavallini, L.; Comito, G.; Giannoni, E.; Folini, M.; Marini, A.; Gandellini, P.; Morandi, A.; Pintus, G.; Raspollini, M.R.; et al. Senescent stroma promotes prostate cancer progression: The role of miR-210. *Mol. Oncol.* **2014**, *8*, 1729–1746. [CrossRef] [PubMed]
28. Hong, X.; Sin, W.C.; Harris, A.L.; Naus, C.C. Gap junctions modulate glioma invasion by direct transfer of microRNA. *Oncotarget* **2015**, *6*, 15566. [CrossRef] [PubMed]
29. Thuringer, D.; Boucher, J.; Jego, G.; Pernet, N.; Cronier, L.; Hammann, A.; Solary, E.; Garrido, C. Transfer of functional microRNAs between glioblastoma and microvascular endothelial cells through gap junctions. *Oncotarget* **2016**, *7*, 73925–73934. [CrossRef] [PubMed]
30. Touil, Y.; Zuliani, T.; Wolowczuk, I.; Kuranda, K.; Prochazkova, J.; Andrieux, J.; Le Roy, H.; Mortier, L.; Vandomme, J.; Jouy, N.; et al. The PI3K/AKT signaling pathway controls the quiescence of the low-Rhodamine123-retention cell compartment enriched for melanoma stem cell activity. *Stem Cells* **2013**, *31*, 641–651. [CrossRef] [PubMed]
31. Barsanti, C.; Trivella, M.G.; D'Aurizio, R.; El Baroudi, M.; Baumgart, M.; Groth, M.; Caruso, R.; Verde, A.; Botta, L.; Cozzi, L.; et al. Differential regulation of microRNAs in end-stage failing hearts is associated with left ventricular assist device unloading. *BioMed Res. Int.* **2015**, *2015*, 592512. [CrossRef] [PubMed]
32. Martin, M. Cutadapt removes adapter sequences from high-throughput sequencing reads. *EMBnet. J.* **2011**, *17*, 10–12. [CrossRef]
33. Wang, W.C.; Lin, F.M.; Chang, W.C.; Lin, K.Y.; Huang, H.D.; Lin, N.S. miRExpress: Analyzing high-throughput sequencing data for profiling microRNA expression. *BMC Bioinform.* **2009**, *10*, 328. [CrossRef] [PubMed]
34. McCarthy, D.J.; Chen, Y.; Smyth, G.K. Differential expression analysis of multifactor RNA-Seq experiments with respect to biological variation. *Nucleic Acids Res.* **2012**, *40*, 4288–4297. [CrossRef] [PubMed]
35. Love, M.I.; Huber, W.; Anders, S. Moderated estimation of fold change and dispersion for RNA-seq data with DESeq2. *Genome Biol.* **2014**, *15*, 550. [CrossRef] [PubMed]

9

The Role of the Neutrophil to Lymphocyte Ratio for Survival Outcomes in Patients with Metastatic Castration-Resistant Prostate Cancer Treated with Abiraterone

Martin Boegemann [1,†,*], Katrin Schlack [1,†], Stefan Thomes [1], Julie Steinestel [1], Kambiz Rahbar [2], Axel Semjonow [1], Andres Jan Schrader [1], Martin Aringer [3] and Laura-Maria Krabbe [1,4]

[1] Department of Urology, Prostate Center, University Hospital Muenster, Albert-Schweitzer-Campus 1, GB A1, D-48149 Muenster, Germany; katrin.schlack@ukmuenster.de (K.S.); s_thom09@uni-muenster.de (S.T.); Julie.steinestel@ukmuenster.de (J.S.); axel.semjonow@ukmuenster.de (A.S.); andresjan.schrader@ukmuenster.de (A.J.S.); laura-maria.krabbe@ukmuenster.de (L.-M.K.)

[2] Department of Nuclear Medicine, Muenster University Medical Center, Albert-Schweitzer-Campus 1, GB A1, D-48149 Muenster, Germany; kambiz.rahbar@ukmuenster.de

[3] Department of Rheumatology, Dresden University Medical Center, Fetscherstraße 74, D-01307 Dresden, Germany; martin.aringer@uniklinikum-dresden.de

[4] Department of Urology, University of Texas Southwestern Medical Center, Dallas, TX 75390-9110, USA

* Correspondence: martin.boegemann@ukmuenster.de

† These authors contributed equally to this work.

Academic Editor: Carsten Stephan

Abstract: The purpose of this study was to examine the prognostic capability of baseline neutrophil-to-lymphocyte-ratio (NLR) and NLR-change under Abiraterone in metastatic castration-resistant prostate cancer patients. The impact of baseline NLR and change after eight weeks of treatment on progression-free survival (PFS) and overall survival (OS) was analyzed using Kaplan-Meier-estimates and Cox-regression. 79 men with baseline NLR <5 and 17 with NLR >5 were analyzed. In baseline analysis of PFS NLR >5 was associated with non-significantly shorter median PFS (five versus 10 months) (HR: 1.6 (95%CI:0.9–2.8); $p = 0.11$). After multivariate adjustment (MVA), ECOG > 0–1, baseline LDH>upper limit of normal (UNL) and presence of visceral metastases were independent prognosticators. For OS, NLR >5 was associated with shorter survival (seven versus 19 months) (HR: 2.3 (95%CI:1.3–4.0); $p < 0.01$). In MVA, ECOG > 0–1 and baseline LDH > UNL remained independent prognosticators. After 8 weeks of Abiraterone NLR-change to <5 prognosticated worse PFS (five versus 12 months) (HR: 4.1 (95%CI:1.1–15.8); $p = 0.04$). MVA showed a trend towards worse PFS for NLR-change to <5 ($p = 0.11$). NLR-change to <5 led to non-significant shorter median OS (seven versus 16 months) (HR: 2.3 (95%CI:0.7–7.1); $p = 0.15$). MVA showed non-significant difference for OS. We concluded baseline NLR <5 is associated with improved survival. In contrast, in patients with baseline NLR >5, NLR-change to <5 after eight weeks of Abiraterone was associated with worse survival and should be interpreted carefully.

Keywords: neutrophil-to-lymphocyte ratio; castration-resistant prostate cancer; prognostic biomarker; treatment response; abiraterone

1. Introduction

Lately, several agents were approved for treatment of metastatic castration-resistant prostate cancer (mCRPC). These include, prior to Docetaxel chemotherapy, Abiraterone [1], Enzalutamide [2] and Sipuleucel-T [3], or after Docetaxel chemotherapy, Abiraterone [4], Enzalutamide [5] and Cabazitaxel [6], or when no chemotherapy is indicated in bone-predominant mCRPC without visceral metastases, radium-223 [7]. All of these medications prolong overall survival (OS). However, there is a shortage of available biomarkers to predict response to each therapy and no data concerning the optimal sequence of therapies. Therefore, the decision which medication to choose is largely based on empirical data, experience, or matters like drug availability or the possibility of reimbursement. Further, early imaging, especially in bone mCRPC can be misleading due to the bone flare phenomenon which can represent a response to treatment, although suggesting progressive disease (PD) [8].

Inflammation is recognized to be a relevant driver of cancer progression [9]. The neutrophil-to-lymphocyte ratio (NLR) as an indicator of cancer-related inflammation has been shown to be predictive for treatment response or even suggested as a marker of therapy control in various tumour entities, for example in renal cell cancer, oesophageal cancer, gastrointestinal cancer, and many others [10–13]. In mCRPC patients treated with Ketoconazole, a NLR cut-off of <3 was identified for differentiation between patients with longer or shorter progression-free survival (PFS) [14]. In the SUN-1120-trial on Sunitinib vs. Placebo in mCRPC Sonpavde found that a NLR > 2.5 and even more so >5 was prognostic of poor OS [15]. And in a post hoc analysis of men treated with Docetaxel within the TAX-327 and VENICE-trials a NLR >than the median of 2, 2.1 was associated with worse survival [16]. A retrospective study on mCRPC patients treated with Abiraterone identified a baseline NLR of <5 in combination with the extent of metastatic spread to be associated with prostate-specific antigen (PSA) response, and overall survival [17].

We hypothesize that in mCRPC patients treated with Abiraterone, the NLR might not only be useable as a predictor of treatment response at baseline, but also as a marker of early treatment response.

2. Results

2.1. Patient Characteristics

The descriptive characteristics of the cohort are presented in Table 1. The study cohort consisted of 96 mCRPC patients, of whom 52 were treated within the pre- and 44 in the post-Docetaxel setting. The median follow-up was 20.0 months (interquartile range (IQR): 11.0–28.0). The median time of Abiraterone treatment was 10.0 months (IQR: 6.0–14.3). No dose modification was necessary for any patient. The median age of the patients was 70.0 years (IQR: 62.0–76.3). Visceral metastases were present in 28.1% at the beginning of Abiraterone treatment. An unfavourable Gleason-Score of $\geq$8 was seen in 59.8% of the men. The median baseline values of PSA, alkaline phosphatase (ALP) and LDH (lactate dehydrogenase) were 134 ng/mL (IQR: 45–349), 126 U/L (IQR: 86–296) and 251 U/L (IQR: 210–358), respectively.

At baseline, a NLR of <5 was present in 79 (82.3%) of the patients. Compared with men with a NLR >5, patients with a NLR <5 had a significantly lower median baseline PSA-level (91 vs. 224 ng/mL; Mann-Whitney *U*-test: $p = 0.04$) and lower baseline median LDH-levels (240 vs. 308 U/L; $p = 0.04$). Further, the baseline LDH was elevated above the upper limit of normal (ULN) at baseline in a larger proportion in the men with a NLR >5 (88.2% vs. 59.5%; χ^2-test: $p = 0.03$). The other baseline characteristics were not statistically different. Bone protective medication (Denosumab or Zoledronic acid) was well balanced between both groups (58.8% vs. 59.5%; χ^2-test: $p = 0.96$) (Table 1).

According to prostate cancer working group 2 (PCWG2)-criteria, PSA-response is defined as a PSA decline of $\geq$50% and was seen in 35.4% of the patients with a baseline NLR >5 compared with 53.2% of the men with a baseline NLR <5 (χ^2-test: $p = 0.18$). A decline of $\geq$90% was found in 5.9% vs. 27.8% (χ^2-test: $p = 0.06$).

Table 1. Characteristics of patients with metastatic castration-resistant prostate cancer (mCRPC) on Abiraterone with a neutrophil-to-lymphocyte-ratio (NLR) <5 and >5.

Variable	All	NLR <5	NLR >5	*p*
Patients (*n*) (%)	96	79 (82.3)	17 (17.7)	
Median NLR Baseline (ng/mL) (IQR)	3.2 (2.5–4.5)			
Age, median (years) (IQR)	70.0 (63.0–76.3)	70.0 (62.0–76.0)	70.0 (65.0–78.0)	0.60
Median follow-up	20.0 (11.0–28.0)	17.5 (11.0–26.8)	29.0 (29.0–29.0)	0.28
Median duration AA therapy (months) (IQR)	10.0 (6.0–14.3)	11.0 (7.0–15.0)	7.0 (5.0–11.5)	0.08
GS ≥8 (*n*) (%)	55 (59.8)	46 (60.5)	9 (56.3)	0.75
Lnn. Metastases (*n*) (%)	61 (63.5)	50 (63.3)	11 (64.7)	0.91
Visceral Metastases (*n*) (%)	27 (28.1)	24 (30.4)	3 (17.6)	0.38
Bone Metastases (*n*) (%)	85 (88.5)	69 (87.3)	16 (94.1)	0.68
Pre CTX (*n*) (%)	52 (54.2)	44 (55.7)	8 (47.1)	0.52
Post CTX (*n*) (%)	44 (45.8)	35 (44.3)	9 (52.9)	
Patients died (*n*) (%)	67 (69.8)	51 (64.6)	16 (94.1)	0.02
ECOG (all) (*n*) (%)				
0	19 (20.0)	16 (20.5)	3 (17.6)	
1	57 (60.0)	47 (60.3)	10 (58.8)	0.91
2	19 (20.0)	15 (19.2)	4 (23.5)	
Antiresorptive therapy (*n*) (%)	57 (59.4)	47 (59.5)	10 (58.8)	0.96
Zoledronic acid (*n*) (%)	40 (41.7)	33 (41.8)	7 (41.2)	0.96
Denosumab (*n*) (%)	19 (19.8)	15 (19.0)	4 (23.5)	0.67
Best clinical outcome (*n*) (%)				
CR	1 (1.1)	1 (1.3)	0 (0)	
PR	54 (56.8)	46 (59.0)	8 (47.1)	0.61
SD	27 (28.4)	20 (25.6)	7 (41.2)	
PD	13 (13.7)	11 (14.1)	2 (11.8)	
PSA red. ≥50% (*n*) (%)	48 (50.0)	42 (53.2)	6 (35.3)	0.18
PSA red. ≥90% (*n*) (%)	23 (24.0)	22 (27.8)	1 (5.9)	0.06
Median PSA Baseline (ng/mL) (IQR)	134 (45–349)	91 (35–334)	224 (107–589)	0.04
Median LDH Baseline (U/L) (IQR)	251 (210–358)	240 (205–357)	308 (245–386)	0.04
LDH BL >UNL (*n*) (%)	62 (64.6)	47 (59.5)	15 (88.2)	0.03
Median ALP Baseline (U/L) (IQR)	126 (86–296)	126 (91–297)	103 (77–266)	0.43

Abbreviations: NLR: neutrophil-to-lymphocyte ratio; IQR: interquartile range; Lnn: lymphonodal; CTX: chemotherapy; CR: complete remission; PR: partial remission; SD: stable disease; PD: progressive disease; ECOG: Easter collaborative Oncology Group; GS: Gleason score; PSA: prostate specific antigen; LDH: lactate dehydrogenase; ALP: alkaline phosphatase; BL: baseline; UNL: upper normal limit.

2.2. *Prognostication of Survival Outcomes at Baseline*

Results of univariate and multivariate analyses for PFS and OS based on baseline NLR (>5 vs. <5) are displayed in Tables 2–4.

Table 2. Univariate analysis for baseline biomarkers for progression-free survival in (a) 96 mCRPC-patients prior to Abiraterone therapy and (b) in 17 patients with a baseline NLR >5 after eight weeks of therapy.

(a) Univariate Analysis PFS at Baseline			**(b) Univariate Analysis of PFS in *n* = 17 Patients with Baseline NLR > 5 after Eight Weeks of Abiraterone**		
Variable	**HR (95%CI)**	***p***	**Variable**	**HR (95%CI)**	***p***
ECOG			ECOG		
0–1	1 (reference)	<0.01	0–1	1 (reference)	0.57
2	2.9 (1.7–4.9)		2	1.4 (0.4–4.8)	
LDH baseline >UNL			LDH baseline >UNL	1 (reference)	
No	1 (reference)	<0.01	No		0.52
Yes	2.6 (1.6–4.3)		Yes	2.0 (0.3–15.4)	
Visceral metastases			Visceral metastases		
No	1 (reference)	0.02	No	1 (reference)	0.85
Yes	2.2 (1.4–3.5)		Yes	0.9 (0.2–3.3)	
ALP baseline >UNL			ALP baseline >UNL		
No	1 (reference)	0.13	No	1 (reference)	0.55
Yes	1.4 (0.9–2.1)		Yes	1.4 (0.5–3.9)	

Table 2. *Cont.*

(a) Univariate Analysis PFS at Baseline			(b) Univariate Analysis of PFS in n = 17 Patients with Baseline NLR > 5 after Eight Weeks of Abiraterone		
Variable	**HR (95%CI)**	***p***	**Variable**	**HR (95%CI)**	***p***
NLR			NLR		
<5	1 (reference)	0.11	No change	1 (reference)	0.04
>5	1.6 (0.9–2.8)		Change to <5	4.1 (1.1–15.8)	
Abiraterone			PSA decline ≥50%		
Pre-Docetaxel	1 (reference)	0.10	Yes	1 (reference)	0.14
Post-Docetaxel	1.4 (0.9–2.2)		No	2.7 (0.7–10.2)	
Gleason Score			Abiraterone		
<8	1 (reference)	0.10	Pre-Docetaxel	1 (reference)	0.41
≥8	1.5 (0.9–2.3)		Post-Docetaxel	1.6 (0.5–4.6)	
Lymphonodal metastases			Gleason Score		
No	1 (reference)	0.77	<8	1 (reference)	0.63
Yes	0.9 (0.6–1.5)		≥8	1.3 (0.4–3.9)	
Bone Metastases			Lymphonodal metastases		
No	1 (reference)	0.82	No	1 (reference)	0.41
Yes	1.1 (0.5–2.2)		Yes	0.6 (0.2–1.9)	

Abbreviations: PFS: progression free survival; HR: hazard ratio; 95%CI: 95% confidence interval; ECOG: Eastern Collaborative Oncology Group; LDH: lactate dehydrogenase; UNL: upper normal limit; PSA: prostate-specific antigen; NLR: neutrophil-to-lymphocyte ratio; ALP: alkaline phosphatase; OS: overall survival.

Table 3. Univariate analysis for baseline biomarkers for overall survival in (a) 96 mCRPC-patients prior to Abiraterone therapy and (b) in 17 patients with a baseline NLR >5 after eight weeks of therapy.

(a) Univariate Analysis OS at Baseline			(b) Univariate Analysis of OS in n = 17 Patients with Baseline NLR >5 after Eight Weeks of Abiraterone		
Variable	**HR (95%CI)**	***p***	**Variable**	**HR (95%CI)**	***p***
ECOG			ECOG		
0–1	1 (reference)	<0.01	0–1	1 (reference)	0.60
2	3.4 (1.9–6.0)		2	1.4 (0.3–4.5)	
LDH baseline >UNL			LDH baseline >UNL		
No	1 (reference)	<0.01	No	1 (reference)	0.65
Yes	3.1 (1.7–5.8)		Yes	0.7 (0.2–3.3)	
Visceral metastases			Visceral metastases		
No	1 (reference)	0.35	No	1 (reference)	0.76
Yes	1.3 (0.8–2.2)		Yes	0.8 (0.2–2.9)	
ALP baseline >UNL			ALP baseline >UNL		
No	1 (reference)	<0.01	No	1 (reference)	0.83
Yes	1.9 (1.2–3.2)		Yes	0.9 (0.3–2.5)	
NLR			NLR		
<5	1 (reference)	<0.01	No change	1 (reference)	0.15
>5	2.3 (1.3–4.0)		Change to <5	2.3 (0.7–7.1)	
Abiraterone			PSA decline ≥50%		
Pre-Docetaxel	1 (reference)	0.06	Yes	1 (reference)	0.08
Post-Docetaxel	1.6 (1.0–2.6)		No	2.9 (0.9–9.4)	
Gleason Score			Abiraterone		
<8	1 (reference)	0.67	Pre-Docetaxel	1 (reference)	0.38
≥8	1.1 (0.7–1.9)		Post-Docetaxel	1.6 (0.6–4.6)	
Lymphonodal metastases			Gleason Score		
No	1 (reference)	0.35	<8	1 (reference)	0.93
Yes	0.8 (0.5–1.3)		≥8	1.1 (0.4–3.0)	
Bone metastases			Lymphonodal metastases		
No	1 (reference)	0.62	No	1 (reference)	0.64
Yes	1.3 (0.5–3.2)		Yes	0.8 (0.3–2.2)	

Abbreviations: PFS: progression-free survival; HR: hazard ratio; 95%CI: 95% confidence interval; ECOG: Eastern Collaborative Oncology Group; LDH: lactate dehydrogenase; UNL: upper normal limit; PSA: prostate-specific antigen; NLR: neutrophil-to-lymphocyte ratio; ALP: alkaline phosphatase; OS: overall survival.

Table 4. Multivariate analysis for significant baseline biomarkers for (a) progression-free and (b) overall survival in 96 mCRPC-patients prior to Abiraterone therapy and (c) progression-free survival and (d) overall survival in 17 patients with a baseline NLR >5 after eight weeks of therapy.

(a) Multivariate Analysis PFS at Baseline

Variable	HR (95%CI)	*p*
ECOG		
0–1	1 (reference)	0.01
2	2.6 (1.5–4.5)	
LDH baseline >UNL		
No	1 (reference)	0.01
Yes	2.2 (1.3–3.8)	
Visceral metastases		
No	1 (reference)	0.04
Yes	1.7 (1.0–2.9)	
ALP baseline >UNL		
No	1 (reference)	0.25
Yes	1.3 (0.8–2.1)	
NLR		
<5	1 (reference)	0.71
>5	1.1 (0.6–2.0)	

(b) Multivariate analysis OS at baseline

Variable	HR (95%CI)	*p*
ECOG		
0–1	1 (reference)	<0.01
2	3.0 (1.6–5.5)	
LDH baseline >UNL		
No	1 (reference)	0.01
Yes	2.4 (1.2–4.6)	
Visceral metastases		
No	1 (reference)	0.56
Yes	1.2 (0.7–2.1)	
ALP baseline >UNL		
No	1 (reference)	0.05
Yes	1.7 (1.0–2.9)	
NLR		
<5	1 (reference)	0.10
>5	1.7 (0.9–3.0)	

(c) Multivariate analysis of PFS in *n* =17 Patients with Baseline NLR >5 after Eight Weeks of Abiraterone

Variable	HR (95%CI)	*p*
NLR		
No change	1 (reference)	0.11
Change to <5	3.4 (0.8–15.2)	
PSA decline ≥50%		
Yes	1 (reference)	0.14
No	1.5 (0.3–6.4)	

(d) Multivariate Analysis of OS in *n* = 17 Patients with Baseline NLR >5 after Eight Weeks of Abiraterone

Variable	HR (95%CI)	*p*
NLR		
No change	1 (reference)	0.47
Change to <5	1.6 (0.5–5.6)	
PSA decline ≥50%		
Yes	1 (reference)	0.25
No	2.2 (0.6–8.1)	

Abbreviations: PFS: progression free survival; HR: hazard ratio; 95%CI: 95% confidence interval; ECOG: Eastern Collaborative Oncology Group; LDH: lactate dehydrogenase; UNL: upper normal limit; PSA: prostate-specific antigen; NLR: neutrophil-to-lymphocyte ratio; ALP: alkaline phosphatase; OS: overall survival.

In univariate analysis (Table 2), baseline LDH >ULN (hazard ratio (HR): 2.6 (95% confidence interval (95%CI): 1.6–4.3); $p < 0.01$), Eastern Collaborative Oncology Group performance status (ECOG) ≥ 2 (HR: 2.9 (95%CI: 1.7–4.9); $p < 0.01$), and the presence of visceral metastases (HR: 2.2 (95%CI: 1.4–3.5); $p = 0.02$) were associated with worse PFS.

At baseline there was a trend for improved median PFS of patients with a NLR <5 (10 months (95%CI: 8.1–11.9)) compared with men with a NLR >5 (five months (95%CI: 1.0–9.0), log-rank $p = 0.09$) (Figure 1a).

After adjusting for the parameters significant in univariate analysis and clinically-important variables, ECOG ≥ 2 (HR: 2.6 (95%CI: 1.5–4.5); $p = 0.01$), baseline LDH >UNL (HR: 2.2 (95%CI: 1.3–3.8); $p = 0.01$) and the presence of visceral metastases (HR: 1.7 (95%CI: 1.0–2.9); $p = 0.04$) remained independent prognosticators of poor PFS (Table 4).

The univariate analysis for OS showed that a baseline NLR >5 (HR: 2.3 (95%CI: 1.3–4.0); $p < 0.01$), ECOG $\geq$2 (HR: 3.4 (95%CI: 1.9–6.0); $p < 0.01$), baseline LDH >UNL (HR: 3.1 (95%CI: 1.7–5.8); $p < 0.01$) and baseline ALP >UNL (HR: 1.9 (95%CI: 1.2–3.2); $p < 0.01$) were associated with worse OS (Table 3).

In Kaplan-Meier analysis the median OS (Figure 1c) of men with a baseline NLR <5 (19 months (95%CI 13.0–25.0) was significantly longer than in patients with a NLR >5 (seven months (95%CI: 4.0–10.0), log-rank $p = 0.04$).

In multivariate analysis of OS (Table 4), only ECOG $\geq$2 (HR: 3.0 (95%CI: 1.6–5.5); $p < 0.01$) and baseline LDH >UNL (HR: 2.4 (95%CI: 1.2–4.6); $p = 0.01$) remained independent prognosticators of worse survival. For NLR >5, OS was reduced but not significantly (HR: 1.7 (95%CI: 0.9–3.0); $p = 0.10$).

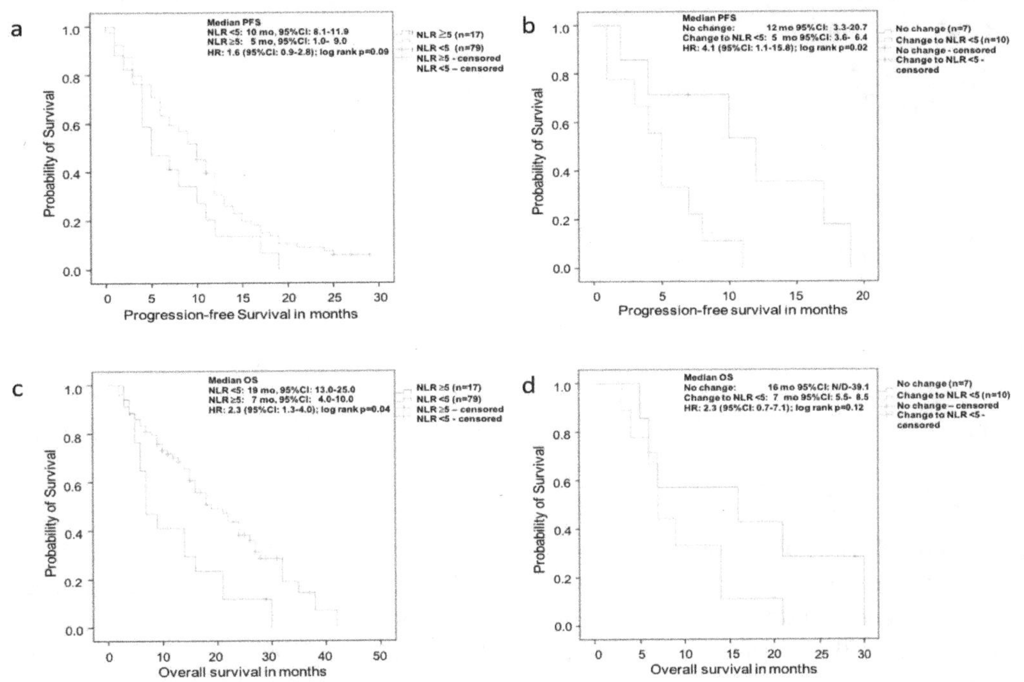

Figure 1. Kaplan-Meier analysis for progression-free survival probability of patients with mCRPC under therapy with Abiraterone (**a**) with baseline neutrophil-to-lymphocyte ratio (NLR) < 5 vs. $\geq$5; (**b**) Patients with or without change of NLR to <5 after eight weeks of therapy and (**c**) overall survival probability with baseline NLR < 5 vs. $\geq$5; and (**d**) patients with or without change of NLR to <5 after eight weeks of therapy.

2.3. *Prognostication of Survival Outcomes with Change of Neutrophil-to-Lymphocyte Ratio (NLR) to <5 in Patients with a Baseline NLR > 5 vs. no Change after Eight Weeks of Abiraterone*

Seventeen men (17.7%) of the whole cohort had a NLR >5 at baseline. In the patients with a change of NLR from >5 to <5 after eight weeks of treatment with Abiraterone ($n = 10$) the neutrophils declined in all but one of the cases in which the lymphocytes increased. Seven patients remained with an NLR of >5 after eight weeks of therapy.

For PFS the univariate Cox-regression analysis (Table 2) showed that change of NLR to <5 at eight weeks of Abiraterone therapy was associated with worse survival (HR: 4.1 (95%CI: 1.1–15.8); $p = 0.04$). All other variables, including decline of PSA $\geq$50%, were no significant prognosticators.

In the Kaplan-Meier analysis of PFS (Figure 1b), equally, the median survival was in favour of no change of NLR (12 months (95%CI 3.3–20.7) compared to change to NLR <5 (five months (95%CI 3.6–6.4), log-rank $p = 0.02$)).

After adjusting for decline of PSA $\geq$50%, there was only a trend for prognostication of worse PFS for change of NLR to <5 (HR: 3.4 (95%CI: 0.8–15.2); $p = 0.11$) (Table 4).

The univariate analysis of OS (Table 3) showed a trend for change of NLR to <5 (HR: 2.3 (95%CI: 0.7–7.1); $p = 0.15$) and no decline of PSA $\geq$50% (HR: 2.9 (95%CI: 0.9–9.4); $p = 0.08$) towards poor survival.

In Kaplan-Meier analysis of OS (Figure 1d) the change of NLR to <5 was associated with a shorter survival of 7 months (95%CI 5.5–8.5) compared with 16 months (95%CI N/D-39.1) in patients with no change of NLR. However, this difference was not statistically significant (log-rank $p = 0.12$).

In multivariate Cox-regression analysis (Table 4) there was no significant difference for the prognostication of worse OS in patients with change of NLR to <5 and no decline of PSA $\geq$50% ($p = 0.47$ and 0.25, respectively).

In Kaplan-Meier analysis of the 79 patients with an initial NLR of <5 at baseline (Figure 2) there was no difference between the subgroup of patients with change of NLR to >5 and in the subgroup with no change of NLR for both PFS and OS (log rank $p = 0.21$, respectively).

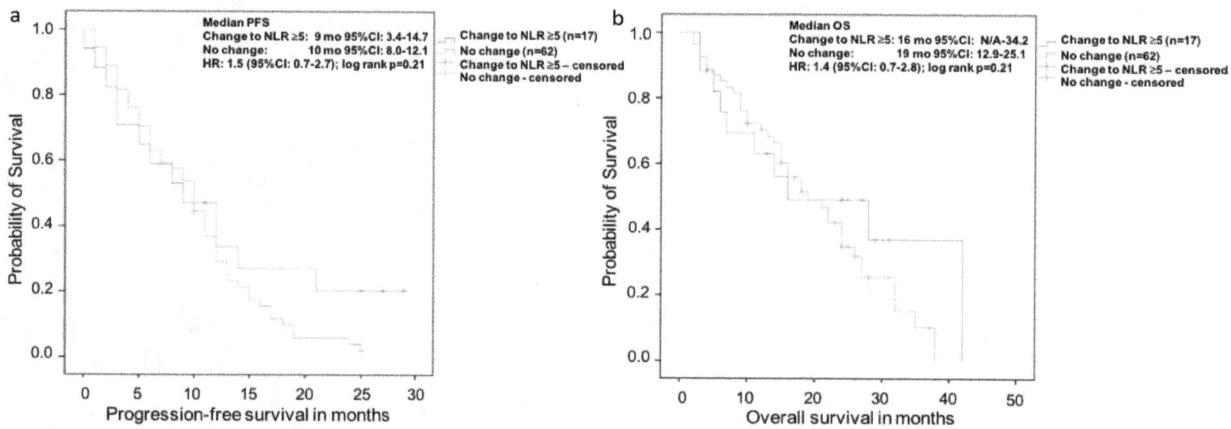

Figure 2. Kaplan-Meier analysis of the subgroup of patients with a NLR <5 at baseline for (**a**) overall survival (OS) and (**b**) progression-free survival (PFS). There was no difference of median survival in the subgroup of patients with a NLR <5 at baseline and change of NLR to >5 vs. no change after eight weeks of Abiraterone therapy (log rank $p = 0.21$). There equally was no difference of median PFS for change of NLR to >5 vs. no change after eight weeks of Abiraterone therapy (log rank $p = 0.21$).

3. Discussion

The NLR was found to be prognostic for survival outcomes and recurrence rate in various tumour entities [18,19]. For prostate cancer, especially in mCRPC, the NLR was equally shown to be prognostic for survival [10,17]. In a study on mCRPC patients treated with Abiraterone, Leibowitz-Amit et al. found that a composite score of baseline NLR <5 and extent of metastatic spread was associated with PSA-response [17]. Our results support these findings. In our cohort of mCRPC patients treated with Abiraterone the baseline NLR with a cut-off of <5 without addition of metastatic spread equally was a prognosticator for prolonged OS. However, after adjustment for other important variables in multivariate analysis there was only a trend towards statistical significance regarding survival. Maybe the limited number of patients with a baseline NLR >5 ($n = 17$) included in this study, precluded reaching significant values in multivariate analyses for survival endpoints.

The underlying immunologic mechanisms are still unclear, but most likely the interactions between tumour cells and immunologic cells and mediators undergo specific changes [9]. An elevated (expected unfavourable) NLR can be caused by rising neutrophils or declining lymphocytes or both. Assuming that a high baseline NLR is prognostic for outcomes under given treatments it would be reasonable to presume that a change of an elevated (expected unfavourable) NLR to a lower (potentially favourable) NLR under treatment could be useful to identify patients with exceptionally good and lasting responses to therapy.

So far, there is very little evidence on NLR as a therapy control marker. For mCRPC there is only one study by Lorente et al., which addressed this matter [10]. Here, in a post hoc analysis of the large registration trial of Cabazitaxel vs. Mitoxantrone, a baseline NLR of <3 was identified to be associated with better survival, better PSA-response and better objective response rate according to RECIST-criteria. Our study is the first to address change of NLR as a treatment response marker in patients treated with Abiraterone. Interestingly, in that study the conversion of an unfavourable NLR of >3 to a favourable NLR < 3 under therapy was independently associated with an improved OS. This result was in line with the expectable. In contrast and most surprisingly, in our study we found that a change of a supposedly unfavourable NLR > 5 to the expected to be favourable NLR <5 after eight weeks of Abiraterone therapy in mCRPC patients was associated with both worse PFS and OS. The reasons for these findings are unclear. One possible explanation could be the immunomodulating effect of Prednisone, which has to be administered to prevent mineral corticoid excess under Abiraterone therapy. In our study, all patients received the recommended dose of 5 mg Prednisone bi-daily with the start of Abiraterone, but no patient had prior prednisone therapy. In the trial of Lorente et al. [10] 45% of the patients had already been on a stable dose of a corticosteroid before initiation of Cabazitaxel-/Mitoxantron-therapy and, thus, at the time when the baseline NLR was determined. The subgroup analysis of patients with or without baseline Prednisone use showed that the patients with Prednisone use had a significantly higher NLR of 3.9 vs. 2.9 ($p < 0.001$) and patients with NLR > 3 were more likely to receive baseline Prednisone ($p = 0.016$). However, Lorente et al. tested for confounding variables and showed that the NLR < 3 was predictive of survival with or without corticosteroid use. This basically supports the role of corticosteroids for elevating the NLR in general. In our study all patients had been treated with Prednisone starting with initiation of Abiraterone therapy. This difference could explain our unexpected findings. Prednisone physiologically leads to an increase of neutrophils first by about 20% by demarginalisation of the intravascular pool, and consecutively, by a greater increase caused by mobilization of the bone marrow neutrophil reserve [20]. Naturally, this effect would be evident for all patients treated with Prednisone and Abiraterone. In the subset of patients with a change of NLR from >5 to <5 after eight weeks of Abiraterone therapy in our study the neutrophils declined in almost all of the cases. An explanation for this may be that these patients had a higher tumour load especially of bone metastases thus leading to a depletion of functioning bone marrow with the production of neutrophils most likely being impaired by bone marrow insufficiency as a result of tumour progression under Abiraterone. The immunomodulating effect of Prednisone under Abiraterone may have a stronger impact due to increasingly depleted bone marrow reserves in case of disease progression.

Recently there were findings that PSA change within four weeks after the start of therapy may be prognostic for survival outcomes. For example, Facchini et al. showed that PSA-change after 15 days of Abiraterone was a surrogate for PFS and OS [21]. Therefore, for future studies, research on change of NLR and the possibility of complement of PSA and change of NLR in this very early setting may be promising.

Our study is limited by problems inherent to the retrospective approach and a relatively small sample size. This holds especially true for the subset of patients with change of NLR to <5. Therefore, our findings need to be validated by prospective studies. The single parameter NLR cut-off of less than, or greater than five needs to be validated as well. We did not do imaging in a per protocol routine fashion and, therefore, could not calculate radiographic PFS.

The underlying effects of the NLR and changes of NLR in relationship to cancer are still unclear and especially our findings concerning unexpected changes under therapy with Prednisone/Abiraterone need to be elucidated.

4. Materials and Methods

4.1. Patients

After ethics committee-approval (2007-467-f-S), we retrospectively reviewed all patients with mCRPC presenting at the Department of Urology in the Muenster University Medical Center between December 2009 and July 2015 and receiving Abiraterone to analyse the impact of the NLR on progression-free and overall survival. All patients gave written informed consent before participating. We performed the study according to the declaration of Helsinki.

The study cohort consisted of confirmed mCRPC patients as defined by PCWG2-criteria [22] in pre- or post-chemotherapy setting. All patients met the requirements for Abiraterone-treatment. The men receiving Abiraterone prior to Docetaxel all had to be asymptomatic or oligo-symptomatic with no need to use opiates and degree of pain of no more than three out of 10 on the numeric-rating-scale. Patients receiving Abiraterone after Docetaxel all had progressive disease on or after chemotherapy. During the reviewed timeframe a total of 96 patients presented with evaluable NLR-data of which 52 patients were treated prior to, and 44 after, chemotherapy, respectively. Five patients (4.8%) had received Enzalutamide prior to Abiraterone. All patients included in the analysis were on a stable dose of anti-bone resorptive medication (Denosumab or Zoledronic acid) at least three months prior to the start of Abiraterone, and during the whole treatment phase, or did not receive antiresorptive medication at all.

The day before start of Abiraterone therapy all patients had blood drawn for baseline analysis of PSA, neutrophils, lymphocytes, and serum chemistry. The analysis of PSA was repeated two and four weeks after initiation of therapy, and four weekly thereafter. Neutrophils and lymphocyte measurements were repeated after eight weeks. PSA-progression was defined according to PCWG2-criteria, i.e., PSA-progression at the date that a 25% or greater increase and an absolute increase of 2 ng/mL or more from the nadir is documented, which is confirmed by a second value obtained three or more weeks later [22].

For documentation of baseline values and changes of soft tissue metastases CT- or MRI-scans of thorax, abdomen and pelvis were performed. For information on bone metastases bone scans were used. Imaging was repeated during the course of the Abiraterone-therapy whenever clinically indicated but not in routine fashion. PD was defined according to RECIST 1.1 criteria for axial cross sectional imaging [23] and by PCWG2 criteria for bone scans [22].

The current response status, i.e., complete remission (CR), partial remission (PR), stable disease (SD) or PD was assessed after each visit. PD was considered evident upon deterioration of general condition or worsening of pain when unequivocally caused be prostate cancer, when PSA-progression occurred or when radiographic progression was detected. The baseline cohort was subdivided according to NLR (group-1 (favorable): NLR < 5; group-2 (non favorable): NLR > 5).

4.2. Statistical Methods

For descriptive statistics we report medians with 95% CI or IQR for continuous variables and as populations and frequencies for categorical variables. We used the χ^2-test, Fisher's exact-test or Mann-Whitney U-test for determining the significance of differences between categorical and continuous variables. For analysis of survival outcomes were applied Kaplan-Meier-analysis. For uni- and multivariate analysis of significance for survival outcomes we used Cox-regression-models. All reported p-values are two-sided and we assumed statistical significance when $p \leq 0.05$. We used SPSS-Statistics V.23 (IBM Inc., Armonk, NY, USA) for statistical assessment.

5. Conclusions

In patients with mCRPC under Abiraterone treatment a pre-treatment NLR < 5 is associated with better survival outcomes. Unexpectedly, after eight weeks of Abiraterone therapy, a change of initially elevated NLR of >5 to <5 was associated with worse survival. The immunomodulating effect of concomitant Prednisone next to Abiraterone combined with insufficient bone marrow reserves in patients with advanced (bony) disease may be the reason for this phenomenon. Thus, a putatively favourable change of NLR to <5 may represent worsening of disease and should be interpreted cautiously. A deeper understanding of the underlying immune mechanisms in this setting is highly warranted. Therefore, larger prospective trials on the matter are needed prior to application of change of NLR in mCRPC.

Author Contributions: Martin Boegemann conceived of the study and participated in its design and coordination, performed part of the statistical analysis and drafted the manuscript. Katrin Schlack helped in acquisition of the data, participated in the study design, performed part of the statistical analysis and participated in critical revision of the manuscript. Stefan Thomes and Julie Steinestel helped in acquisition of the data and participated in critical revision of the manuscript. Kambiz Rahbar participated in critical revision of the manuscript. Axel Semjonow and Andres Jan Schrader participated in critical revision of the manuscript. Martin Aringer helped in drafting and participated in critical revision of the manuscript. Laura-Maria Krabbe helped in acquisition of the data, in statistical analysis and critical revision of the manuscript. All authors read and approved the final manuscript.

Abbreviations

mCRPC	Metastatic castration resistant prostate cancer
OS	Overall survival
PD	Progressive disease
NLR	Neutrophil-to-lymphocyte ratio
PFS	Progression-free survival
PSA	Prostate specific antigen
IQR	Interquartile range
ALP	Alkaline phosphatase
LDH	Lactate dehydrogenase
ULN	Upper normal limit
PCWG2	Prostate cancer working group 2
HR	Hazard ratio
95%CI	95% confidence interval
ECOG	Eastern Collaborative Oncology Group Performance Status
CR	Complete remission
PR	Partial remission
SD	Stable disease

References

1. Ryan, C.J.; Smith, M.R.; Fizazi, K.; Saad, F.; Mulders, P.F.; Sternberg, C.N.; Miller, K.; Logothetis, C.J.; Shore, N.D.; Small, E.J.; et al. Abiraterone acetate plus prednisone versus placebo plus prednisone in chemotherapy-naive men with metastatic castration-resistant prostate cancer (COU-AA-302): Final overall survival analysis of a randomised, double-blind, placebo-controlled phase 3 study. *Lancet Oncol.* **2015**, *16*, 152–160. [CrossRef]
2. Beer, T.M.; Tombal, B. Enzalutamide in metastatic prostate cancer before chemotherapy. *N. Engl. J. Med.* **2014**, *371*, 1755–1756. [CrossRef] [PubMed]
3. Kantoff, P.W.; Higano, C.S.; Shore, N.D.; Berger, E.R.; Small, E.J.; Penson, D.F.; Redfern, C.H.; Ferrari, A.C.; Dreicer, R.; Sims, R.B.; et al. Sipuleucel-T immunotherapy for castration-resistant prostate cancer. *N. Engl. J. Med.* **2010**, *363*, 411–422. [CrossRef] [PubMed]
4. Fizazi, K.; Scher, H.I.; Molina, A.; Logothetis, C.J.; Chi, K.N.; Jones, R.J.; Staffurth, J.N.; North, S.; Vogelzang, N.J.; Saad, F.; et al. Abiraterone acetate for treatment of metastatic castration-resistant prostate cancer: Final overall survival analysis of the COU-AA-301 randomised, double-blind, placebo-controlled phase 3 study. *Lancet Oncol.* **2012**, *13*, 983–992. [CrossRef]
5. Scher, H.I.; Fizazi, K.; Saad, F.; Taplin, M.E.; Sternberg, C.N.; Miller, K.; de Wit, R.; Mulders, P.; Chi, K.N.; Shore, N.D.; et al. Increased survival with enzalutamide in prostate cancer after chemotherapy. *N. Engl. J. Med.* **2012**, *367*, 1187–1197. [PubMed]

6. De Bono, J.S.; Oudard, S.; Ozguroglu, M.; Hansen, S.; Machiels, J.P.; Kocak, I.; Gravis, G.; Bodrogi, I.; Mackenzie, M.J.; Shen, L.; et al. Prednisone plus cabazitaxel or mitoxantrone for metastatic castration-resistant prostate cancer progressing after docetaxel treatment: A randomised open-label trial. *Lancet* **2010**, *376*, 1147–1154. [CrossRef]
7. Parker, C.; Nilsson, S.; Heinrich, D.; Helle, S.I.; O'Sullivan, J.M.; Fossa, S.D.; Chodacki, A.; Wiechno, P.; Logue, J.; Seke, M.; et al. α emitter radium-223 and survival in metastatic prostate cancer. *N. Engl. J. Med.* **2013**, *369*, 213–223. [CrossRef] [PubMed]
8. Ryan, C.J.; Shah, S.; Efstathiou, E.; Smith, M.R.; Taplin, M.E.; Bubley, G.J.; Logothetis, C.J.; Kheoh, T.; Kilian, C.; Haqq, C.M.; et al. Phase II study of abiraterone acetate in chemotherapy-naive metastatic castration-resistant prostate cancer displaying bone flare discordant with serologic response. *Clin. Cancer Res.* **2011**, *17*, 4854–4861. [CrossRef] [PubMed]
9. Hanahan, D.; Weinberg, R.A. Hallmarks of cancer: The next generation. *Cell* **2011**, *144*, 646–674. [CrossRef] [PubMed]
10. Lorente, D.; Mateo, J.; Templeton, A.J.; Zafeiriou, Z.; Bianchini, D.; Ferraldeschi, R.; Bahl, A.; Shen, L.; Su, Z.; Sartor, O.; et al. Baseline neutrophil-lymphocyte ratio (NLR) is associated with survival and response to treatment with second-line chemotherapy for advanced prostate cancer independent of baseline steroid use. *Ann. Oncol.* **2015**, *26*, 750–755. [CrossRef] [PubMed]
11. Luo, Y.; She, D.L.; Xiong, H.; Fu, S.J.; Yang, L. Pretreatment Neutrophil to Lymphocyte Ratio as a Prognostic Predictor of Urologic Tumors: A Systematic Review and Meta-Analysis. *Medicine* **2015**, *94*, e1670. [CrossRef] [PubMed]
12. Xin-Ji, Z.; Yong-Gang, L.; Xiao-Jun, S.; Xiao-Wu, C.; Dong, Z.; Da-Jian, Z. The prognostic role of neutrophils to lymphocytes ratio and platelet count in gastric cancer: A meta-analysis. *Int. J. Surg.* **2015**, *21*, 84–91. [CrossRef] [PubMed]
13. Yodying, H.; Matsuda, A.; Miyashita, M.; Matsumoto, S.; Sakurazawa, N.; Yamada, M.; Uchida, E. Prognostic significance of neutrophil-to-lymphocyte ratio and platelet-to-lymphocyte ratio in oncologic outcomes of esophageal cancer: A systematic review and meta-analysis. *Ann. Surg. Oncol.* **2016**, *23*, 646–654. [CrossRef] [PubMed]
14. Keizman, D.; Gottfried, M.; Ish-Shalom, M.; Maimon, N.; Peer, A.; Neumann, A.; Rosenbaum, E.; Kovel, S.; Pili, R.; Sinibaldi, V.; et al. Pretreatment neutrophil-to-lymphocyte ratio in metastatic castration-resistant prostate cancer patients treated with ketoconazole: Association with outcome and predictive nomogram. *Oncologist* **2012**, *17*, 1508–1514. [CrossRef] [PubMed]
15. Sonpavde, G.; Pond, G.R.; Armstrong, A.J.; Clarke, S.J.; Vardy, J.L.; Templeton, A.J.; Wang, S.L.; Paolini, J.; Chen, I.; Chow-Maneval, E.; et al. Prognostic impact of the neutrophil-to-lymphocyte ratio in men with metastatic castration-resistant prostate cancer. *Clin. Genitourin. Cancer* **2014**, *12*, 317–324. [CrossRef] [PubMed]
16. Van Soest, R.J.; Templeton, A.J.; Vera-Badillo, F.E.; Mercier, F.; Sonpavde, G.; Amir, E.; Tombal, B.; Rosenthal, M.; Eisenberger, M.A.; Tannock, I.F.; et al. Neutrophil-to-lymphocyte ratio as a prognostic biomarker for men with metastatic castration-resistant prostate cancer receiving first-line chemotherapy: Data from two randomized phase III trials. *Ann. Oncol.* **2015**, *26*, 743–749. [CrossRef] [PubMed]
17. Leibowitz-Amit, R.; Templeton, A.J.; Omlin, A.; Pezaro, C.; Atenafu, E.G.; Keizman, D.; Vera-Badillo, F.; Seah, J.A.; Attard, G.; Knox, J.J.; et al. Clinical variables associated with PSA response to abiraterone acetate in patients with metastatic castration-resistant prostate cancer. *Ann. Oncol.* **2014**, *25*, 657–662. [CrossRef] [PubMed]
18. Donskov, F. Immunomonitoring and prognostic relevance of neutrophils in clinical trials. *Semin. Cancer Biol* **2013**, *23*, 200–207. [CrossRef] [PubMed]
19. Guthrie, G.J.; Charles, K.A.; Roxburgh, C.S.; Horgan, P.G.; McMillan, D.C.; Clarke, S.J. The systemic inflammation-based neutrophil-lymphocyte ratio: Experience in patients with cancer. *Crit. Rev. Oncol. Hematol.* **2013**, *88*, 218–230. [CrossRef] [PubMed]
20. Nakagawa, M.; Terashima, T.; D'Yachkova, Y.; Bondy, G.P.; Hogg, J.C.; van Eeden, S.F. Glucocorticoid-induced granulocytosis: Contribution of marrow release and demargination of intravascular granulocytes. *Circulation* **1998**, *98*, 2307–2313. [CrossRef] [PubMed]
21. Facchini, G.; Caffo, O.; Ortega, C.; D'Aniello, C.; Di Napoli, M.; Cecere, S.C.; Della Pepa, C.; Crispo, A.; Maines, F.; Ruatta, F.; et al. Very Early PSA Response to Abiraterone in mCRPC Patients: A Novel Prognostic Factor Predicting Overall Survival. *Front. Pharmacol.* **2016**, *7*, 123. [CrossRef] [PubMed]

22. Scher, H.I.; Halabi, S.; Tannock, I.; Morris, M.; Sternberg, C.N.; Carducci, M.A.; Eisenberger, M.A.; Higano, C.; Bubley, G.J.; Dreicer, R.; et al. Design and end points of clinical trials for patients with progressive prostate cancer and castrate levels of testosterone: Recommendations of the Prostate Cancer Clinical Trials Working Group. *J. Clin. Oncol.* **2008**, *26*, 1148–1159. [CrossRef] [PubMed]
23. Eisenhauer, E.A.; Therasse, P.; Bogaerts, J.; Schwartz, L.H.; Sargent, D.; Ford, R.; Dancey, J.; Arbuck, S.; Gwyther, S.; Mooney, M.; et al. New response evaluation criteria in solid tumours: Revised RECIST guideline (version 1.1). *Eur. J. Cancer* **2009**, *45*, 228–247. [CrossRef] [PubMed]

10

RNase L Suppresses Androgen Receptor Signaling, Cell Migration and Matrix Metalloproteinase Activity in Prostate Cancer Cells

Shubham Dayal, Jun Zhou, Praveen Manivannan, Mohammad Adnan Siddiqui, Omaima Farid Ahmad, Matthew Clark, Sahezeel Awadia, Rafael Garcia-Mata, Lirim Shemshedini and Krishnamurthy Malathi *

Department of Biological Sciences, 2801 W. Bancroft St., University of Toledo, Toledo, OH 43606, USA; Shubham.Dayal@rockets.utoledo.edu (S.D.); Jun.zhou@rockets.utoledo.edu (J.Z.); Praveen.Manivannan@rockets.utoledo.edu (P.M.); Mohammad.Siddiqui@rockets.utoledo.edu (M.A.S.); Omaima.Ahmad@rockets.utoledo.edu (O.F.A.); clark.matt11@gmail.com (M.C.); Sahezeel.Awadia@rockets.utoledo.edu (S.A.); Rafael.GarciaMata@utoledo.edu (R.G.-M.); Lirim.Shemshedini@utoledo.edu (L.S.)

* Correspondence: Malathi.Krishnamurthy@utoledo.edu

Academic Editor: Carsten Stephan

Abstract: The interferon antiviral pathways and prostate cancer genetics converge on a regulated endoribonuclease, RNase L. Positional cloning and linkage studies mapped Hereditary Prostate Cancer 1 (*HPC1*) to *RNASEL*. To date, there is no correlation of viral infections with prostate cancer, suggesting that RNase L may play additional roles in tumor suppression. Here, we demonstrate a role of RNase L as a suppressor of androgen receptor (AR) signaling, cell migration and matrix metalloproteinase activity. Using RNase L mutants, we show that its nucleolytic activity is dispensable for both AR signaling and migration. The most prevalent HPC1-associated mutations in RNase L, R462Q and E265X, enhance AR signaling and cell migration. RNase L negatively regulates cell migration and attachment on various extracellular matrices. We demonstrate that RNase L knockdown cells promote increased cell surface expression of integrin β1 which activates Focal Adhesion Kinase-Sarcoma (FAK-Src) pathway and Ras-related C3 botulinum toxin substrate 1-guanosine triphosphatase (Rac1-GTPase) activity to increase cell migration. Activity of matrix metalloproteinase (MMP)-2 and -9 is significantly increased in cells where RNase L levels are ablated. We show that mutations in RNase L found in HPC patients may promote prostate cancer by increasing expression of AR-responsive genes and cell motility and identify novel roles of RNase L as a prostate cancer susceptibility gene.

Keywords: RNase L; androgen receptor; filamin A; prostate cancer

1. Introduction

RNase L is an interferon-regulated endoribonuclease that provides cellular defense against virus infections by targeting diverse RNA substrates [1,2]. Other non-canonical roles of RNase L in regulating barrier function, cellular differentiation, senescence, development of diabetes, lipid storage and demyelination of axons indicate broader roles than the established antiviral functions [3–7]. Genetic association of Hereditary Prostate Cancer 1 (*HPC1*) to *RNASEL* expands the role of RNase L to include tumor suppression [8]. However, beyond the established antiviral effect via nucleolytic function, little is known about the antitumor function of RNase L. Four germline mutations in *HPC1/RNASEL* have been identified in hereditary prostate cancer cases: M1I (start codon substitution), E265X (stop codon at 265), 471ΔAAAG (deletion causing a frameshift and stop codon) and R462Q (missense mutation at 462) [8–11]. The variant RNase L R462Q, which is defective in inducing apoptosis and has a three-fold decrease in enzymatic activity, was reported in 43% of early onset cases of hereditary prostate cancer [12]. However, in some studies, no clear correlation of prostate cancer with RNase L R462Q mutation has been observed indicating heterogeneous disease with more complex etiology involving multiple genes and factors [13–15]. Previous studies show that prostate cancer cells depleted of RNase L were resistant to apoptosis by the combined treatment of anti-cancer drugs, TNF-related apoptosis-inducing ligand (TRAIL) and Camptothecin, suggesting that mutations in RNase L may render tumor cells refractory to cell death by conventional therapies [16].

RNase L is expressed in all cell types as a latent enzyme. It is activated by a unique and specific oligonucleotide ligand, 2–5A, that is produced from cellular adenosine 5′-triphosphate (ATP) by oligoadenylate synthetase (OAS) and double-strand RNA (dsRNA) during interferon exposure or viral infections [2,17]. In the absence of 2–5A, RNase L exists as an inactive monomer. Binding to the activator, 2–5A, induces conformational change and dimerization to produce an active endoribonuclease which cleaves diverse RNA substrates. The cleaved RNA products amplify interferon production [18], activate inflammasome [19] and promote a switch from autophagy to apoptosis [20]. Recent reports show that RNase L negatively regulates cell migration and downregulates messenger RNAs (mRNAs) for cell adhesion [21,22]. While these established roles of RNase L may contribute to tumor development, they do not provide understanding of how mutations in RNase L predispose to prostate cancer.

RNase L interacts with several cellular proteins like Filamin A, IQ (isoleucineglutamine) motif containing GTPase activating protein 1 (IQGAP1), ligand of numb protein X (LNX), androgen receptor (AR), extracellular matrix (ECM) and cytoskeletal proteins that may provide alternative mechanisms by which it mediates biological functions [3,23–26]. Recently, we have shown a nuclease-independent role of RNase L in regulating actin dynamics by interacting with an actin-binding protein, Filamin A, to regulate virus entry [3]. RNase L was also reported to interact with AR in breast cancer cells [25]. Filamin A interacts with AR, and a cleaved fragment of Filamin A colocalizes with AR in the nucleus to repress AR-responsive gene expression suggesting important roles for these interactions in regulating androgen signaling [27–29]. Several studies demonstrate the importance of microtubules and actin cytoskeleton in shuttling of AR from cytoplasm to the nucleus in cell lines and in clinical samples of prostate cancers [30–32]. Considering the requirement of AR to promote prostate cancer and the association of RNase L with genetic predisposition to HPC, we explored the mechanisms that underlie tumor suppression. In this study, we demonstrate the role of RNase L, which did not rely on enzyme activity, as a suppressor of AR signaling, cell migration and matrix metalloproteinase activity. The most prevalent HPC1-associated mutations in RNase L, R462Q and E265X, enhanced AR signaling and cell migration and our studies identify a novel role of RNase L as a prostate cancer susceptibility gene.

2. Results

2.1. RNase L Negatively Regulates Androgen Signaling

Mutations in RNase L correlate with HPC and RNase L interacts with AR and Filamin A (FLNA) [3,25]. To determine the role of RNase L in HPC, we first examined the effect of androgen, R1881, on the interaction of RNase L with AR and FLNA. Androgen-responsive LNCaP cells were transfected with Flag-RNase L and treated with R1881 (1 nM), and the interaction with AR and FLNA was analyzed by coimmunoprecipitation. In untreated cells, Flag-RNase L interacts with AR and FLNA (Figure 1A). Following treatment with R1881 for 1 h, AR dissociates from Flag-RNase L and there was reduced FLNA associated with Flag-RNase L which decreased further at 24 h. In the absence of ligand, AR remains in the cytoplasm and translocates to the nucleus on binding to androgens to regulate transcription of androgen-responsive genes [33,34]. To determine the impact of RNase L on AR subcellular localization, RNase L was depleted in LNCaP cells using short hairpin RNA (shRNA) and stimulated with R1881 (1 nM) for 24 h and analyzed by confocal microscopy. Increased nuclear AR staining was observed only after R1881 treatment (Figure 1B, top) as quantified by measuring fluorescence intensity from three or more fields from three independent experiments (Figure 1B, bottom). Since RNase L interacts with FLNA in addition to AR, we knocked-down expression of FLNA or both RNase L and FLNA in LNCaP cells (Figure 1E) and stimulated with R1881 for 24 h. Cells lacking FLNA expression showed increased nuclear AR staining which was further increased when both RNase L and FLNA were depleted (Figure 1B). To test if the effect of RNase L on AR nuclear accumulation impacts AR-responsive gene expression, mRNA levels of AR target genes *PSA*, *ETV1* and *sGCα1* were determined in response to R1881 (Figure 1C). The effect of RNase L on AR-transcriptional activity was determined in cells expressing prostate specific antigen (PSA)-luciferase reporter construct, which has copies of AR-response elements fused to luciferase reporter, after stimulating with R1881 (Figure 1D). Increased expression of AR-responsive genes and AR-transcriptional activity correlated with increase in AR nuclear localization in cells lacking RNase L or FLNA and the effect was potentiated in cells lacking both RNase L and FLNA. These results suggest that RNase L negatively regulates androgen signaling and these effects may be mediated, in part, by interaction with FLNA.

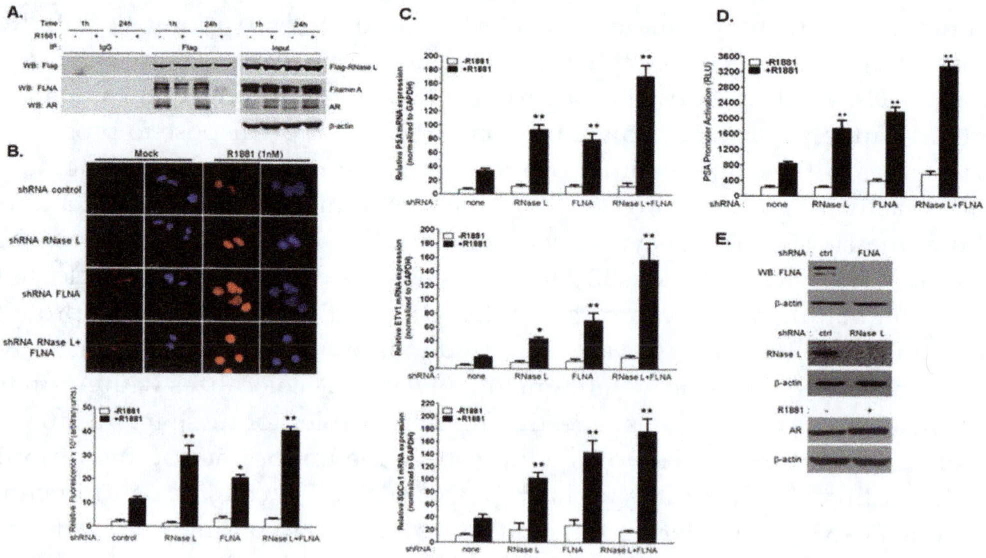

Figure 1. RNase L negatively regulates androgen signaling. (**A**) RNase L interacts with androgen receptor (AR) and Filamin A (FLNA) and dissociates on androgen treatment. LNCaP cells expressing Flag-RNase L were treated with vehicle or R1881 (1 nM) for 1 h or 24 h and immunoprecipitated with Flag-M2 agarose beads or isotype control immunoglobulin G (IgG) beads. The samples were separated on sodium dodecyl sulfate-polyacrylamide gel electrophoresis (SDS-PAGE), and the presence of AR or FLNA was determined using specific antibodies by Western blot analysis (WB). (**B**) Localization of endogenous AR in LNCaP cells expressing short hairpin RNA (shRNA) to knockdown RNase L, Filamin A or both compared to control shRNA. Cells grown in 2% charcoal stripped serum media were treated with vehicle (mock) or R1881 (1 nM) for 24 h, stained with AR antibody followed by Alexa 647-conjugated secondary antibodies and analyzed under confocal microscope. Images are representative of experiments performed in triplicate. AR localization in the nucleus (stained with diamidino-2-phenylindole (DAPI) in blue) was quantitated by measuring fluorescence intensity using Image J software. More than 10 cells (from at least three fields) were analyzed from three independent experiments. RNase L inhibits AR-mediated gene expression. LNCaP cells expressing shRNAs (as in B) were treated or mock-treated and (**C**) quantitative reverse transcriptase-polymerase chain reaction (RT-PCR) of messenger RNA (mRNA) levels of *PSA*, *ETV1* and *sGCα1* was determined and normalized to glyceraldehyde-3-phosphate dehydrogenase (*GAPDH*) mRNA levels. (**D**) Prostate specific antigen (PSA)-luciferase promoter activity was determined 18 h after R1881 treatment and normalized to β-galactosidase levels. Data shown are mean values ± standard deviation (SD) of experiments performed in triplicate from three independent experiments. Student's *t*-test was used to determine *p*-values. * $p < 0.01$, ** $p < 0.001$ and compared to cells expressing control shRNA and treated with R1881. (**E**) Cell lysates were analyzed on immunoblots for knockdown of RNase L or Filamin A and increase in AR on R1881 treatment normalized to β-actin levels. Scale bar 10 μm; Magnification ×63.

RNase L has an N-terminal ankyrin repeat domain, a pseudokinase domain in the middle and a C-terminal ribonuclease domain. RNase L binds to its activator, 2–5A, via the ankyrin repeat and pseudokinase domains allowing dimerization which is required for nuclease activity. To identify the region of RNase L that is required for suppression of androgen signaling, we over-expressed full-length Flag-RNase L (FL 1–741), N-terminal 1–335 amino acid residues (lacking nuclease domain (ΔC (1–335)) or C-terminal 386–741 amino acid residues (lacking ankyrin repeats (ΔN (386–741)) or vector alone in LNCaP cells (Figure 2B) and stimulated with R1881 for 24 h. Compared to cells expressing endogenous levels of RNase L (Figure 2, labeled as none), over-expression of RNase L suppressed AR nuclear localization two-fold (Figure 2A) which correlated with decrease in expression of AR-responsive genes (Figure 2C) and AR-transcriptional activity (Figure 2D). Interestingly, the N-terminal domain of RNase L which lacks nuclease activity suppressed androgen signaling, whereas expression of C-terminal domain alone increased AR nuclear localization, mRNA levels of AR target genes as well as AR-transcriptional activity (Figure 2A–D). Taken together, our results show that RNase L suppresses androgen signaling in LNCaP cells and the N-terminal ankyrin repeat domain is required for this effect.

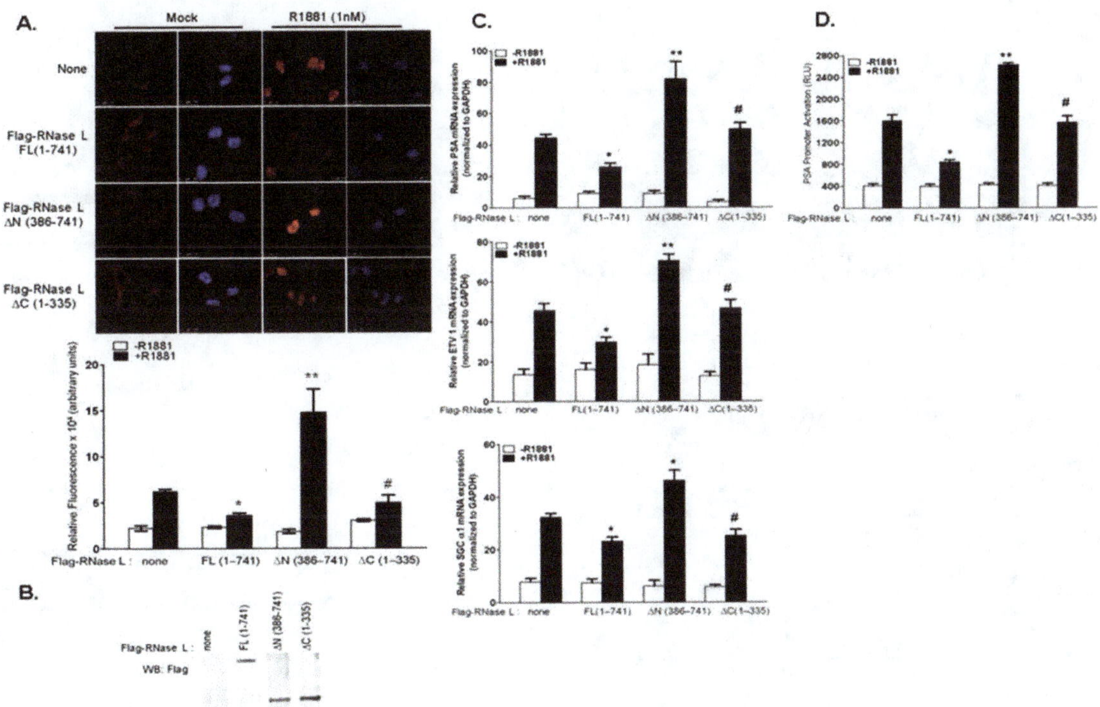

Figure 2. Over-expression of RNase L suppresses AR signaling. (**A**) LNCaP cells expressing full-length Flag-RNase L (FL 1–741), Flag-RNase L lacking N-terminal 385 amino acid residues (ΔN 386–741), Flag-RNase L lacking C-terminal 336–741 amino acid residues (ΔC 1–335) or vector alone (none) were grown in 2% charcoal stripped serum containing media and treated with R1881 or vehicle for 24 h, analyzed under confocal microscope for AR nuclear localization and quantitated as in Figure 1B. (**B**) Cell lysates were analyzed on immunoblots for expression of Flag-RNase L (full-length and truncated proteins) and normalized to β-actin levels. LNCaP cells overexpressing full-length or truncated RNase L mutants as above were treated with R1881 or mock-treated and (**C**) quantitative RT-PCR of mRNA levels of *PSA*, *ETV1* and *sGCα1* was determined and normalized to *GAPDH* mRNA levels. (**D**) PSA-luciferase promoter activity was determined 18 h after R1881 treatment and normalized to β-galactosidase levels. Data shown are mean values ± SD of experiments performed in triplicate from three independent experiments. Student's *t*-test was used to determine *p*-values. * $p < 0.01$, ** $p < 0.001$, # not significant, and compared to cells expressing vector alone and treated with R1881. Scale bar 10 μm; Magnification ×63.

2.2. *The Effect of RNase L on AR Signaling Is Not Due to Altered AR Stability*

Our results show that knockdown of endogenous RNase L increased AR signaling and over-expression of RNase L in LNCaP cells resulted in marked reduction of nuclear AR levels. We analyzed the subcellular distribution of AR in cells with endogenous levels of RNase L and FLNA, knockdown of either RNase L or FLNA and knockdown of both RNase L and FLNA by cellular fractionation following R1881 treatment. We validated the knockdown of RNase L and or FLNA and induction of AR expression in response to R1881 in immunoblots (Figure 3A). Cytosolic and nuclear extracts of cells with and without R1881 treatment were analyzed for AR protein levels. Consistent with our imaging experiments (Figure 1B), treatment of cells with R1881 resulted in translocation of AR from the cytosolic to the nuclear fraction. Quantitation of immunoblots for AR protein shows that depleting RNase L or FLNA increased AR nuclear-to-cytoplasmic ratio (N/C ratio), and depleting both resulted in further increase in nuclear AR levels (Figure 3B).

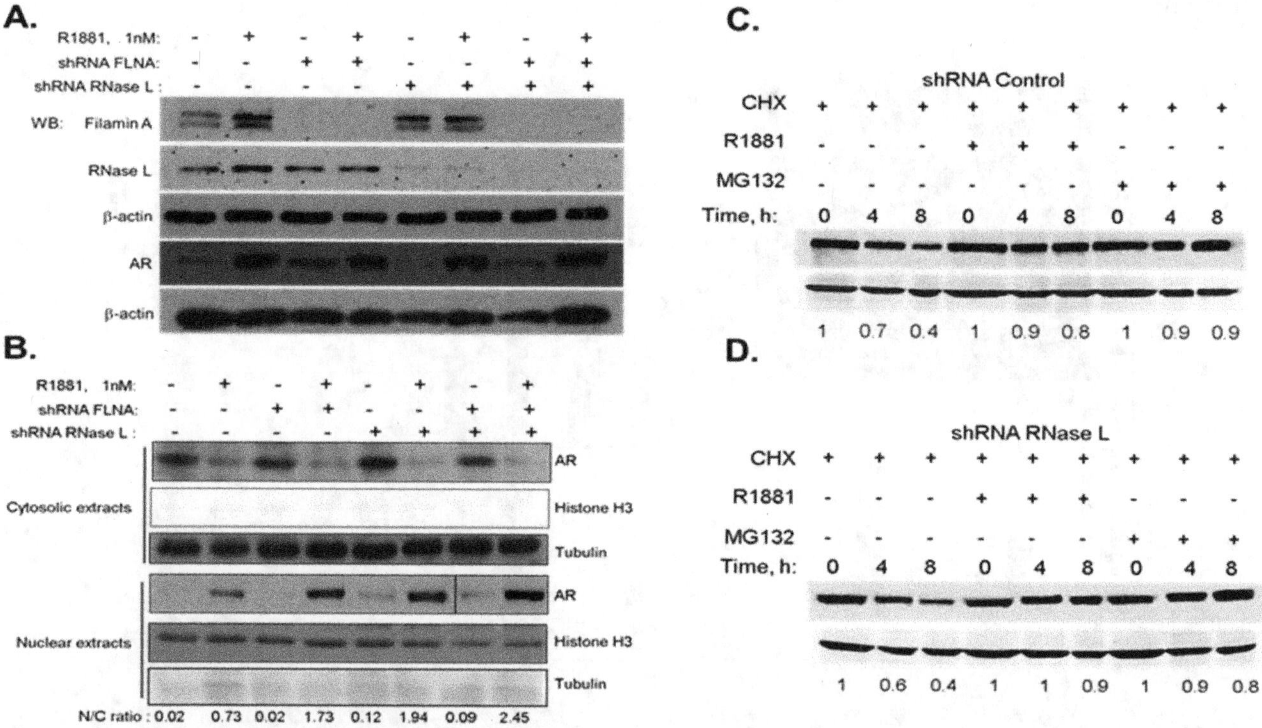

Figure 3. Increased AR localization in the nucleus in RNase L-depleted cells is not due to altered AR stability. LNCaP cells expressing shRNA to knockdown RNase L, FLNA or both and control shRNA were grown in 2% charcoal-stripped serum containing media and treated with vehicle or R1881 and (**A**) Cell lysates were analyzed on immunoblots for knockdown and AR expression levels. (**B**) Cells were fractionated and AR from nuclear (N) and cytosolic (C) extracts were analyzed by immunoblotting with anti-AR, histone H3 (marker for nuclear extract), α-tubulin (marker for cytosolic extract) antibodies. Nuclear-to-cytoplasmic (N/C) ratio of AR protein with or without R1881 was determined by densitometric analysis of band intensities using Image J software. LNCaP cells with control shRNA (**C**) or RNase L shRNA (**D**) in growth medium were treated with cycloheximide (CHX, 50 μg/mL) alone or combined with MG132 (20 μM) or R1881 (1 nM) for 4 h or 8 h. Cell lysates were prepared in 2% SDS and levels of AR were normalized on immunoblots with β-actin and relative changes in AR levels compared to CHX treatment for 0 h (band intensity set as 1) was determined. Similar results were observed in three independent experiments.

Due to the inhibitory effect of RNase L on AR nuclear accumulation, we tested the possibility that RNase L may affect AR protein stability. Control and RNase L shRNA expressing LNCaP cells were treated with cycloheximide (CHX) for the indicated times to block *de novo* protein translation and combined with either proteasome inhibitor, MG132, to block AR degradation or R1881 to induce AR protein levels. As demonstrated by other studies, AR protein levels declined in cells treated with CHX alone [35] and the reduced levels were comparable in cells depleted or expressing RNase L (Figure 3C,D). No differences in MG132 stabilized AR was observed in both cells suggesting that RNase L does not alter AR stability.

2.3. Hereditary Prostate Cancer 1 (HPC1)-Associated Mutants of RNase L Enhance AR Transcriptional Activity

To understand how mutations in RNase L contribute to HPC, we examined the effect of HPC1-associated RNase L mutants on androgen signaling. To further address if RNase L enzyme activity is required for androgen signaling, other mutations in RNase L were generated by site-directed mutagenesis of Flag-RNase L construct including R667A (nuclease-dead), K166E (reduced enzyme activity), K240/274N (defective 2–5A binding and lacks enzyme activity), Y312A (defective 2–5A binding and lacks enzyme activity). Expression of Flag-RNase L Wild type (WT) and mutant proteins is shown in immunoblots (Figure 4E). RNase L activity of the WT and mutant constructs was determined by rRNA cleavage in response to PolyI:C transfection in HeLa cells which lack detectable RNase L activity (Figure 4F) [36,37]. As endogenous RNase L may mask some of the effects of mutants we express, we used a knockdown/rescue approach in which endogenous RNase L levels were depleted in LNCaP cells with shRNA targeting the 3′-UTR (Figure 1E) and reconstituted with Flag-RNase L (WT) or RNase L mutants and stimulated with R1881 for 24 h. We then monitored the subcellular localization of AR by confocal microscopy (Figure 4A) and quantitated the amount of nuclear AR (Figure 4B). Expression of WT RNase L suppressed nuclear translocation of AR as we observed in Figure 2. However, cells expressing HPC1-associated mutants, R462Q and E265X showed increased AR in the nucleus. Since both mutants compromised RNase L enzyme activity, we tested other RNase L mutants which had reduced activity (K166E), lacked enzyme activity due to defect in binding the activator 2–5A (K240/274N and Y312A) or in the nuclease domain (R667A) to determine if enzyme activity of RNase L was required for androgen signaling. In contrast with other mutants, RNase L Y312A, which is defective in 2–5A binding and lacks enzyme activity, was able to suppress nuclear AR localization like WT RNase L (Figure 4A, arrows). We did not observe any change in AR subcellular localization in the absence of R1881. The increase in nuclear AR correlated with mRNA levels of AR target genes and AR-transcriptional activity (Figure 4C,D). Together, these results suggest that HPC1-associated RNase L mutants may contribute to HPC by regulating androgen signaling. Further, the effect of RNase L on androgen signaling appears to be independent of nucleolytic functions (Figure 4F).

2.4. Cell Migration Is Increased in Cells with Reduced Levels of RNase L

Our published observation that RNase L interacts with the actin-binding protein, FLNA, to regulate actin dynamics [3] suggests that RNase L may have additional roles in HPC besides regulating androgen signaling. The ability of RNase L to modulate actin cytoskeleton prompted us to explore whether RNase L affected cell migration in prostate cancer cells. To investigate the role of RNase L in prostate cancer cell motility, RNase L levels were knocked-down using shRNA in DU145, PC3 and LNCaP cells and compared to cells expressing endogenous RNase L levels (expressing control non-targeting shRNA) (Figure 5B, inset). Confluent monolayer of cells in serum-free media were scratched and replaced with growth media. Cell migration to close the wound was imaged (Figure 5A) and quantitated (Figure 5B) over time as indicated. In all three prostate cancer cells, depletion of RNase L had marked effect (1.5–2-fold) in enhancing cell migration and the effect was most significant at 24 h experimental endpoint. No significant difference in cell proliferation was observed between control and knockdown cells over the 24 h time course of the experiment (data not shown). The difference in cell migration was quantitated by transwell cell migration assays in response to serum (Figure 5C). Consistent with scratch wound healing assays, RNase L knockdown cells migrated significantly more (1.5–2-fold) through fibronectin-coated filters in response to serum.

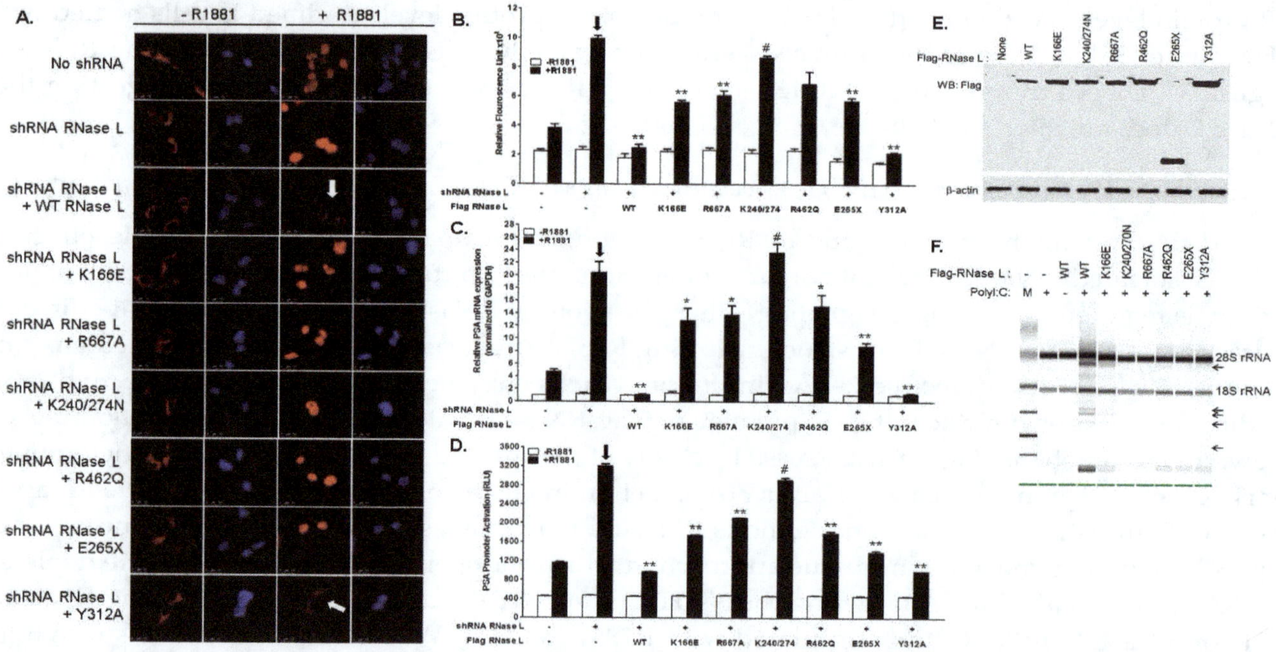

Figure 4. Hereditary Prostate Cancer 1-associated mutants of RNase L enhance AR transcriptional activity. (**A**) Endogenous RNase L-knockdown LNCaP cells were reconstituted with Flag-Wild-type (WT) or mutated RNase L as indicated and treated with vehicle (−R1881) or R1881 (1 nM) for 24 h. AR nuclear localization was analyzed under confocal microscope; and (**B**) quantitated by measuring fluorescence intensity using Image J software as described in Figure 1B. White arrows point to lack of nuclear localization in WT and RNase L Y312A mutant expressing cells. AR transcriptional activity was monitored in LNCaP cells reconstituted with WT and RNase L mutants treated with vehicle or R1881 by (**C**) quantitative RT-PCR of mRNA levels of *PSA*, *ETV1* and *sGCα1* normalized to *GAPDH* mRNA levels. (**D**) PSA-luciferase promoter activity 18 h after R1881 treatment and normalized to β-galactosidase levels. Data shown are mean values ± SD of experiments performed in triplicate from three independent experiments. Student's *t*-test was used to determine *p*-values. * $p < 0.01$, ** $p < 0.001$, # not significant, and compared to RNase L knockdown cells (shown with arrow on graphs) treated with R1881. (**E**) Cell lysates were analyzed for expression of Flag-RNase L (WT) and mutants as indicated using anti-Flag antibodies and normalized to β-actin levels. (**F**) HeLa cells were transfected with Flag-RNase L (WT) and RNase L mutants and enzyme activity was determined by monitoring rRNA cleavage (shown by arrows) as determined in RNA chips by transfecting cells with PolyI:C (2 μg/mL) and isolation of total RNA. Scale bar 10 μm, Magnification ×63.

To further demonstrate that the increased cell migration was due to lack of RNase L, we used WT and *Rnase l*$^{-/-}$ (RNase L KO) primary mouse embryonic fibroblasts (MEFs) and monitored wound closure by wound healing assays and cell migration in transwell assays. Migration of RNase L KO MEFs was enhanced 2–3-fold in response to serum or fibronectin compared to WT MEFs (Figure 5D–F). In addition, we reconstituted RNase L expression in DU145 or PC3 RNase L knockdown cells and compared wound closure in cells with endogenous levels of RNase L, depleted of RNase L or over-expressing RNase L (Figure 6A,C). Expression of RNase L is shown in immunoblots as inset in Figure 6B,D. At 24 h experimental endpoint wound closure was 47% in DU145 cells with endogenous RNase L (WT), 76% in RNase L-depleted cells and 29% in over-expressing cells. In PC3 cells, endogenous RNase L expressing cells (WT) showed 45%, RNase L-depleted cells showed 68%

and over-expressing cells showed 27% wound closure. To determine the consequence of RNase L activation on cell migration, DU145 cells were transfected with activator, 2–5A which causes RNase L dimerization, or mock transfected and wound closure was imaged and quantitated (Figure 6E,F). 2–5A treatment of cells decreased migration of DU145 cells by 48% compared to mock transfected cells. Taken together, these results demonstrate that RNase L inhibits cell migration in prostate cancer and primary cells. Furthermore, activation of RNase L by 2–5A, which results in conformational change and dimerization of RNase L, also suppresses cell migration.

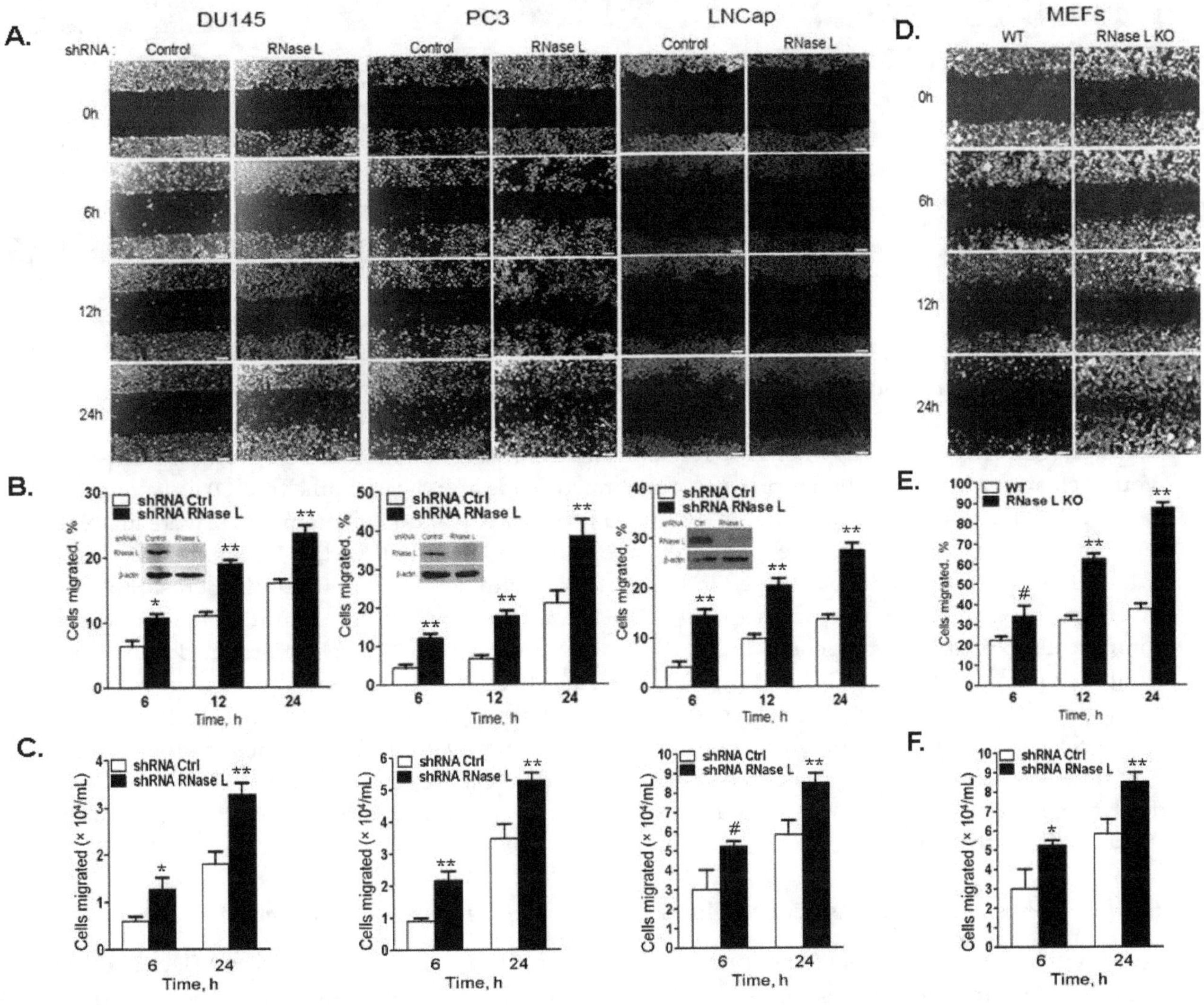

Figure 5. Cell migration is increased in cells with reduced RNase L levels. DU145, PC3 or LNCaP cells expressing control or RNase L shRNA (**A–C**) and WT or RNase L KO mouse embryonic fibroblasts (MEFs) (**D–F**) were grown to confluence. (**A**,**D**) The cell monolayer was scratched and wound closure was imaged under phase-contrast microscope at indicated times. (**B**,**E**) Cells migrated (%) to close the wound was quantitated by Image J software. Knock-down of RNase L on immunoblots is shown as inset in (**B**). (**C**,**F**) Transwell chambers coated with fibronectin were used to measure cell migration at 6 h and 24 h in response to growth medium with 10% serum by counting cells that migrated to the lower surface of the filters from experiments performed in triplicate. Data shown are mean values ± SD of experiments performed in triplicate from three independent experiments. Student's t-test was used to determine p-values. * $p < 0.01$, ** $p < 0.001$, # not significant, and compared to cells expressing control shRNA (**A–C**) and compared to WT MEFs (**D–F**). Scale bar 100 μm, Magnification ×10.

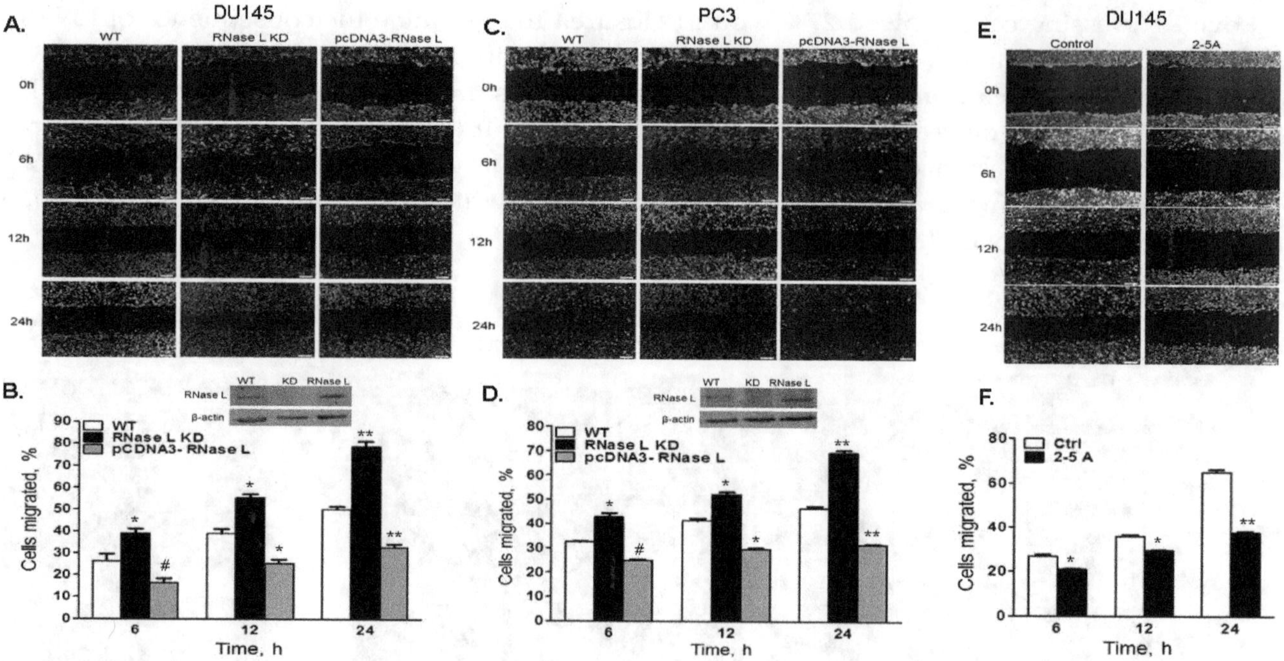

Figure 6. Over-expression or activation of RNase L inhibits cell migration. DU145 (**A,B**) or PC3 (**C,D**) cells expressing control shRNA and expressing endogenous levels of RNase L (WT), shRNA to knockdown RNase L (RNase L KD) or overexpressing RNase L after knockdown of endogenous RNase L (pcDNA3-RNase L) were grown to confluence. (**A,C**) Cell monolayers were scratched and wound closure was imaged under phase-contrast microscope at indicated times. (**B,D**) Cells migrated (%) to close the wound was quantitated by Image J software. RNase L protein levels were analyzed on immunoblots using anti-RNase L antibody and shown as inset in B and D. Data shown are mean values $\pm$ SD of experiments performed in triplicate from three independent experiments. Student's t-test was used to determine p-values. * $p < 0.01$, ** $p < 0.001$, # not significant, and compared to control cells expressing endogenous levels (WT) of RNase L. (**E**) DU145 cells were mock transfected (control) or transfected with 2–5A (10 μM) to activate RNase L. The monolayer was scratched and wound closure was imaged under phase-contrast microscope at indicated times. (**F**) Cells migrated (%) to close the wound was quantitated by Image J software. Data shown are mean values $\pm$ SD of experiments performed in triplicate from three independent experiments. Student's t-test was used to determine p-values. * $p < 0.01$, ** $p < 0.001$, and compared to mock-treated (control) cells (**E,F**). Scale bar 100 μm, Magnification ×10.

2.5. *Hereditary Prostate Cancer-Associated Mutants of RNase L Promote Cell Migration*

We have shown that RNase L suppresses AR signaling and cell migration. Because the most common RNase L mutations associated with HPC enhance AR signaling, we investigated whether these RNase L mutants also affect cell migration. To further explore if RNase L enzyme activity is required for cell migration, we also tested the RNase L mutants we generated that have reduced enzyme activity (K166E) or lack enzyme activity due to mutation in the nuclease domain (R667A) or defect in binding the activator, 2–5A (K240/274N, Y312A). Loss of heterozygosity of RNase L has been observed in HPC1 prostate tumors [8]. Therefore, we depleted RNase L in DU145 and PC3 cells and reconstituted with vector alone (none), Flag-RNase L (WT) or Flag-RNase L mutants as indicated (Figure 7A–F). Confluent monolayers of cells were scratched and wound closure was imaged (Figure 7A,C) and quantitated (Figure 7B,D). Differences in cell migration between cells expressing various RNase L mutants were also quantitated by transwell assays through fibronectin coated filters in response to serum (Figure 7E,F). Consistent with our observations, RNase L knockdown cells showed increased migration and expression of WT RNase L suppressed cell migration. HPC1-associated RNase L mutants, R462Q and E265X, showed increase in cell migration compared to cells expressing WT

RNase L (shown by arrows in Figure 7B,D–F). RNase L K166E, which has reduced enzyme activity, R667A, which is nuclease-dead, and K240/274N which lacks enzyme activity showed 1.5–2-fold increase in migration compared to WT expressing cells. In contrast with other RNase L mutants which lack enzyme function, the Y312A mutant which also lacks enzyme activity due to its inability to bind 2–5A, suppressed cell migration (shown by arrows in Figure 7B,D–F). This effect was comparable to WT RNase L indicating that different regions of RNase L, presumably through interacting proteins, may contribute to cell migration rather than enzyme activity.

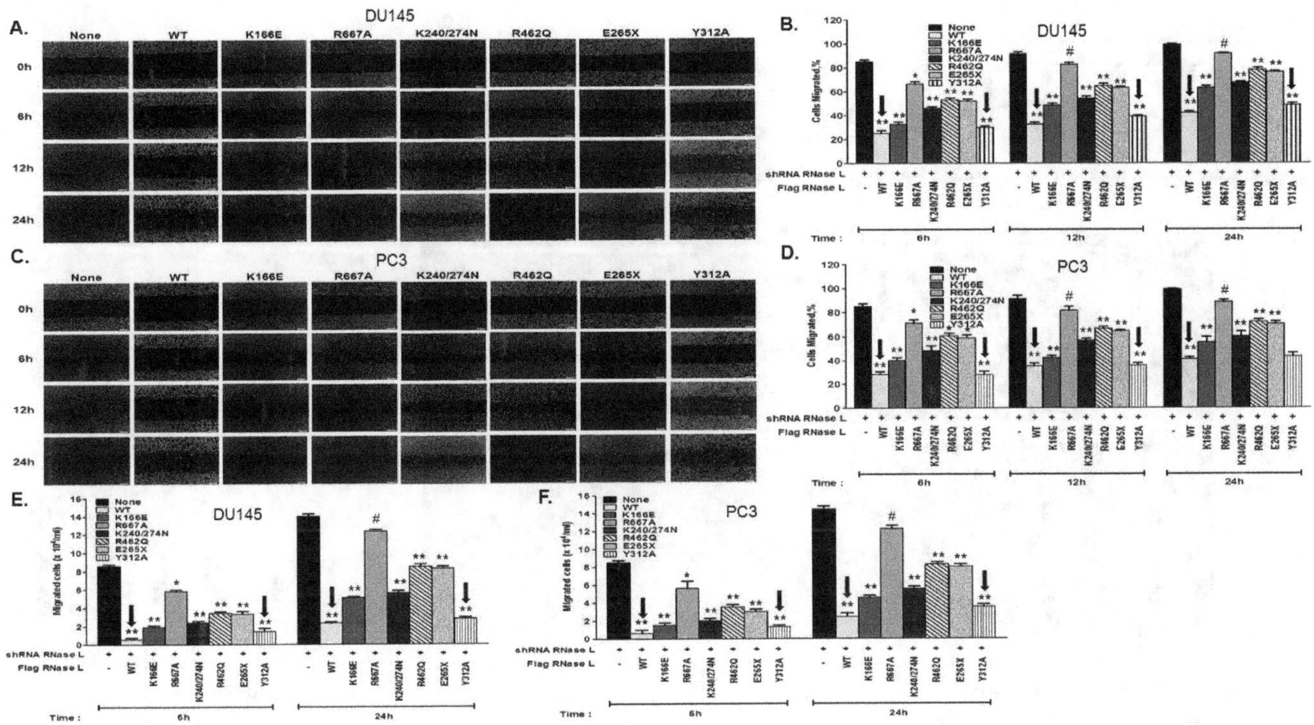

Figure 7. Hereditary prostate cancer-associated mutants of RNase L promote cell migration. Endogenous RNase L was knocked down in DU145 or PC3 cells and reconstituted with Flag vector (none), Flag-RNase L (WT) or Flag-RNase L mutants as indicated. (**A**,**C**) Cell monolayers were scratched and wound closure was imaged under phase-contrast microscope at indicated times. (**B**,**D**) Cells migrated (%) to close the wound was quantitated by Image J software. (**E**,**F**) Transwell chambers coated with fibronectin were used to measure cell migration at 6 h and 24 h in response to growth medium with 10% serum by counting cells that migrated to the lower surface of the filters from experiments performed in triplicate. Arrows are used to highlight RNase L mutants that suppress migration as WT RNase L. Data shown are mean values ± SD of experiments performed in triplicate from three independent experiments. Student's t-test was used to determine p-values. * $p < 0.01$, ** $p < 0.001$, # not significant, and compared to cells expressing shRNA to knockdown RNase L. Scale bar 100 μm, Magnification ×10.

2.6. *RNase L-Depletion Increases Cell Attachment and Cell Spreading*

Interaction of the cell with extracellular matrix (ECM) causes engagement of specific transmembrane receptors and signaling molecules which modulate cytoskeletal organization resulting in distinct cell morphology, attachment and migration [38]. To characterize the consequence of RNase L on cell attachment, RNase L was knocked-down using shRNA in DU145, PC3 or LNCaP cells and compared to control shRNA expressing cells. Cells were allowed to attach to dishes coated with fibronectin (FN), laminin (LN), collagen I (C I), collagen IV (C IV) or vitronectin (VN) for 1 h. Wells were then washed and attached cells were quantitated by staining. Knockdown of RNase L in all three prostate cancer cell lines tested showed increase in cell attachment to all the ECM substrates, and the difference was 2–2.5-fold greater in response to fibronectin (Figure 8A–C). We monitored DU145 and PC3 cells for both shape and cell spreading after incubation on FN substrates. Expression of RNase L appeared to result in the presence of more rounded cells which spread slowly. In contrast RNase L-depleted cells tend to spread rapidly and the cell area increased in a time-dependent manner (Figure 8D,E). Both the rate and extent of cell spreading were significantly lower at all the time points in RNase L expressing cells. These results suggest that RNase L inhibits cell attachment and cell spreading.

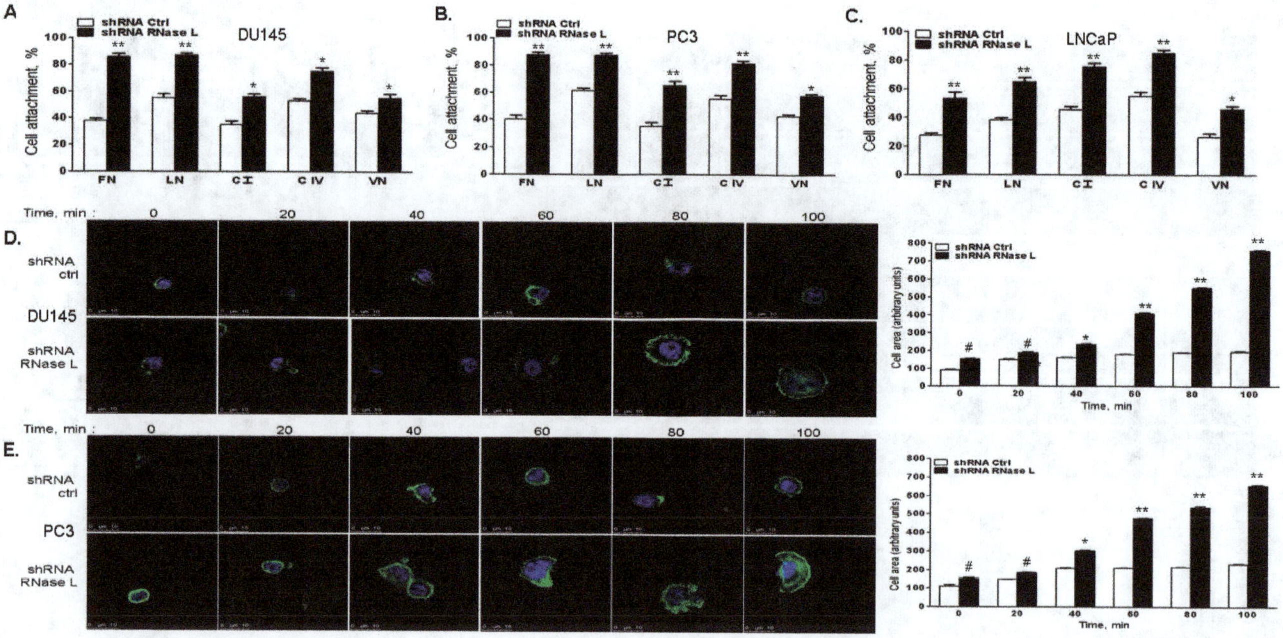

Figure 8. RNase L depletion increases cell attachment to extracellular matrix substrates and cell spreading. (**A**) DU145; (**B**) PC3; or (**C**) LNCaP cells expressing control shRNA or RNase L shRNA were allowed to attach to wells coated with 10 μg/mL each of fibronectin (FN), laminin (LN), collagen I (C I), collagen IV (C IV) or vitronectin (VN) for 1 h. Plates were washed and attached cells were stained. Cell attachment (%) was determined from means ± SD of experiments performed in triplicate from three separate experiments. (**D**) DU145; or (**E**) PC3 expressing control shRNA or RNase L shRNA were allowed to attach and spread on surfaces coated with fibronectin (10 μg/mL) at various time points, fixed and F-actin was labeled with Alexa 488-labeled phalloidin and imaged by confocal microscope. Areas of individual cells from at least 30 measurements were determined by Image J software. Data shown represent the mean of cell area ± standard error of mean (SEM) of three experiments performed in triplicate. Student's *t*-test was used to determine *p*-values. * $p < 0.01$, ** $p < 0.001$, # not significant, and compared to cells expressing control shRNA. Scale bar 10 μm, Magnification ×63.

2.7. Depletion of RNase L Promotes Integrin Activation and FAK-Src Signaling in Response to Fibronection

Integrins are transmembrane receptors that physically link ECM to intracellular actin cytoskeleton [39]. Trafficking and recycling of integrin β1 to the cell membrane and clustering is required for cell attachment, spreading and migration [40]. Clustering of integrins activates signaling events involving focal adhesion kinase (FAK) and Src [41,42]. Since RNase L regulates cell attachment and migration, we investigated if the effects were mediated by integrin-regulated Focal Adhesion Kinase-Sarcoma (FAK-Src) signaling pathways. To assess the role of RNase L in regulating integrin β1 expression and activation, prostate cancer cells depleted of RNase L or WT were allowed to spread on FN and cell suspensions were fixed and incubated with integrin β1 antibodies to label cell surface integrin β1. Flow cytometric analysis showed that cell surface integrin β1 was increased 1.5–3-fold following knockdown of RNase L (Figure 9A–C). No changes in protein levels of integrin β1 were observed between WT and RNase L knockdown cells. Consistent with roles in cell migration, attachment and spreading, RNase L is important for activation of integrin β1. Activation of RNase L with 2–5A which promotes dimerization, inhibits cell migration (Figure 6E,F) and we observed decrease in cell surface integrin β1 expression in DU145, PC3 and LNCaP cells transfected with 2–5A and this effect was not due to decrease in integrin β1 protein levels (Figure 10A–C).

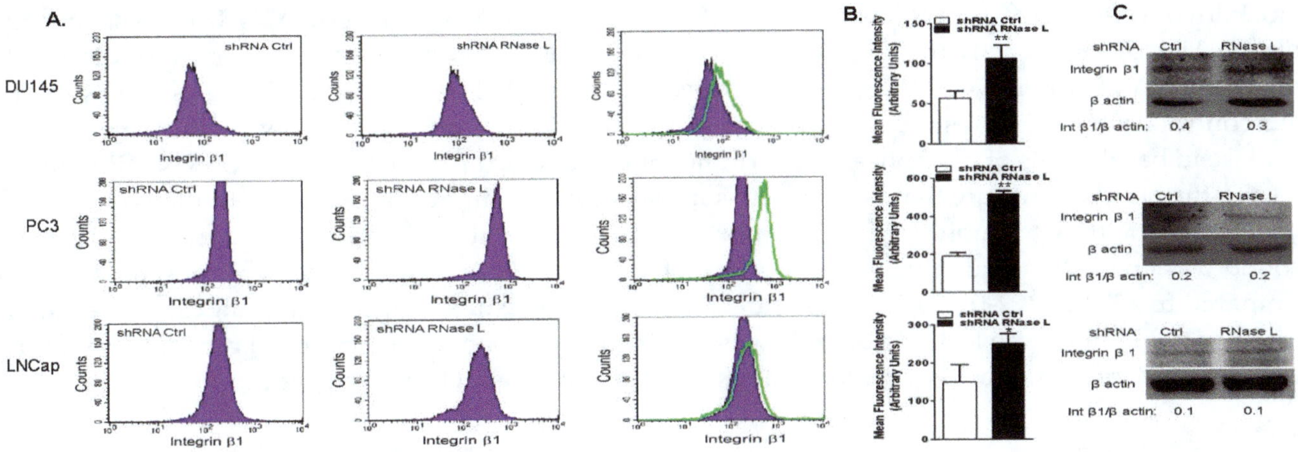

Figure 9. Cells with reduced levels of RNase L exhibit increased surface expression of integrin β1. DU145, PC3 or LNCaP cells expressing control shRNA or RNase L shRNA were plated on fibronectin-coated dishes and analyzed by flow cytometry for surface staining with antibodies against integrin β1 and Alexa-488 conjugated secondary antibodies. (**A**) Representative histograms; and (**B**) bar graphs for the mean fluorescence intensity of at least three independent experiments for integrin β1 are shown. Student's *t*-test was used to determine *p*-values. * $p < 0.01$, ** $p < 0.001$ and compared to cells expressing control shRNA. (**C**) Expression of integrin β1 in cell lysates was determined on immunoblots and normalized to levels of β-actin.

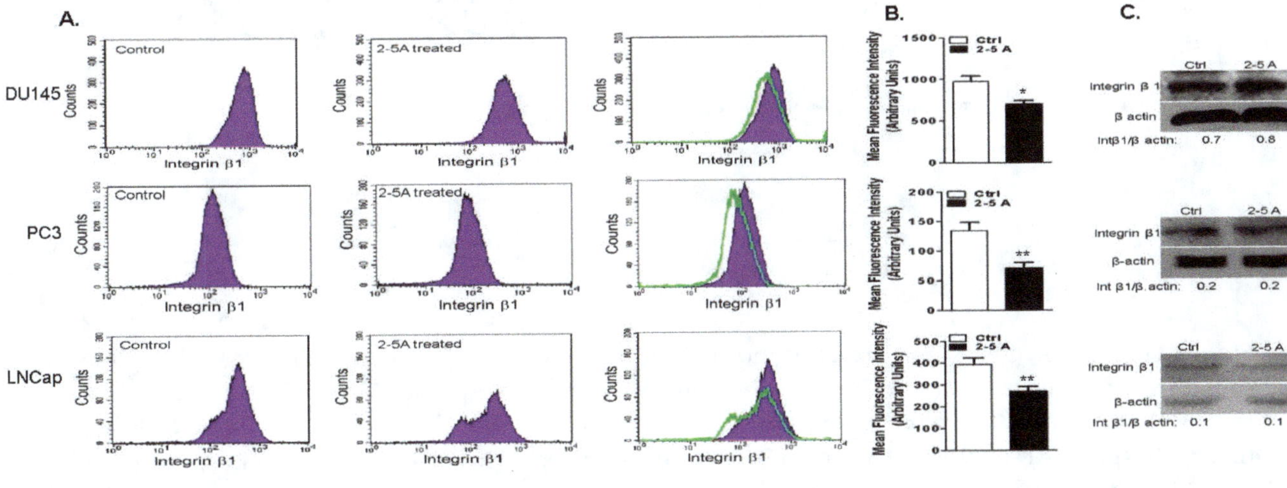

Figure 10. Activation of RNase L reduces surface expression of integrin β1. DU145, PC3 or LNCaP cells were mock-treated (control) or transfected with 2–5A (10 μM) to activate RNase L and plated on fibronectin-coated dishes and analyzed by flow cytometry for surface staining with antibodies against integrin β1 and Alexa-488 conjugated secondary antibodies. (**A**) Representative histograms; and (**B**) bar graphs for the mean fluorescence intensity of at least three independent experiments for integrin β1 are shown. Student's *t*-test was used to determine *p*-values. * $p < 0.01$, ** $p < 0.001$ and compared to mock-treated cells. (**C**) Expression of integrin β1 in cell lysates was determined on immunoblots and normalized to levels of β-actin.

FAK is recruited to sites of integrin clustering and activated by autophosphorylation at Y397 which in turn facilitates Src binding [43–45]. Phosphorylation of Src at Y416 can lead to formation of FAK-Src signaling complex which acts with downstream regulators including RhoGTPases to control cell shape and turnover of focal adhesion during cell migration [46,47]. We tested FAK activation after integrin β1 clustering in response to FN in PC3 cells with endogenous or knockdown of RNase L and in WT and RNase L KO MEFs. FAK Y397 phosphorylation was increased 43% in PC3 RNase L knockdown cells and 48% in RNase L KO MEFs compared to PC3 control or WT MEFs, respectively (Figure 11A,B). Src is activated by binding to pY397-FAK and we observed a corresponding 60% increase in pY416 Src in PC3 RNase L knockdown cells and 70% in RNase L KO MEFs compared to PC3 control or WT MEFs respectively (Figure 11A,B). In PC3 RNase L knockdown cells, we observed increase in basal levels of phospho-FAK and phospho-Src which increased further on FN stimulation.

To further demonstrate that Src activity is involved in cell migration, RNase L-depleted PC3 cells were treated with Src inhibitor, PP2, and monolayers were scratched and cell migration to close the wound was imaged and quantitated. In mock-treated cells 85% of wound closure was observed at 24 h compared to 43% in PP2-treated cells (Figure 11C,D). These results suggest that integrin clustering in response to FN in RNase L-depleted cells was significantly enhanced over control cells which in turn reflected in increased phosphorylation of FAK and Src which effects cell migration.

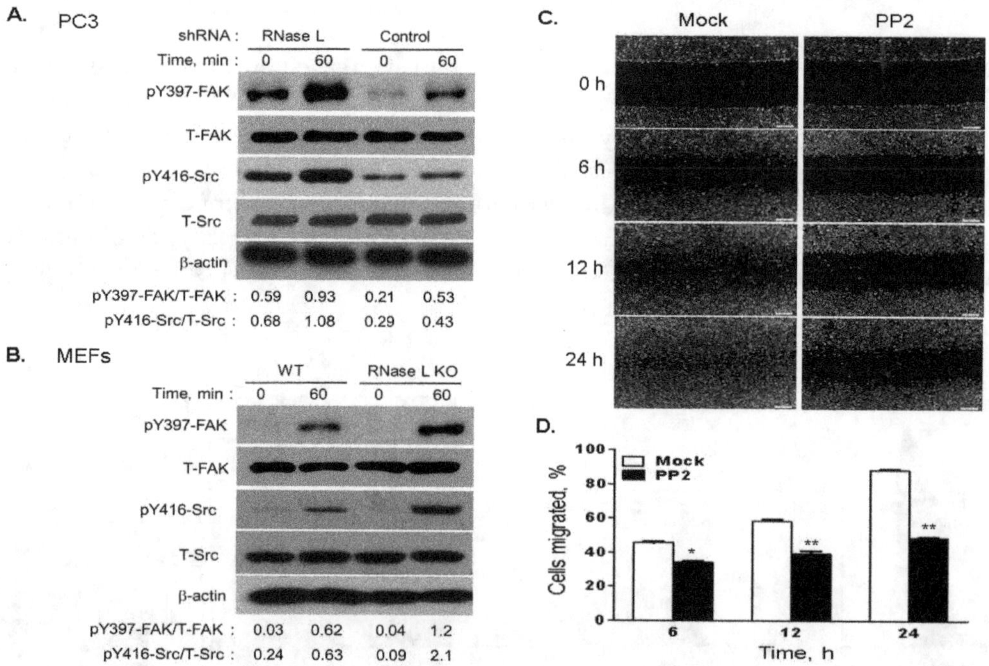

Figure 11. Increased FAK and Src phosphorylation in response to fibronectin in RNase L-depleted cells effects cell migration. (**A**) PC3 cells expressing control or RNase L shRNA; and (**B**) WT and *Rnase* $l^{-/-}$ (RNase L KO) MEFs were serum starved and plated on fibronectin-coated plates for indicated times. Phospho-FAK (Y397) and phospho-Src (Y416) was detected in cell lysates using phospho-specific antibodies on immunoblots followed by Western blotting with anti-FAK, anti-Src antibodies and β-actin for loading control. (pY397)-FAK and (pY416)-Src intensity values were normalized to total-FAK and total-Src intensities respectively using Image J software. Representative immunoblots from experiments performed in triplicate are shown. (**C**) PC3 RNase L-depleted cells growing in confluent monolayers were pretreated with vehicle (mock) or Src inhibitor (PP2, 10 μM) for 1 h. Cell monolayers were scratched and wound closure was imaged under phase-contrast microscope at indicated times in growth medium containing PP2 inhibitor. (**D**) Cells migrated (%) to close the wound was quantitated by Image J software. Data shown are mean values ± SD of experiments performed in triplicate from three independent experiments. Student's *t*-test was used to determine *p*-values. * $p < 0.01$, ** $p < 0.001$, and compared to vehicle-treated (mock) cells. Scale bar 100 μm, Magnification ×10.

2.8. Increased Rac1 Activity Mediates Enhanced Cell Migration in RNase L-Depleted Cells

Signaling pathways triggered by integrins regulate FAK-Src activity and involve Rho GTPases which are crucial for remodeling cytoskeleton and cell mobility [48,49]. To investigate which of the Rho family, GTPases-RhoA, Cdc42 or Rac1, mediate RNase L-dependent migration, RNase L-depleted DU145 or PC3 cells were transfected with empty vector (mock), or dominant-negative forms of RhoA (T19N), Cdc42 (T17N) or Rac1 (T17N) [50]. Expression of the proteins on immunoblots is shown in Figure S1. Monolayers of cells were scratched and wound closure was imaged and quantitated at indicated times (Figure 12A–D). Expression of the dominant-negative Rac1 significantly inhibited migration of RNase L-depleted cells whereas RhoA (T19N) and Cdc42 (T17N) had marginal effects. To examine the effect of reduced RNase L levels on Rac1 activity in response to FN, we measured Ras-related C3 botulinum toxin substrate 1 (Rac1) activity by precipitating active GTP-bound Rac1 with GST-PAK-binding domain (GST-PBD) and estimating the abundance relative to total levels of Rac1 protein. In both DU145 (Figure 13A,B) and PC3 (Figure 13C,D), adhesion to FN stimulated a rapid and transient increase in Rac1 activity which peaked at 30 min and declined by 1 h. In contrast, RNase L knockdown cells had higher basal level of Rac1 which increased further on FN stimulation and was sustained at 1 h (Figure 13A–D). Our data support the observation that increased integrin and FAK-Src signaling in response to FN in RNase L knockdown cells contributes to increased Rac1 activity and cell migration.

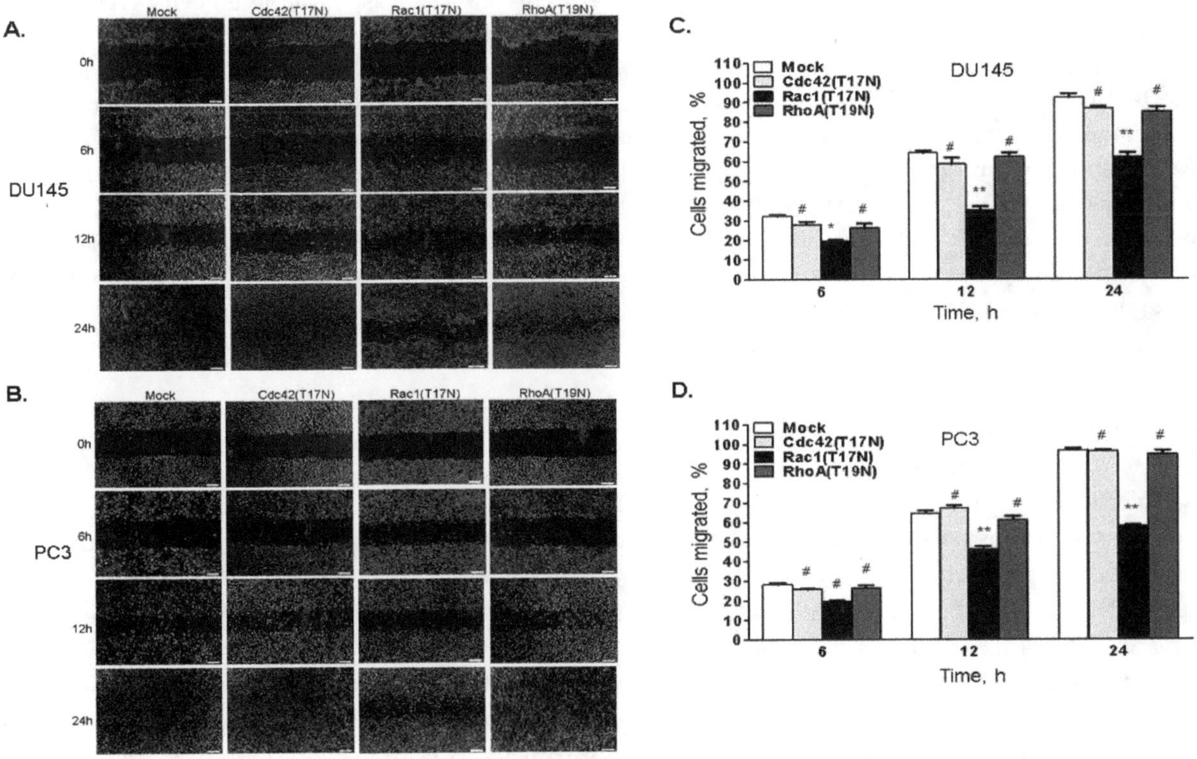

Figure 12. Ras-related C3 botulinum toxin substrate 1 (Rac1) mediates enhanced cell migration in RNase L-depleted cells. RNase L shRNA expressing (**A**) DU145 cells; or (**B**) PC3 cells were transfected with empty vector (mock), dominant negative Cdc42 (T17N), dominant negative Rac1 (T17N) or dominant negative RhoA (T19N) expressing plasmids. After 24 h, cell monolayers were scratched and wound closure was imaged under phase-contrast microscope at indicated times. (**C**,**D**) Cells migrated (%) to close the wound was quantitated by Image J software. Data shown are mean values ± SD of experiments performed in triplicate from three independent experiments. Student's *t*-test was used to determine *p*-values. * $p < 0.01$, ** $p < 0.001$, # not significant, and compared to RNase L-depleted cells mock transfected with empty vector. Scale bar 100 μm, Magnification ×10.

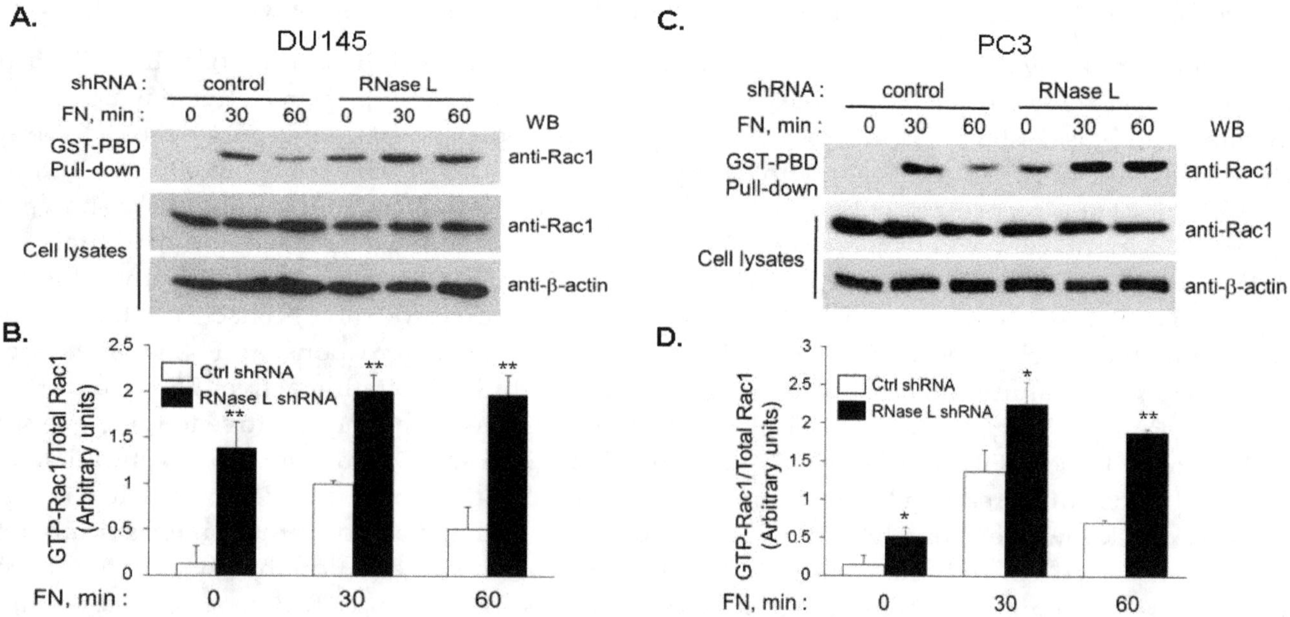

Figure 13. Rac1 activity in response to fibronectin is increased in RNase L-depleted cells. (**A**) DU145; or (**C**) PC3 cells expressing control or RNase L shRNA were plated on fibronectin-coated dishes for indicated times. Cell lysates were incubated with agarose-immobilized GST-PAK1 binding domain (GST-PBD) and co-precipitated proteins were subject to immunoblotting with anti-Rac1 antibodies to detect the amount of GTP-bound Rac1 (active Rac1) and compared to expression of Rac1 in cell lysates. Representative immunoblots from experiments performed in triplicate are shown. (**B**,**D**) Activity of Rac1 was quantitated by comparing the intensities of active Rac1 with those of total Rac1 in each lane using Image J software. Data are mean values ± SEM expressed as increase in Rac1 activity from three independent experiments. Student's *t*-test was used to determine *p*-values. * $p < 0.01$, ** $p < 0.001$, and compared to control shRNA expressing cells.

2.9. RNase L Regulates MMP-2 and MMP-9 Activities

Matrix metalloproteinases (MMPs) remodel the ECM and play a critical role in cell migration, invasion, tissue metastasis and impact tumor progression [51]. Elevated levels of MMP-2 and MMP-9 are observed in prostate cancer and correlate with increased metastasis [52,53]. To determine if activity of MMP-2 and -9 are regulated by RNase L, culture supernatants of control and RNase L knockdown DU145, PC3 and LNCaP cells were analyzed for activity of secreted MMP-2 and -9 by gelatin zymography. MMP-2 and -9 gelatinase activity, observed by cleared areas on gels, was higher in RNase L-depleted cells than in control cells (1.5–5-fold increase in MMP-2 activity compared to control cells and 1.5–2-fold increase in MMP-9 activity compared to control cells) (Figure 14A,B). Similar increase in MMP-2 and -9 activities was also observed in RNase L KO MEFs compared to WT MEFs (Figure S2). Activation of RNase L by transfecting 2–5A inhibited cell migration (Figure 6E,F) and we observed a decrease in MMP-2 and -9 activity in culture supernatants following 2–5A transfection compared to control cells (Figure 14A,C). Taken together, these results demonstrate that depleting RNase L leads to increased activity of MMP-2 and -9 in prostate cancer cells which correlates with increased cell migration. Silencing of RNase L or activation of RNase L did not affect expression of *MMP-9* mRNA (Figure S3).

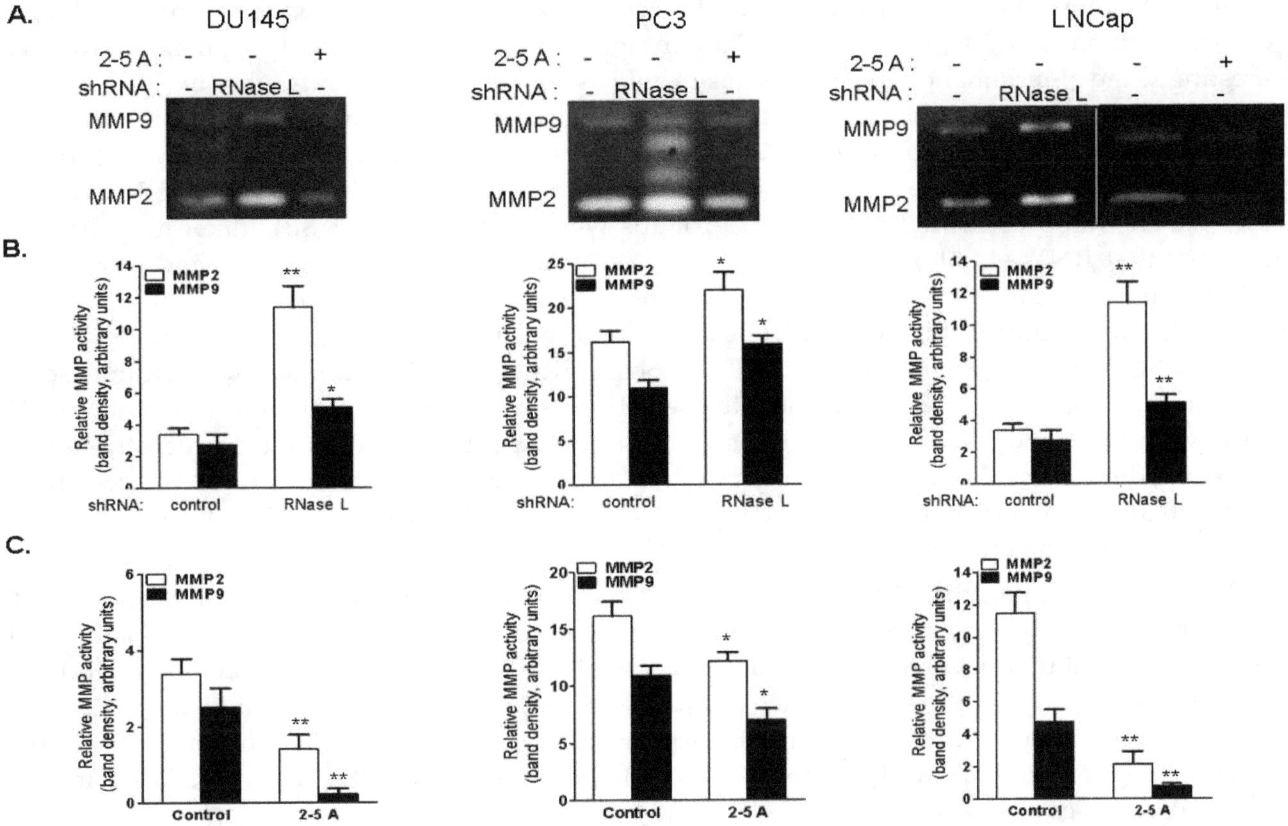

Figure 14. RNase L regulates matrix metalloproteinases (MMP) -2 and MMP-9 activities. (**A**) Gelatin zymography analysis of MMP-2 and MMP-9 activities in conditioned media harvested from DU145, PC3 or LNCaP cells expressing control or RNase L shRNA or transfected with 2–5A complexed with lipofectamine 2000 and added to cells to activate RNase L. Data shown are representative of three independent experiments. Quantitative analysis of MMP-2 and MMP-9 activities in (**B**) Cells expressing RNase L shRNA compared to control shRNA, and (**C**) Cells transfected with 2–5A to activate RNase L compared to control cells. Data shown are mean values ± SEM from three independent experiments. Student's t-test was used to determine p-values. * $p < 0.01$, ** $p < 0.001$, and compared to control shRNA expressing cells (**B**); and control cells (**C**).

3. Discussion

In the present study, we demonstrate the role of RNase L as a suppressor of AR signaling, cell migration and activity of matrix metalloproteinases identifying an unrecognized role of RNase L in prostate cancer. Importantly, the nuclease function of RNase L was not required for suppression. The relevance of the HPC1 (*RNASEL*) mutations in prostate cancer is poorly understood. We provide evidence that the most prevalent HPC1-associated mutations in RNase L, R462Q substitution and E265X truncation, enhance AR nuclear translocation, transcriptional activity and cell migration. This study not only identifies Androgen Receptor as a target of RNase L regulation, but also demonstrates that the effect of HPC1-associated mutations on AR signaling and cell migration is amenable to regulation by physiological conditions that exist in prostate cancer cells.

In androgen-treated cells, the interaction between RNase L, Filamin A and AR is disrupted and AR translocates to the nucleus to induce AR-responsive gene expression. In LNCaP cells lacking RNase L significantly higher nuclear AR was observed, similar to FLNA-depleted cells, and cells lacking both proteins showed further increase in nuclear AR which was reflected by increase in AR transcriptional activity, and expression of AR target genes (Figure 1). Increased nuclear AR was only observed in cells treated with R1881 indicating that RNase L effect on AR is ligand-dependent. As would be expected for a dynamic interaction, over-expression of full-length RNase L suppressed AR nuclear localization and AR nuclear activities. In other studies, over-expression of Filamin A inhibited AR transcriptional activity on androgen treatment indicating common underlying mechanisms [27]. Interestingly, the N-terminal fragment of RNase L which interacted with FLNA inhibited AR signaling similar to the full-length protein, while the C-terminal nuclease domain that fails to interact with FLNA, enhanced AR signaling (Figure 2) [3]. Analysis of subcellular AR distribution following R1881 treatment demonstrated increase in nuclear/cytoplasmic ratio in cells lacking RNase L or FLNA which was exacerbated when both proteins were lacking (Figure 3B). Taken together, our data show that RNase L, along with FLNA, may sequester AR in the cytoplasm and in response to R1881 the dissociation of the complex facilitates nuclear localization of AR. In the absence of the ligand, AR remains in the cytoplasm as a part of a multiprotein complex that includes HSP70 and HSP90 [54–56]. We have not ruled out the possibility that RNase L may alter AR interaction with HSP proteins. However, given that RNase L has been shown to regulate actin dynamics [3], interact with ECM and cytoskeletal proteins [24,26] and, importantly, inhibition of microtubule and cytoskeletal dynamics inhibits androgen-dependent AR nuclear translocation and AR transcriptional activity [30,31,57,58]; together these data suggest significant involvement of RNase L-regulated actin dynamics in AR translocation.

Sustained signaling through AR is a hallmark of castration-resistant prostate cancer (CRPC) and alternative splicing variants of AR (AR-Vs) that lack ligand-binding domain and constitutively active are reported to be upregulated [59–61]. It is established that AR-Vs upregulate transcription of canonical AR-responsive genes and other unique set of target genes [60,62]. Unlike full-length AR, transcriptional activities of the constitutively active AR-Vs are refractory to treatment with taxanes which do not block nuclear translocation of AR-V [63]. Future studies will address if RNase L impacts AR-V-mediated signaling activity.

In addition to transcriptional regulation, AR activity and abundance is regulated at the level of protein degradation and stability [64]. Inhibition of ubiquitin-proteasome degradation pathway has been reported to increase AR levels and several ubiquitin ligases bind to AR and regulate AR functions [65–67]. AR levels decreased to similar levels in WT and RNase L knockdown LNCaP cells (Figure 3) in the absence of ligand, R1881, when *de novo* protein translation is inhibited by cycloheximide treatment. Furthermore, inhibiting proteasome-mediated AR degradation by treating cells with MG132 did not result in altered stability of AR protein when RNase L was depleted. Thus, the inhibitory effect of RNase L on AR signaling does not appear to be due to the effect on AR degradation or stability. These observations support the notion that the final activity of AR in any given cell may eventually reflect balance and coordination of several regulators, including RNase L.

HPC1-associated mutations in RNase L have been studied in the context of RNase L enzyme activity and inducing apoptosis [12] as possible explanation for HPC, but do not address how the mutations contribute specifically to prostate cancer. RNase L R462Q mutant had reduced ability to dimerize into an active enzyme and had three-fold reduced activity and E265X produced a truncated protein which lacked the nuclease domain [12]. Since both mutants compromised RNase L enzyme activity, we raised the possibility that nuclease activity may be important. Recent description of RNase L structure allowed identification of residues critical for recognition of 2–5A, dimerization and nuclease function and we designed mutants based on the structural predictions and tested the ribonuclease activity (Figure 4E,F) [37,68]. In addition to the HPC1-associated mutants, we analyzed the RNase L mutants we generated that either lacked enzyme activity due to mutations in nuclease domain (R667A), or have reduced enzyme activity (K166E) or lack activity due to defects in binding activator, 2–5A (Y312A, K240/274N) for effects on AR signaling. The Y312A mutant lacks enzyme activity like the K240/274N and R667A mutations; however it can suppress AR signaling like WT RNase L indicating that enzyme activity may be dispensable (Figure 4). We conclude that in normal prostate cells RNase L is a negative regulator of AR signaling and loss of RNase L function in HPC can enhance AR signaling which is a hallmark of most prostate cancers.

RNase L regulates actin dynamics suggesting a possible role in cell migration [3]. Our results, consistent with other published data [21,22], shows that prostate cancer cells depleted of RNase L show greater migration in wound healing and transwell migration assays in response to fibronectin and serum (Figure 5). In reconstitution experiments, over-expression of RNase L suppressed cell migration compared to both endogenous levels and knockdown cells while activation of RNase L, which requires RNase L dimerization, inhibited cell migration (Figure 6). Unlike WT RNase L, HPC1-associated mutants, R462Q and E265X supported enhanced cell migration. Other RNase L mutants which have reduced activity (K166E) or lack activity (R667A and K240/274N) show enhanced cell migration. RNase L Y312A is an exception in that it lacks enzyme activity but suppresses cell migration like WT RNase L. The difference in the effect of K240/274N and Y312A may reflect the roles each of the residues play in contacting 2–5A versus disrupting domain interactions. K240 and K274 are critical residues in the P-loop motifs in the ankyrin repeats and may disrupt ankyrin repeat-protein kinase domain interaction and prevent 2–5A binding thereby affecting RNase activity [69]. It is possible that K240/274N mutant alters binding of proteins that contact RNase L through ankyrin repeats and the pseudokinase domains. Y312 is one of the residues that have been shown to provide direct contact with 2–5A and Y312A substitution may therefore lack activity while possibly retaining folding [37]. The precise mechanism by which these mutants affect interactions with other proteins will be addressed in future studies.

The mutations we have tested for AR signaling and cell migration span all the functional domains of RNase L. Mutations in the N-terminal ankyrin repeat domain, which serves as protein interaction domain, have variable effects on nuclear AR and cell migration and mutation in the C-terminal catalytic domain fails to suppress like WT. Biochemical studies showed that RNase L associated with the cytoskeleton assumes an inactive conformation and exists as a monomer while retaining the ability to bind with interacting proteins [24,70]. 2–5A binds to ankyrin repeat 2 and 4 and the pseudokinase domain facilitating dimerization and enzymatic activation. Activation of RNase L may cause dramatic conformational change and dimerization that induces its release from interacting proteins. Based on our results, we propose that the effect of RNase L on AR signaling and cell migration is mediated, in part, by protein-protein interactions and does not require enzymatic activity. Several proteins like Filamin A, LNX and or other cytoskeletal proteins may contribute to both these effects by interacting with RNase L [3,24,26]. Additional studies are required to investigate if the effect of the RNase L mutants is mediated by altered interaction with any of these interacting proteins. RNase L also inhibits cell attachment to ECM substrates and cell spreading on fibronectin. An earlier report showed that activity of RNase L downregulates transcripts involved in cell adhesion both transcriptionally and post-transcriptionally [22]. In contrast, we observed the suppressive effect of RNase L on cell migration in cells expressing endogenous RNase L in the absence of activation or with mutants that lacked enzyme activity.

We explored the underlying mechanisms for increased cell migration in RNase L-depleted cells by analyzing activation of integrin β1 which is primarily involved in adhesion to fibronectin. Increased cell surface expression of integrin β1 in RNase L-depleted cells corresponded with increase in cell migration and decrease correlated with activation of RNase L and inhibition of cell migration (Figures 9 and 10). Further, in androgen responsive LNCap cells, treatment with R1881 resulted in increase in cell surface expression of integrin β1 and RNase L-depleted cells treated with R1881 showed a corresponding increase in integrin β1 expression on cell surface (Figure S4). Activated integrins recruit and induce phosphorylation of FAK and Src which initiate signaling events to activate Rho GTPases to control cell shape and motility [41,42,47]. Accordingly, increase in integrin-stimulated FAK and Src phosphorylation was observed in RNase L-depleted cells and RNase L KO MEFs in response to fibronectin. Inhibiting Src activity with PP2 inhibitor in RNase L-depleted cells decreased cell migration compared to mock-treated cells demonstrating the involvement of the pathway for cell migration. Activity of Rho GTPases is required for cell migration and our testing of small Rho GTPases revealed that expression of dominant-negative form of Rac1 (T17N) significantly inhibited migration of RNase L-depleted cells, whereas dominant-negative Cdc42 (T17N) or RhoA (T19N) did not. Rac1 activity is regulated by Src in many cell types and elevated expression of Rac1 is observed in prostate cancer cells and tumors [71,72]. Our results show higher activity of Rac1 in response to fibronectin in RNase L-depleted cells compared to control cells although total levels of Rac1 protein were very similar. This is the first evidence of regulation of Rac1 activity by RNase L. Interestingly, the two proteins that interact with RNase L, namely, Filamin A and IQGAP1 are reported to regulate Rac1 activity [73]. Based on these observations and published data, RNase L appears to regulate cytoskeletal events, including AR signaling and cell migration, by virtue of its association and interaction with cytoskeletal and motor assembly proteins [26]. Apart from effects on cell migration, RNase L regulates activity of MMP-2 and MMP-9. Knockdown of RNase L increases gelatinase activity of both MMP-2 and -9 (Figure 14) which can enhance ECM remodeling and invasive potential of cells. Consistent with our observations, activation of RNase L inhibited integrin activation, cell migration as well as activity of MMP-2 and -9. MMP activities can be regulated at the level of transcription and post-transcriptionally by activators and inhibitors [74]. Levels of *MMP-9* mRNA did not change in knockdown cells and while not explored here, RNase L may affect MMP activity by regulating natural MMP inhibitors, tissue inhibitors of metalloproteinases (TIMPs).

Collectively, the results presented here identify RNase L as a suppressor of AR signaling, cell migration and MMP activity. Using RNase L mutants we show that nucleolytic activity is dispensable for both AR signaling and migration. HPC1-associated mutations in RNase L enhance AR signaling and cell migration and our study has identified a novel role of RNase L as a prostate cancer susceptibility gene. It is likely that RNase L mutations identified as risk factors in other types of cancers may affect cell migration and contribute to tumor development extending the antitumor role of RNase L beyond prostate cancer.

4. Materials and Methods

4.1. Chemicals, Reagents and Antibodies

Chemicals, unless indicated otherwise, were from Sigma Aldrich (St. Louis, MO, USA). Synthetic androgen R1881 was from Sigma Aldrich, extracellular matrices fibronectin, vitronectin, laminin, collagen I, collagen IV and Src inhibitor PP2 were from Millipore (Billerica, MA, USA). Cycloheximide (Sigma-Aldrich) and MG132 (EMD-Millipore, Billerica, MA, USA) were used at indicated concentrations. Antibodies to AR (N-20), Integrin β1 (M-106) and Filamin A were from Santa Cruz Biotechnology (Santa Cruz, CA, USA), Rac-1 (clone 102) was from BD Biosciences (San Jose, CA, USA). Total FAK, phospho-FAK (Y397), total Src, phospho-Src (Y416) were from Cell Signaling, Inc. (Danvers, MA, USA). RNase L monoclonal antibody was kindly provided by Robert Silverman (Cleveland Clinic). Antibodies to β-actin, monoclonal and polyclonal antibodies to Flag tag, Flag-M2 agarose beads were from Sigma Aldrich. Anti-mouse IgG and anti-rabbit IgG HRP linked secondary antibodies were from Cell Signaling, Inc. (Danvers, MA, USA) and ECL reagents were from GE Healthcare (Piscataway, NJ, USA) and Boston Bioproducts (Ashland, MA, USA). Alexa 488-labeled Phalloidin, and Alexa fluor 647 donkey anti-rabbit IgG were from Life Technologies, Carlsbad, CA, USA.

4.2. Cell Culture and Transfections

DU145, PC3 cells, WT and Rnasel$^{-/-}$ MEFs ((RNase L KO) primary and transformed with SV40 large T antigen, kindly provided by R.H. Silverman, Cleveland Clinic) and LNCaP cells (ATCC, Manassas, VA, USA) were grown in Roswell Park Memorial Institute (RPMI) 1640 supplemented with 100 μg/mL penicillin/streptomycin, 2 mM L-glutamine and 10% heat-inactivated fetal bovine serum (Sigma-Aldrich, St. Louis, MO, USA). For experiments involving androgen treatment, cells were transferred to phenol red-free medium supplemented with 2% charcoal-stripped serum (Hyclone, Logan, UT, USA) at least 24 h prior to addition of the synthetic androgen R1881 (1 nM) or ethanol vehicle (0.01%). Cells were maintained in 95% air, 5% CO_2 at 37 °C. RNase L-silencing (targeting the 3′-UTR), Filamin-A silencing, and non-silencing shRNAs were generated as suggested by the manufacturer using a GIPZ-lentiviral shRNA system and knock down cells or controls were selected with 1 μg/mL of puromycin as described previously [3] (Open Biosystems, Thermo Scientific, PA, USA). In some experiments, RNase L was knocked down using shRNA plasmid as described previously [16]. Knock-down of endogenous proteins was determined by western blotting. Transfection of 2–5A (10 μM) was performed using lipofectamine 2000 (Invitrogen, Thermo Fisher Scientific, Waltham, MA, USA) according to the manufacturer's protocol as described previously [75]. Briefly, cells were plated 1 day before transfection, so that the cells are 80%–90% confluent at the time of transfection. 2–5A was diluted into serum-free media and then mixed with lipofectamine 2000 reagent for 15 min before being added to cells in growth media. Preparation of 2–5A using ATP and recombinant 2–5A synthetase (a generous gift from Rune Hartmann, University of Aarhus, Aarhus, Denmark) has been described previously [75]. PolyI:C (2 μg/mL) was transfected into cells using Polyjet reagent (SignaGen Laboratories, Gaithersburg, MD, USA). Activity of RNase L in intact cells was determined in HeLa cells reconstituted with Flag-RNase L mutant constructs as described previously [75]. In experiments involving inhibitors, cells were preincubated with inhibitor for 1 h prior to treatment and then replaced with growth medium.

4.3. Plasmids

Plasmids Flag-RNase L, Flag-RNase L R667A, Flag-RNase L (1–335, ΔC), Flag-RNase L (386–741, ΔN) (kindly provided by Robert Silverman, Cleveland Clinic) were transfected using lipofectamine 2000 as per manufacturer's instructions. The Flag-RNase L mutants were constructed by site-directed mutagenesis using the primers listed in Table 1 and QuikChange Lightning Multi Site-Directed Mutagenesis Kit (Agilent Technologies, Santa Clara, CA, USA). The constructs were sequenced to confirm the mutations and expression confirmed by immunoblot analysis. The dominant negative Myc-tagged RhoA (T19N), Rac1 (T17N) and Cdc42 (T17N) eukaryotic expression constructs were described previously [50].

Table 1. List of primers used for mutagenesis.

Primer Name	Sequence of Primer
K274N R	5′-CAAGCAGCAGTGCTGTATTGCCATCACTGTCTGTG-3′
K274N F	5′-CACAGACAGTGATGGCAATACAGCACTGCTGCTTG-3′
K240N R	5′-GGATCAGGGGAGTATTCCCTCTTTCTCCCC-3′
K240N F	5′-GGGGAGAAAGAGGGAATACTCCCCTGATCC-3′
R667A R	5′-CAATGTGTTCTCCCAAATTCGCGATGAACTTTAGCAGATCAC-3′
R667A F	5′-GTGATCTGCTAAAGTTCATCGCGAATTTGGGAGAACACATTG-3′
R462Q R	5′-TAAATATAGATGACAGGACATTTTGGGCAAATTCATCTTCCTCATTT-3′
R462Q F	5′-AAATGAGGAAGATGAATTTGCCCAAAATGTCCTGTCATCTATATTTA-3′
E265X R	5′-CTGTGTCATTAATCTATATGTGCTCTTGCTCCAGAAGC-3′
E265X F	5′-GCTTCTGGAGCAAGAGCACATATAGATTAATGACACAG-3′
K166E F	5′-AGAGCGGCTGAGGGAGGGAGGGGCCACAG-3′
K166E R	5′-CTGTGGCCCCTCCCTCCCTCAGCCGCTCT-3′
Y312A R	5′-CAAGGGAATGGTCAGCATTCCGCCTCGCTGTCATAACAAGAT-3′
Y312A F	5′-ATCTTGTTATGACAGCGAGGCGGAATGCTGACCATTCCCTTG-3′

4.4. Co-Immunoprecipitation and Immunoblotting

LNCaP cells expressing Flag-RNase L plasmid were either not treated, treated with R1881 (1 nM) for 1 h or 24 h and harvested. Cells were washed with ice cold PBS and lysed in buffer containing 0.5% NP-40, 90 mM KCl, 5 mM magnesium acetate, 20 mM Tris, pH 7.5, 5 mM β mercaptoethanol, 0.1 M phenylmethylsulfonyl fluoride (PMSF), 0.2 mM sodium orthovanadate, 50 mM NaF, 10 mM glycerophosphate, protease inhibitor (Roche Diagnostics, Indianapolis, IN, USA) on ice for 20 min. The lysates were clarified by centrifugation at 10,000× *g* (at 4 °C for 20 min). Clarified cell lysates were precleared and mixed with control IgG or FlagM2-agarose beads and rotated end-to-end 1 h or overnight at 4 °C. The beads were collected and washed five times in lysis buffer. The immunoprecipitated proteins were dissociated by boiling in Laemmli sample buffer, separated on 10% SDS-polyacrylamide gels, transferred to nitrocellulose membrane (Biorad, Hercules, CA, USA) and subjected to immunoblotting. Membranes were probed with different primary antibodies according to the manufacturer's protocols. Membranes were washed with Tris Buffered Saline (TBS) with 1% Tween 20 and incubated with goat anti-mouse or goat anti-rabbit antibody tagged with horseradish peroxidase (Cell Signaling, Danvers, MA, USA) for 1 h. Proteins in the blots were detected by enhanced chemiluminesence (GE Healthcare). Cell extracts from LNCaP cells treated with cycloheximide (50 μg/mL) alone or combined with MG132 (20 μM) or R1881 (1 nM) were prepared in 2% sodium dodecyl sulphate (SDS) and subjected to immunoblotting. PC3 (control and RNase L knockdown) cells or WT and RNase LKO MEFs were serum starved for 16 h and plated on fibronectin coated dishes for 1 h. FAK and Src phosphorylation was detected by immunoblotting using anti-phospho FAK (Y397) or anti-phospho Src (Y416) antibodies (Cell Signaling, Danvers, MA, USA).

4.5. Immunofluorescence Assays

LNCaP cells (WT, RNase L knockdown, Filamin A knockdown or RNase L and Filamin A knockdown) on glass coverslips were treated with phenol red-free RPMI medium supplemented with 2% charcoal-stripped serum (Hyclone, Logan, UT, USA) at least 24 h prior to addition of the synthetic androgen R1881 (1 nM) or ethanol vehicle (0.01%) for 24 h. In some experiments, LNCaP RNase L-knockdown cells were reconstituted with Flag-RNase L (WT) or various Flag-RNase L mutants and plated on coverslips and treated as described above. Cells were fixed in 4% paraformaldehyde (Boston Bioproducts, MA, USA) for 15 min and permeabilized with 5% goat serum, 0.3% Triton-X-100 in PBS for 1 h. After washing and blocking in 1% Bovine Serum Albumin (BSA) in PBS, the cells were reacted with anti-AR antibody (N-20, Santa Cruz Biotechnology, CA, USA, 1:200 in 1% BSA, 0.3% Triton-X-100 in PBS) at 4 °C for 16 h followed by washing and incubation with fluorescent dye-conjugated secondary antibodies, Alexa-647 Goat anti-rabbit IgG (1:200, 1 h at 4 °C, Molecular probes, CA, USA). Cells were mounted in Vectashield with DAPI to stain the nucleus (Vector Labs, Burlingame, CA, USA). Fluorescence and confocal microscopy assessments were performed with Leica CS SP5 multi-photon laser scanning confocal microscope (Leica Microsystems, Weitzler, Germany) and quantitated using Image J software (National Institutes of Health). Images were processed using Adobe Photoshop CS4 (Adobe, San Jose, CA, USA). More than 10 cells (from at least three fields) were analyzed for each condition from three independent experiments.

4.6. Luciferase Reporter Gene Assays

LNCaP cells (WT, RNase L knockdown, Filamin A knockdown or RNase L and Filamin A knockdown) were transfected with AR-responsive PSA-luciferase [76] (1.0 μg), and plasmid pCH110 expressing β-galactosidase (0.1 μg) to normalize transfection efficiency in phenol red-free RPMI medium supplemented with 2% charcoal-stripped serum (Hyclone, Logan, UT, USA) at least 24 h prior to addition of the synthetic androgen R1881 (1 nM) or ethanol vehicle (0.01%). Cells were harvested in luciferase lysis buffer 24 h after treatment, and luciferase activity was determined using luciferase assay kit (Promega, Madison, WI, USA) and normalized to β-galactosidase levels. Experiments were performed in triplicate, and the results are representative of three independent experiments and shown as ± SD.

4.7. RNA Isolation and Quantitative Real Time Polymerase Chain Reaction

RNA was isolated using Trizol reagent (Invitrogen, Thermo Fisher Scientific,) as per the manufacturer's instructions and used for cDNA synthesis using random decamers and a RETROscript cDNA synthesis kit (Life Technologies; Thermo Fisher Scientific). Expression of androgen-responsive genes was determined by quantitative reverse transcription polymerase chain reaction (qRT-PCR) using

SYBR Green PCR Master Mix (Bio-Rad Laboratories Inc., Hercules, CA, USA) using the gene-specific primers and normalized to *GAPDH* expression. Primer sequences used are listed in Table 2 below. Experiments were performed in triplicate, and the results are representative of three independent experiments and shown as ± SD.

Table 2. List of primers for quantitative real-time polymerase chain reaction.

Primer Name	Sequence of Primer
PSA F	5′-GCAGCATTGAACCAGAGGAG-3′
PSA R	5′-CCCATGACGTGATACCCTGA-3′
sGCα1 F	5′-CTGCCTCATTTGCTTCATCA-3′
sGCα1 R	5′-TTGCCATGCTGAGCTGTTTA-3′
ETV1 F	5′-CACTGGGTCGTGGTACTCCT-3′
ETV1 R	5′-TACCCCATGGACCACAGATT-3′
MMP9 F	5′-GCCATTCACGTCGTCCTTAT-3′
MMP9 R	5′-TTGACAGCGACAAGAAGTGG-3′

4.8. Cell Fractionation

LNCaP cells (WT, RNase L knockdown, Filamin A knockdown or RNase L and Filamin A knockdown) were treated with R1881 or vehicle for 24 h and harvested. Twenty-five percent of the cells were saved as input, and the remaining portion was fractionated into nuclear and cytosolic fractions using Nuclear/Cytosol Fractionation Kit (MBL International Corp., Woburn, MA, USA). The fractions were then subjected to immunoblotting as described above to measure AR levels and quantitated using NIH Image J software.

4.9. Wound Healing Assay

Confluent monolayers of cells in 6-well plates were incubated in serum-free medium for 24 h. Monolayers were scratched with a micropipette tip and washed in phosphate buffer saline (PBS), and replaced with complete growth medium. Migration of cells to close the wound was monitored at indicated times and phase-contrast images were acquired on an Olympus IX81 inverted microscope using a 10× objective lens and a XM10 camera (Olympus, Tokyo, Japan). Wound closure was calculated from at least three independent experiments using NIH Image J software. Data shown are representative of three independent experiments and quantitation is shown as ± SD.

4.10. Cell Migration Assay

Transwell cell migration assays were performed using a modified Boyden chamber (Corning Inc., Corning, NY, USA) containing a fibronectin-coated polycarbonate membrane filter (6.5 mm diameter, 8 µm pore size) in growth medium. DU145, PC3 or LNCaP cells (2×10^5) cells (control or RNase L knockdown) and WT or RNase L KO MEFs were incubated in serum-free medium for 24 h and plated in the upper chamber and allowed to migrate for indicated times to lower chamber that contained growth medium with 10% fetal bovine serum (FBS). Non-migrated cells on the upper chamber were scraped with a cotton swab, and migrated cells on the bottom surface were trypsinized and counted with a hemocytometer. Experiments were performed in triplicate, and the results are representative of three independent experiments and shown as mean ± SEM.

4.11. Cell Spreading Assay

DU145 or PC3 (control or RNase L-knockdown) were plated on fibronectin-coated coverslips for indicated times up to 100 min. Attached and spread cells were fixed with 3.7% paraformaldehyde in PBS (Boston Bioproducts, Ashland, MA, USA) for 10 min and permeabilized with 0.1% Triton-X-100 for 5 min. F-actin was labeled with Alexa 488-labeled phalloidin (Life Technologies, CA, USA) and mounted in Vectashield with DAPI (4′,6-diamidino-2-phenylindole, Vector Laboratories, Burlingame,

CA, USA). Cells were imaged by the use of a Leica TCS SP5 multiphoton laser scanning confocal microscope (Leica Microsystems, Weitzler, Germany), and cell area was quantitated using NIH Image J software. Experiments were repeated in triplicate with at least 30 measurements per time point for each experiment. Data are shown as mean area at indicated time points $\pm$ SEM.

4.12. Cell Attachment Assay

To quantitate cell attachment to different extracellular matrix substrates, 96-well plates were coated with 10 μg/mL each of fibronectin, vitronectin, laminin, collagen I or collagen IV (EMD Millipore, Billerica, MA, USA). Prior to use, the wells were treated with 1% BSA in 1$\times$ PBS (pH 7.4). Cells (2×10^5) in single cell suspension in serum-free medium were added per well in triplicate and incubated at 37 °C for 1 h. Wells were washed three times with PBS, fixed in 95% ethanol and stained with 0.1% crystal violet for 30 min at room temperature. The wells were washed extensively to remove excess stain. Cells were lysed in 0.2% Triton-X-100 and absorbance measured at 570 nm. Percent cell attachment was determined from three independent experiments performed in triplicate and shown as mean $\pm$ SEM.

4.13. Flow Cytometry and Analysis

DU145, PC3 or LNCaP cells (control or RNase L-knockdown) were grown in 100 mm dishes to 80%–90% confluence and then plated on dishes coated with 10 μg/mL fibronectin for 2 h. Cells were harvested and resuspended in ice-cold HEPES-buffer (20 mM HEPES, 125 mM NaCl, 45 mM glucose, 5 mM KCl, 0.1% albumin, pH 7.4) and incubated with anti-integrin β1 antibodies (Santa Cruz Biotechnologies, Santa Cruz, CA, USA) for 1 h. Isotype-specific antibodies were used as controls. Cells were washed three times in HEPES-buffer and incubated with Alexa-fluor-488 labeled secondary antibodies. Flow cytometry was performed using a FACSCalibur System (BectonDickinson, Heidelberg, Germany) equipped with Cell Quest software (Becton-Dickinson, San Jose, CA, USA). In some experiments, cells were transfected with 2–5A (10 μM) for 4 h and subject to flow cytometry analysis.

4.14. Rac Activity Assays

DU145 or PC3 cells (control and RNase L knockdown) were plated on dishes coated with 10 μg/mL fibronectin for 30 min or 1 h. Assays for GTP-bound Rac1 were performed as described [77]. Cells were lysed and precipitated using GST-PBD (PAK-binding domain) beads for pulling down active Rac1. Bead bound proteins (for active Rac1) and cell lysates (total Rac1) were resolved on a 13% SDS-PAGE gel and transferred onto nitrocellulose membranes and probed with primary antibodies against Rac1. The levels of active Rac1 were calculated by comparing the intensities of the active Rac1 bands with those of the total Rac1 bands in each lane using Image J software (National Institutes of Health). Data are expressed as fold increase in Rac1 activity over control and are representative of three independent experiments.

4.15. Gelatin Zymography

Gelatin zymography was performed under non-reducing conditions on 8% polyacrylamide gels copolymerized with 0.1% gelatin (Sigma-Aldrich, St. Louis, MO, USA). Activity of MMP-9 and -2 was determined in culture supernatants of control and RNase L knockdown cells (2×10^5 cells) treated or not with 2–5A (10 μM) as described previously [78]. Clear bands representing MMP-9 and -2 activities were imaged and quantitated using Image J software (National Institute of Health). Data shown are representative of three independent experiments and quantitation is shown mean as $\pm$ SD.

4.16. Statistical Analysis

All values are presented as mean $\pm$ SEM from at least three independent experiments or are representative of three independent experiments performed in triplicate and shown as mean $\pm$ SD.

Student's t-tests were used for determining statistical significance between groups. p-values are shown for all experiments and $p < 0.05$ was considered significant.

5. Conclusions

In this study, we demonstrate a role of RNase L as a suppressor of Androgen Receptor (AR) signaling, cell migration and matrix metalloproteinase activity. Using RNase L mutants, we show that its nucleolytic activity is dispensable for both AR signaling and migration. The most prevalent HPC1-associated mutations in RNase L, R462Q and E265X, enhanced AR signaling and cell migration and our studies identify a novel role of RNase L as a prostate cancer susceptibility gene.

Acknowledgments: This work was supported by National Institutes of Health (NIH) Grants AI089518 (Krishnamurthy Malathi), AI119980-01A1 (Krishnamurthy Malathi), 1R21CA194776-01A1 (Rafael Garcia-Mata), 1R15CA199101-01A1 (Rafael Garcia-Mata), internal grants (Krishnamurthy Malathi) and startup funds from University of Toledo (Krishnamurthy Malathi). We thank Sushovita Mukherjee for data in the preliminary studies and technical help. We thank Robert Silverman (Cleveland Clinic) for RNase L KO MEFs, RNase L antibody and Flag-RNase L plasmids. We thank Douglas Leaman (University of Toledo) and Travis Taylor (University of Toledo) for valuable discussions through the course of this work.

Author Contributions: Krishnamurthy Malathi and Lirim Shemshedini conceived and designed the experiments; Shubham Dayal, Jun Zhou, Praveen Manivannan, Mohammad Adnan Siddiqui, Omaima Farid Ahmad, Matthew Clark and Krishnamurthy Malathi performed the experiments; Krishnamurthy Malathi, Rafael Garcia-Mata and Lirim Shemshedini analyzed the data; Rafael Garcia-Mata, Sahezeel Awadia contributed important reagents and materials; and Krishnamurthy Malathi wrote the paper.

References

1. Borden, E.C.; Sen, G.C.; Uze, G.; Silverman, R.H.; Ransohoff, R.M.; Foster, G.R.; Stark, G.R. Interferons at age 50: Past, current and future impact on biomedicine. *Nat. Rev. Drug Discov.* **2007**, *6*, 975–990. [CrossRef] [PubMed]
2. Silverman, R.H. Viral encounters with 2′,5′-oligoadenylate synthetase and RNase L during the interferon antiviral response. *J. Virol.* **2007**, *81*, 12720–12729. [CrossRef] [PubMed]
3. Malathi, K.; Siddiqui, M.A.; Dayal, S.; Naji, M.; Ezelle, H.J.; Zeng, C.; Zhou, A.; Hassel, B.A. RNase L interacts with filamin a to regulate actin dynamics and barrier function for viral entry. *mBio* **2014**, *5*, e02012. [CrossRef] [PubMed]
4. Al-Ahmadi, W.; Al-Haj, L.; Al-Mohanna, F.A.; Silverman, R.H.; Khabar, K.S. RNase L downmodulation of the rna-binding protein, hur, and cellular growth. *Oncogene* **2009**, *28*, 1782–1791. [CrossRef] [PubMed]
5. Zeng, C.; Yi, X.; Zipris, D.; Liu, H.; Zhang, L.; Zheng, Q.; Malathi, K.; Jin, G.; Zhou, A. RNase L contributes to experimentally induced type 1 diabetes onset in mice. *J. Endocrinol.* **2014**, *223*, 277–287. [CrossRef] [PubMed]
6. Fabre, O.; Salehzada, T.; Lambert, K.; Boo Seok, Y.; Zhou, A.; Mercier, J.; Bisbal, C. RNase L controls terminal adipocyte differentiation, lipids storage and insulin sensitivity via Chop10 mRNA regulation. *Cell Death Differ.* **2012**, *19*, 1470–1481. [CrossRef] [PubMed]
7. Ireland, D.D.; Stohlman, S.A.; Hinton, D.R.; Kapil, P.; Silverman, R.H.; Atkinson, R.A.; Bergmann, C.C. RNase L mediated protection from virus induced demyelination. *PLoS Pathog.* **2009**, *5*, e1000602. [CrossRef] [PubMed]
8. Carpten, J.; Nupponen, N.; Isaacs, S.; Sood, R.; Robbins, C.; Xu, J.; Faruque, M.; Moses, T.; Ewing, C.; Gillanders, E.; et al. Germline mutations in the ribonuclease l gene in families showing linkage with Hpc1. *Nat. Genet.* **2002**, *30*, 181–184. [CrossRef] [PubMed]
9. Casey, G.; Neville, P.J.; Plummer, S.J.; Xiang, Y.; Krumroy, L.M.; Klein, E.A.; Catalona, W.J.; Nupponen, N.; Carpten, J.D.; Trent, J.M.; et al. RNase L arg462gln variant is implicated in up to 13% of prostate cancer cases. *Nat. Genet.* **2002**, *32*, 581–583. [CrossRef] [PubMed]
10. Rennert, H.; Bercovich, D.; Hubert, A.; Abeliovich, D.; Rozovsky, U.; Bar-Shira, A.; Soloviov, S.; Schreiber, L.; Matzkin, H.; Rennert, G.; et al. A novel founder mutation in the *RNASEL* gene, 471delaaag, is associated with prostate cancer in Ashkenazi jews. *Am. J. Hum. Genet.* **2002**, *71*, 981–984. [CrossRef] [PubMed]

11. Rokman, A.; Ikonen, T.; Seppala, E.H.; Nupponen, N.; Autio, V.; Mononen, N.; Bailey-Wilson, J.; Trent, J.; Carpten, J.; Matikainen, M.P.; et al. Germline alterations of the *RNASEL* gene, a candidate *Hpc1* gene at 1q25, in patients and families with prostate cancer. *Am. J. Hum. Genet.* **2002**, *70*, 1299–1304. [CrossRef] [PubMed]
12. Xiang, Y.; Wang, Z.; Murakami, J.; Plummer, S.; Klein, E.A.; Carpten, J.D.; Trent, J.M.; Isaacs, W.B.; Casey, G.; Silverman, R.H. Effects of *RNASEL* mutations associated with prostate cancer on apoptosis induced by 2′,5′-oligoadenylates. *Cancer Res.* **2003**, *63*, 6795–6801. [PubMed]
13. Maier, C.; Haeusler, J.; Herkommer, K.; Vesovic, Z.; Hoegel, J.; Vogel, W.; Paiss, T. Mutation screening and association study of *RNASEL* as a prostate cancer susceptibility gene. *Br. J. Cancer* **2005**, *92*, 1159–1164. [CrossRef] [PubMed]
14. Orr-Urtreger, A.; Bar-Shira, A.; Bercovich, D.; Matarasso, N.; Rozovsky, U.; Rosner, S.; Soloviov, S.; Rennert, G.; Kadouri, L.; Hubert, A.; et al. *RNASEL* mutation screening and association study in Ashkenazi and non-Ashkenazi prostate cancer patients. *Cancer Epidemiol. Biomark. Prev.* **2006**, *15*, 474–479. [CrossRef] [PubMed]
15. Wiklund, F.; Jonsson, B.A.; Brookes, A.J.; Stromqvist, L.; Adolfsson, J.; Emanuelsson, M.; Adami, H.O.; Augustsson-Balter, K.; Gronberg, H. Genetic analysis of the *RNASEL* gene in hereditary, familial, and sporadic prostate cancer. *Clin. Cancer Res.* **2004**, *10*, 7150–7156. [CrossRef] [PubMed]
16. Malathi, K.; Paranjape, J.M.; Ganapathi, R.; Silverman, R.H. Hpc1/*RNASEL* mediates apoptosis of prostate cancer cells treated with 2′,5′-oligoadenylates, topoisomerase i inhibitors, and tumor necrosis factor-related apoptosis-inducing ligand. *Cancer Res.* **2004**, *64*, 9144–9151. [CrossRef] [PubMed]
17. Silverman, R.H. A scientific journey through the 2–5A/RNase L system. *Cytokine Growth Factor Rev.* **2007**, *18*, 381–388. [CrossRef] [PubMed]
18. Malathi, K.; Dong, B.; Gale, M., Jr.; Silverman, R.H. Small self-RNA generated by RNase L amplifies antiviral innate immunity. *Nature* **2007**, *448*, 816–819. [CrossRef] [PubMed]
19. Chakrabarti, A.; Banerjee, S.; Franchi, L.; Loo, Y.M.; Gale, M., Jr.; Nunez, G.; Silverman, R.H. RNase L activates the NLRP3 inflammasome during viral infections. *Cell Host Microbe* **2015**, *17*, 466–477. [CrossRef] [PubMed]
20. Siddiqui, M.A.; Mukherjee, S.; Manivannan, P.; Malathi, K. RNase L cleavage products promote switch from autophagy to apoptosis by caspase-mediated cleavage of Beclin-1. *Int. J. Mol. Sci.* **2015**, *16*, 17611–17636. [CrossRef] [PubMed]
21. Banerjee, S.; Li, G.; Li, Y.; Gaughan, C.; Baskar, D.; Parker, Y.; Lindner, D.J.; Weiss, S.R.; Silverman, R.H. RNase L is a negative regulator of cell migration. *Oncotarget* **2015**, *6*, 44360–44372.
22. Rath, S.; Donovan, J.; Whitney, G.; Chitrakar, A.; Wang, W.; Korennykh, A. Human RNase L tunes gene expression by selectively destabilizing the microrna-regulated transcriptome. *Proc. Natl. Acad. Sci. USA* **2015**, *112*, 15916–15921. [CrossRef] [PubMed]
23. Sato, A.; Naito, T.; Hiramoto, A.; Goda, K.; Omi, T.; Kitade, Y.; Sasaki, T.; Matsuda, A.; Fukushima, M.; Wataya, Y.; et al. Association of RNase L with a ras gtpase-activating-like protein IQGAP1 in mediating the apoptosis of a human cancer cell-line. *FEBS J.* **2010**, *277*, 4464–4473. [CrossRef] [PubMed]
24. Ezelle, H.J.; Malathi, K.; Hassel, B.A. The roles of RNase L in antimicrobial immunity and the cytoskeleton-associated innate response. *Int. J. Mol. Sci.* **2016**, *17*, E74. [CrossRef] [PubMed]
25. Bettoun, D.J.; Scafonas, A.; Rutledge, S.J.; Hodor, P.; Chen, O.; Gambone, C.; Vogel, R.; McElwee-Witmer, S.; Bai, C.; Freedman, L.; et al. Interaction between the androgen receptor and RNase L mediates a cross-talk between the interferon and androgen signaling pathways. *J. Biol. Chem.* **2005**, *280*, 38898–38901. [CrossRef] [PubMed]
26. Gupta, A.; Rath, P.C. Expression of mrna and protein-protein interaction of the antiviral endoribonuclease RNase L in mouse spleen. *Int. J. Biol. Macromol.* **2014**, *69*, 307–318. [CrossRef] [PubMed]
27. Loy, C.J.; Sim, K.S.; Yong, E.L. Filamin-a fragment localizes to the nucleus to regulate androgen receptor and coactivator functions. *Proc. Natl. Acad. Sci. USA* **2003**, *100*, 4562–4567. [CrossRef] [PubMed]
28. Mooso, B.A.; Vinall, R.L.; Tepper, C.G.; Savoy, R.M.; Cheung, J.P.; Singh, S.; Siddiqui, S.; Wang, Y.; Bedolla, R.G.; Martinez, A.; et al. Enhancing the effectiveness of androgen deprivation in prostate cancer by inducing Filamin A nuclear localization. *Endocr. Relat. Cancer* **2012**, *19*, 759–777. [CrossRef] [PubMed]
29. Savoy, R.M.; Ghosh, P.M. The dual role of filamin a in cancer: Can't live with (too much of) it, can't live without it. *Endocr. Relat. Cancer* **2013**, *20*, R341–356. [CrossRef] [PubMed]

30. Zhu, M.L.; Horbinski, C.M.; Garzotto, M.; Qian, D.Z.; Beer, T.M.; Kyprianou, N. Tubulin-targeting chemotherapy impairs androgen receptor activity in prostate cancer. *Cancer Res.* **2010**, *70*, 7992–8002. [CrossRef] [PubMed]
31. Darshan, M.S.; Loftus, M.S.; Thadani-Mulero, M.; Levy, B.P.; Escuin, D.; Zhou, X.K.; Gjyrezi, A.; Chanel-Vos, C.; Shen, R.; Tagawa, S.T.; et al. Taxane-induced blockade to nuclear accumulation of the androgen receptor predicts clinical responses in metastatic prostate cancer. *Cancer Res.* **2011**, *71*, 6019–6029. [CrossRef] [PubMed]
32. Ting, H.J.; Chang, C. Actin associated proteins function as androgen receptor coregulators: An implication of androgen receptor's roles in skeletal muscle. *J. Steroid Biochem. Mol. Biol.* **2008**, *111*, 157–163. [CrossRef] [PubMed]
33. Taplin, M.E.; Balk, S.P. Androgen receptor: A key molecule in the progression of prostate cancer to hormone independence. *J. Cell. Biochem.* **2004**, *91*, 483–490. [CrossRef] [PubMed]
34. Karantanos, T.; Evans, C.P.; Tombal, B.; Thompson, T.C.; Montironi, R.; Isaacs, W.B. Understanding the mechanisms of androgen deprivation resistance in prostate cancer at the molecular level. *Eur. Urol.* **2015**, *67*, 470–479. [CrossRef] [PubMed]
35. Lee, D.K.; Chang, C. Endocrine mechanisms of disease: Expression and degradation of androgen receptor: Mechanism and clinical implication. *J. Clin. Endocrinol. Metab.* **2003**, *88*, 4043–4054. [CrossRef] [PubMed]
36. Malathi, K.; Paranjape, J.M.; Bulanova, E.; Shim, M.; Guenther-Johnson, J.M.; Faber, P.W.; Eling, T.E.; Williams, B.R.; Silverman, R.H. A transcriptional signaling pathway in the IFN system mediated by 2′-5′-oligoadenylate activation of RNase L. *Proc. Natl. Acad. Sci. USA* **2005**, *102*, 14533–14538. [CrossRef]
37. Huang, H.; Zeqiraj, E.; Dong, B.; Jha, B.K.; Duffy, N.M.; Orlicky, S.; Thevakumaran, N.; Talukdar, M.; Pillon, M.C.; Ceccarelli, D.F.; et al. Dimeric structure of pseudokinase RNase L bound to 2–5A reveals a basis for interferon-induced antiviral activity. *Mol. Cell* **2014**, *53*, 221–234. [CrossRef] [PubMed]
38. Juliano, R.L.; Haskill, S. Signal transduction from the extracellular matrix. *J. Cell Biol.* **1993**, *120*, 577–585. [CrossRef] [PubMed]
39. Guo, W.; Giancotti, F.G. Integrin signalling during tumour progression. *Nat. Rev. Mol. Cell Biol.* **2004**, *5*, 816–826. [CrossRef] [PubMed]
40. Boudreau, N.J.; Jones, P.L. Extracellular matrix and integrin signalling: The shape of things to come. *Biochem. J.* **1999**, *339*, 481–488. [CrossRef] [PubMed]
41. Schlaepfer, D.D.; Hunter, T. Signal transduction from the extracellular matrix–a role for the focal adhesion protein-tyrosine kinase fak. *Cell Struct. Funct.* **1996**, *21*, 445–450. [CrossRef] [PubMed]
42. Mitra, S.K.; Schlaepfer, D.D. Integrin-regulated FAK-Src signaling in normal and cancer cells. *Curr. Opin. Cell Biol.* **2006**, *18*, 516–523. [CrossRef] [PubMed]
43. Hamadi, A.; Bouali, M.; Dontenwill, M.; Stoeckel, H.; Takeda, K.; Ronde, P. Regulation of focal adhesion dynamics and disassembly by phosphorylation of FAK at tyrosine 397. *J. Cell Sci.* **2005**, *118*, 4415–4425. [CrossRef] [PubMed]
44. Schlaepfer, D.D.; Mitra, S.K.; Ilic, D. Control of motile and invasive cell phenotypes by focal adhesion kinase. *Biochim. Biophys. Acta* **2004**, *1692*, 77–102. [CrossRef] [PubMed]
45. Arias-Salgado, E.G.; Lizano, S.; Sarkar, S.; Brugge, J.S.; Ginsberg, M.H.; Shattil, S.J. Src kinase activation by direct interaction with the integrin beta cytoplasmic domain. *Proc. Natl. Acad. Sci. USA* **2003**, *100*, 13298–13302. [CrossRef] [PubMed]
46. Palazzo, A.F.; Eng, C.H.; Schlaepfer, D.D.; Marcantonio, E.E.; Gundersen, G.G. Localized stabilization of microtubules by integrin- and FAK-facilitated rho signaling. *Science* **2004**, *303*, 836–839. [CrossRef] [PubMed]
47. Lawson, C.D.; Burridge, K. The on-off relationship of Rho and Rac during integrin-mediated adhesion and cell migration. *Small GTPases* **2014**, *5*, e27958. [CrossRef] [PubMed]
48. Nobes, C.D.; Hawkins, P.; Stephens, L.; Hall, A. Activation of the small GTP-binding proteins Rho and Rac by growth factor receptors. *J. Cell Sci.* **1995**, *108*, 225–233. [PubMed]
49. Hall, A. Small GTP-binding proteins and the regulation of the actin cytoskeleton. *Annu. Rev. Cell Biol.* **1994**, *10*, 31–54. [CrossRef] [PubMed]
50. Boulter, E.; Garcia-Mata, R.; Guilluy, C.; Dubash, A.; Rossi, G.; Brennwald, P.J.; Burridge, K. Regulation of Rho GTPase crosstalk, degradation and activity by Rhogdi1. *Nat. Cell Biol.* **2010**, *12*, 477–483. [CrossRef] [PubMed]

51. Kessenbrock, K.; Plaks, V.; Werb, Z. Matrix metalloproteinases: Regulators of the tumor microenvironment. *Cell* **2010**, *141*, 52–67. [CrossRef] [PubMed]
52. Morgia, G.; Falsaperla, M.; Malaponte, G.; Madonia, M.; Indelicato, M.; Travali, S.; Mazzarino, M.C. Matrix metalloproteinases as diagnostic (MMP-13) and prognostic (MMP-2, MMP-9) markers of prostate cancer. *Urol. Res.* **2005**, *33*, 44–50. [CrossRef] [PubMed]
53. Incorvaia, L.; Badalamenti, G.; Rini, G.; Arcara, C.; Fricano, S.; Sferrazza, C.; Di Trapani, D.; Gebbia, N.; Leto, G. MMP-2, MMP-9 and Activin A blood levels in patients with breast cancer or prostate cancer metastatic to the bone. *Anticancer Res.* **2007**, *27*, 1519–1525. [PubMed]
54. Fang, Y.; Fliss, A.E.; Robins, D.M.; Caplan, A.J. Hsp90 regulates androgen receptor hormone binding affinity in vivo. *J. Biol. Chem.* **1996**, *271*, 28697–28702. [CrossRef] [PubMed]
55. Schneider, C.; Sepp-Lorenzino, L.; Nimmesgern, E.; Ouerfelli, O.; Danishefsky, S.; Rosen, N.; Hartl, F.U. Pharmacologic shifting of a balance between protein refolding and degradation mediated by hsp90. *Proc. Natl. Acad. Sci. USA* **1996**, *93*, 14536–14541. [CrossRef] [PubMed]
56. He, B.; Bai, S.; Hnat, A.T.; Kalman, R.I.; Minges, J.T.; Patterson, C.; Wilson, E.M. An androgen receptor NH2-terminal conserved motif interacts with the cooh terminus of the hsp70-interacting protein (chip). *J. Biol. Chem.* **2004**, *279*, 30643–30653. [CrossRef] [PubMed]
57. Mistry, S.J.; Oh, W.K. New paradigms in microtubule-mediated endocrine signaling in prostate cancer. *Mol. Cancer Ther.* **2013**, *12*, 555–566. [CrossRef] [PubMed]
58. Yuan, X.; Cai, C.; Chen, S.; Chen, S.; Yu, Z.; Balk, S.P. Androgen receptor functions in castration-resistant prostate cancer and mechanisms of resistance to new agents targeting the androgen axis. *Oncogene* **2014**, *33*, 2815–2825. [CrossRef] [PubMed]
59. Dehm, S.M.; Schmidt, L.J.; Heemers, H.V.; Vessella, R.L.; Tindall, D.J. Splicing of a novel androgen receptor exon generates a constitutively active androgen receptor that mediates prostate cancer therapy resistance. *Cancer Res.* **2008**, *68*, 5469–5477. [CrossRef] [PubMed]
60. Guo, Z.; Yang, X.; Sun, F.; Jiang, R.; Linn, D.E.; Chen, H.; Chen, H.; Kong, X.; Melamed, J.; Tepper, C.G.; et al. A novel androgen receptor splice variant is up-regulated during prostate cancer progression and promotes androgen depletion-resistant growth. *Cancer Res.* **2009**, *69*, 2305–2313. [CrossRef] [PubMed]
61. Hu, R.; Dunn, T.A.; Wei, S.; Isharwal, S.; Veltri, R.W.; Humphreys, E.; Han, M.; Partin, A.W.; Vessella, R.L.; Isaacs, W.B.; et al. Ligand-independent androgen receptor variants derived from splicing of cryptic exons signify hormone-refractory prostate cancer. *Cancer Res.* **2009**, *69*, 16–22. [CrossRef] [PubMed]
62. Hu, R.; Lu, C.; Mostaghel, E.A.; Yegnasubramanian, S.; Gurel, M.; Tannahill, C.; Edwards, J.; Isaacs, W.B.; Nelson, P.S.; Bluemn, E.; et al. Distinct transcriptional programs mediated by the ligand-dependent full-length androgen receptor and its splice variants in castration-resistant prostate cancer. *Cancer Res.* **2012**, *72*, 3457–3462. [CrossRef] [PubMed]
63. Zhang, G.; Liu, X.; Li, J.; Ledet, E.; Alvarez, X.; Qi, Y.; Fu, X.; Sartor, O.; Dong, Y.; Zhang, H. Androgen receptor Splice variants circumvent ar blockade by microtubule-targeting agents. *Oncotarget* **2015**, *6*, 23358–23371. [CrossRef] [PubMed]
64. Gioeli, D.; Paschal, B.M. Post-translational modification of the androgen receptor. *Mol. Cell. Endocrinol.* **2012**, *352*, 70–78. [CrossRef] [PubMed]
65. Lin, H.K.; Wang, L.; Hu, Y.C.; Altuwaijri, S.; Chang, C. Phosphorylation-dependent ubiquitylation and degradation of androgen receptor by Akt require MDM2 E3 ligase. *EMBO J.* **2002**, *21*, 4037–4048. [CrossRef] [PubMed]
66. Qi, J.; Tripathi, M.; Mishra, R.; Sahgal, N.; Fazli, L.; Ettinger, S.; Placzek, W.J.; Claps, G.; Chung, L.W.; Bowtell, D.; et al. The e3 ubiquitin ligase siah2 contributes to castration-resistant prostate cancer by regulation of androgen receptor transcriptional activity. *Cancer Cell* **2013**, *23*, 332–346. [CrossRef] [PubMed]
67. Xu, K.; Shimelis, H.; Linn, D.E.; Jiang, R.; Yang, X.; Sun, F.; Guo, Z.; Chen, H.; Li, W.; Chen, H.; et al. Regulation of androgen receptor transcriptional activity and specificity by Rnf6-induced ubiquitination. *Cancer Cell* **2009**, *15*, 270–282. [CrossRef]
68. Han, Y.; Donovan, J.; Rath, S.; Whitney, G.; Chitrakar, A.; Korennykh, A. Structure of human RNase L reveals the basis for regulated RNA decay in the IFN response. *Science* **2014**, *343*, 1244–1248. [CrossRef] [PubMed]
69. Zhou, A.; Hassel, B.A.; Silverman, R.H. Expression cloning of 2–5a-dependent RNaase: A uniquely regulated mediator of interferon action. *Cell* **1993**, *72*, 753–765. [CrossRef]

70. Tnani, M.; Aliau, S.; Bayard, B. Localization of a molecular form of interferon-regulated RNase l in the cytoskeleton. *J. Interferon Cytokine Res.* **1998**, *18*, 361–368. [CrossRef] [PubMed]
71. Timpson, P.; Jones, G.E.; Frame, M.C.; Brunton, V.G. Coordination of cell polarization and migration by the rho family GTPases requires src tyrosine kinase activity. *Curr. Biol. CB* **2001**, *11*, 1836–1846. [CrossRef]
72. Engers, R.; Ziegler, S.; Mueller, M.; Walter, A.; Willers, R.; Gabbert, H.E. Prognostic relevance of increased Rac GTPase expression in prostate carcinomas. *Endocr. Relat. Cancer* **2007**, *14*, 245–256. [CrossRef] [PubMed]
73. Jacquemet, G.; Morgan, M.R.; Byron, A.; Humphries, J.D.; Choi, C.K.; Chen, C.S.; Caswell, P.T.; Humphries, M.J. Rac1 is deactivated at integrin activation sites through an Iqgap1-Filamin-A-Racgap1 pathway. *J. Cell Sci.* **2013**, *126*, 4121–4135. [CrossRef] [PubMed]
74. Gong, Y.; Chippada-Venkata, U.D.; Oh, W.K. Roles of matrix metalloproteinases and their natural inhibitors in prostate cancer progression. *Cancers* **2014**, *6*, 1298–1327. [CrossRef] [PubMed]
75. Siddiqui, M.A.; Malathi, K. Rnase L induces autophagy via c-Jun N-terminal kinase and double-stranded RNA-dependent protein kinase signaling pathways. *J. Biol. Chem.* **2012**, *287*, 43651–43664. [CrossRef] [PubMed]
76. Cai, C.; Hsieh, C.L.; Omwancha, J.; Zheng, Z.; Chen, S.Y.; Baert, J.L.; Shemshedini, L. *Etv1* is a novel androgen receptor-regulated gene that mediates prostate cancer cell invasion. *Mol. Endocrinol.* **2007**, *21*, 1835–1846. [CrossRef] [PubMed]
77. Guilluy, C.; Dubash, A.D.; Garcia-Mata, R. Analysis of RhoA and Rho gef activity in whole cells and the cell nucleus. *Nat. Protoc.* **2011**, *6*, 2050–2060. [CrossRef] [PubMed]
78. Mukherjee, S.; Siddiqui, M.A.; Dayal, S.; Ayoub, Y.Z.; Malathi, K. Epigallocatechin-3-gallate suppresses proinflammatory cytokines and chemokines induced by toll-like receptor 9 agonists in prostate cancer cells. *J. Inflamm. Res.* **2014**, *7*, 89–101. [PubMed]

11

An Automated Micro-Total Immunoassay System for Measuring Cancer-Associated α2,3-linked Sialyl *N*-Glycan-Carrying Prostate-Specific Antigen May Improve the Accuracy of Prostate Cancer Diagnosis

Tomokazu Ishikawa [1,2], Tohru Yoneyama [1,3,*], Yuki Tobisawa [1], Shingo Hatakeyama [1], Tatsuo Kurosawa [2], Kenji Nakamura [2], Shintaro Narita [4], Koji Mitsuzuka [5], Wilhelmina Duivenvoorden [6], Jehonathan H. Pinthus [6], Yasuhiro Hashimoto [3], Takuya Koie [1], Tomonori Habuchi [4], Yoichi Arai [5] and Chikara Ohyama [1,3]

1 Department of Urology, Hirosaki University Graduate School of Medicine, Hirosaki 036-8562, Japan; ishikawa.tomokazu@wako-chem.co.jp (T.I.); tobisawa@hirosaki-u.ac.jp (Y.T.); shingoh@hirosaki-u.ac.jp (S.H.); goodwin@hirosaki-u.ac.jp (T.K.); coyama@hirosaki-u.ac.jp (C.O.)
2 Diagnostics Research Laboratories, Wako Pure Chemical Industries, Hyogo 661-0963, Japan; kurosawa.tatsuo@wako-chem.co.jp (T.K.); nakamura.kenji@wako-chem.co.jp (K.N.)
3 Department of Advanced Transplant and Regenerative Medicine, Hirosaki University Graduate School of Medicine, Hirosaki 036-8562, Japan; bikkuri@opal.plala.or.jp
4 Department of Urology, Akita University Graduate School of Medicine, Akita 010-8543, Japan; narishin@doc.med.akita-u.ac.jp (S.N.); thabuchi@doc.med.akita-u.ac.jp (T.H.)
5 Department of Urology, Tohoku University Graduate School of Medicine, Sendai 980-8574, Japan; mitsuzuka@uro.med.tohoku.ac.jp (K.M.); yarai@uro.med.tohoku.ac.jp (Y.A.)
6 Department of Surgery, McMaster University, Hamilton, ON L8S4L8, Canada; duiven@mcmaster.ca (W.D.); pinthusj@hhsc.ca (J.H.P.)
* Correspondence: tohruyon@hirosaki-u.ac.jp

Academic Editor: Carsten Stephan

Abstract: The low specificity of the prostate-specific antigen (PSA) for early detection of prostate cancer (PCa) is a major issue worldwide. The aim of this study to examine whether the serum PCa-associated α2,3-linked sialyl *N*-glycan-carrying PSA (S2,3PSA) ratio measured by automated micro-total immunoassay systems (μTAS system) can be applied as a diagnostic marker of PCa. The μTAS system can utilize affinity-based separation involving noncovalent interaction between the immunocomplex of S2,3PSA and *Maackia amurensis* lectin to simultaneously determine concentrations of free PSA and S2,3PSA. To validate quantitative performance, both recombinant S2,3PSA and benign-associated α2,6-linked sialyl *N*-glycan-carrying PSA (S2,6PSA) purified from culture supernatant of PSA cDNA transiently-transfected Chinese hamster ovary (CHO)-K1 cells were used as standard protein. Between 2007 and 2016, fifty patients with biopsy-proven PCa were pair-matched for age and PSA levels, with the same number of benign prostatic hyperplasia (BPH) patients used to validate the diagnostic performance of serum S2,3PSA ratio. A recombinant S2,3PSA- and S2,6PSA-spiked sample was clearly discriminated by μTAS system. Limit of detection of S2,3PSA was 0.05 ng/mL and coefficient variation was less than 3.1%. The area under the curve (AUC) for detection of PCa for the S2,3PSA ratio (%S2,3PSA) with cutoff value 43.85% (AUC; 0.8340) was much superior to total PSA (AUC; 0.5062) using validation sample set. Although the present results are preliminary, the newly developed μTAS platform for measuring %S2,3PSA can achieve the required assay performance specifications for use in the practical and clinical setting and may improve the accuracy of PCa diagnosis. Additional validation studies are warranted.

Keywords: prostate-specific antigen; α2,3-linked sialyl *N*-glycan; *Maackia amurensis* lectin (MAA) lectin; biomarker

1. Introduction

Serum prostate-specific antigen (PSA) is widely used as a powerful biomarker for detecting prostate cancer (PCa) [1,2]. However, PSA-based PCa screening has resulted in over-diagnosis, leading to unnecessary prostate biopsies and overtreatment of indolent cancer [3–5]. Therefore, novel, more specific screening methods are urgently needed, especially for young healthy men. Of the various molecular isoforms of PSA, proPSA is one of the most promising potential biomarkers [6–10]. A multi-biomarker test for identifying aggressive prostate cancer that combines total PSA, free PSA, intact PSA, and human kallikrein-2 has been developed [11,12]. In contrast, we focused on the cancer-associated glycan alterations that have frequently been observed during carcinogenesis [13,14]. More importantly, some glycans, for example α-fetoprotein [15] and human chorionic gonadotropin [16], have been found to have specific cancer-associated carbohydrate alterations compared with their normal counterparts. The glycoprotein PSA has an *N*-glycosylation site on its 45th amino acid from the N-terminus. In a prior study, we cleaved a PSA-specific sequence (Ile-Arg-Asn-Lys, IRNK) that includes the glycosylated-Asn (N) and performed an intensive structural analysis of the glycan profile of PSA using matrix-assisted laser desorption/ionization time-of-flight (MALDI-TOF) mass spectrometry [17]. This resulted in our identification of a PCa-associated aberrant glycosylation of PSA, which produces α2,3-linked sialyl *N*-glycan that is readily observed on free PSA (S2,3PSA), whereas α2,6-linked sialyl *N*-glycan on free PSA (S2,6PSA) is exclusive to benign prostatic hyperplasia (BPH) [18] (Figure 1).

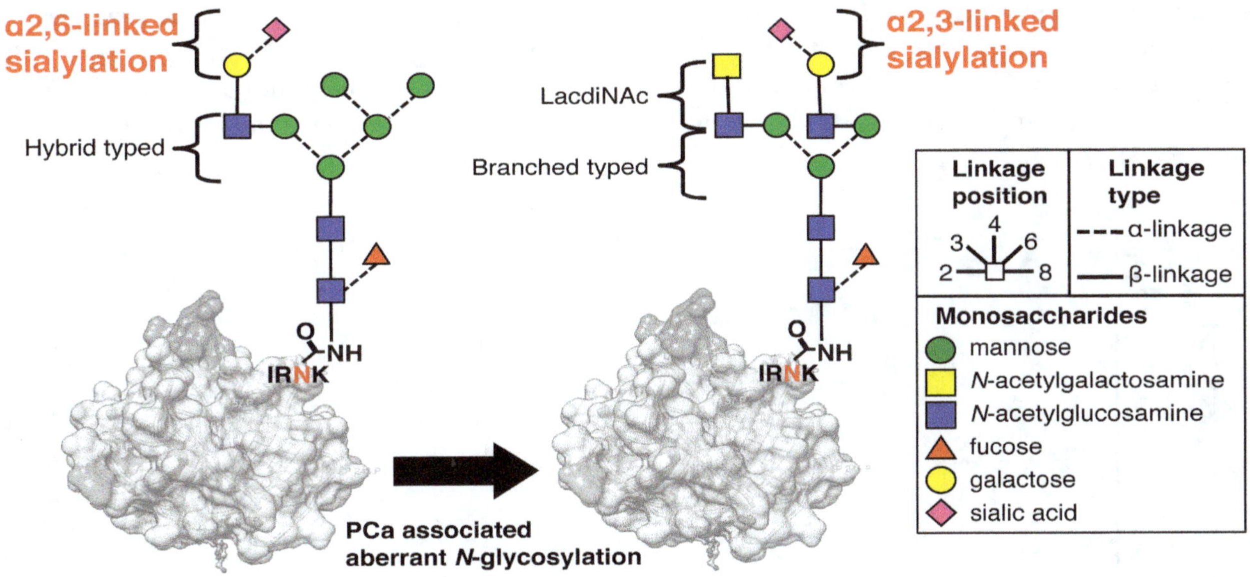

Figure 1. Prostate cancer-associated aberrant glycosylation of *N*-glycan on prostate-specific antigen (PSA). In normal PSA, the terminal sialic acids link to galactose residues with an α2,6 linkage whereas in prostate cancer (PCa)-associated PSA, the linkage between the terminal sialic acid and galactose residues is an α2,3 linkage [18]. Carbon linkage positions are denoted by the bond position drawn on each monosaccharide. Ile-Arg-Asn-Lys, (IRNK): *N*-glycosylation site of PSA.

We have also previously developed a magnetic bead-based S2,3PSA assay (Luminex method) that more accurately diagnoses early PCa than the conventional PSA test [19]. However, this method cannot measure benign S2,6PSA and does not have enough quantitative capability for clinical application. With the aim of overcoming these issues, we investigated using microfluidic technology, also referred to as micro-total analysis systems (μTAS system) [20–23], to quantitate both S2,6PSA and S2,3PSA in patient serum samples with a one-time measurement. μTAS immunoassays incorporating an automated platform can achieve the required assay performance specifications in clinical laboratories more efficiently than existing methodologies. In this study, we developed an automated μTAS system for measuring serum S2,3PSA ratio (%S2,3PSA) in clinical settings.

2. Results

2.1. Preparation of FLAG-Tag-Fused Recombinat S2,3 and S2,6 PSA in Chinese Hamster Ovary (CHO) Cells

To construct S2,3PSA and S2,6PSA recombinant standard protein, FLAG-tag-fused human PSA cDNA (PSA–FLAG) was transiently transfected into CHO cells. Results of immunoblotting of PSA–FLAG-transfected CHO culture supernatant are shown in Figure 2a. Using an *Agrocybe cylindracea* (ACG) lectin affinity column and gel filtration column chromatography, S2,3PSA and S2,6PSA containing asialo-type *N*-glycan carrying recombinant PSA standard protein was purified from culture supernatants of human PSA expressed by CHO cells (Figure 2b,c). Lectin array analysis then revealed the putative glycan structure of purified S2,3 and S2,6PSA recombinant standard (Figure 2d). Signal intensity of recombinant S2,3PSA against *Mackkia amurensis* lectin (MAL) that preferentially bound the sialic acid α2,3-linked galactose structure was much higher than that of recombinant S2,6PSA. Signal intensity of recombinant S2,3PSA against *Sambucus Nigra* lectin (SNA) and *Sambucus Sieboldiana* lectin (SSA) that preferentially bound the sialic acid α2,6-linked galactose structure was much lower than that of recombinant S2,6PSA. These results suggest that the culture supernatant of PSA–FLAG-transfected CHO cells contained both α2,3- and α2,6-linked sialyl *N*-glycan-carrying recombinant PSA and could be utilized as a standard protein of μTAS system measuring S2,3PSA ratio (%S2,3PSA).

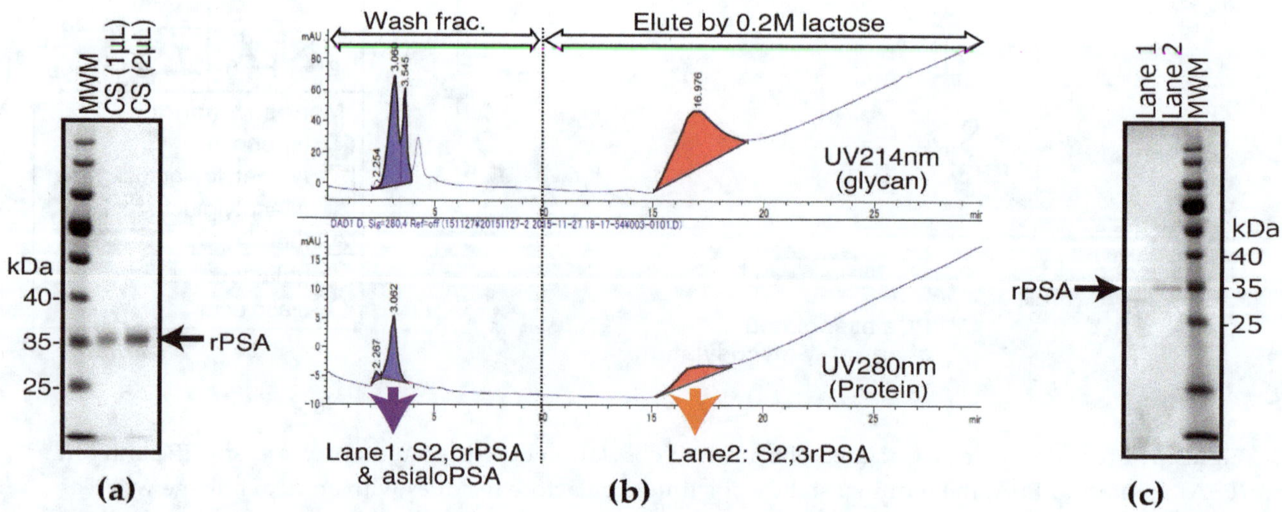

Figure 2. *Cont.*

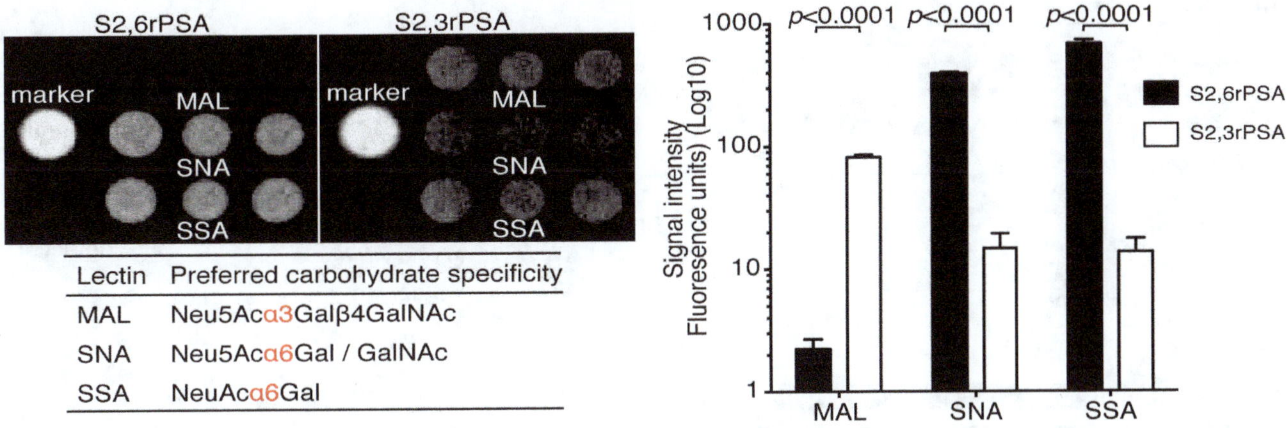

(d)

Figure 2. Preparation of α2,3-linked sialyl *N*-glycan-carrying PSA (S2,3PSA) and α2,6-linked sialyl *N*-glycan-carrying PSA (S2,6PSA) in Chinese hamster ovary (CHO)-K1 cells transfected with PSA–FLAG. CHO-K1 cells were transfected with FLAG-tag-fused human PSA cDNA (PSA–FLAG). (**a**) Culture supernatant (CS) with serum free media were blotted onto polyvinylidene fluoride (PVDF) membrane and probed with anti-FLAG antibodies; (**b**) Chromatograms obtained using *Agrocybe cylindracea* (ACG) lectin column chromatography for α2,3-linked sialyl *N*-glycan-carrying recombinant PSA (S2,3rPSA) collected from 0.2 M lactose eluted fraction and other glyco-isoform free PSA containing α2,6-linked sialyl *N*-glycan (S2,6rPSA) or asialo-type *N*-glycan collected from washed fraction. S2,3rPSA and S2,6PSA was further purified by gel filtration column chromatography; (**c**) Washed fraction (lane 1) and 0.2 M lactose-eluted fraction (lane 2) (indicating chromatogram) (**b**) were blotted onto PVDF membrane and probed with anti-FLAG antibodies; (**d**) Lectin array profiling of S2,3rPSA and S2,6rPSA proteins. Purified S2,3rPSA and S2,6rPSA was applied to the lectin array, including triplicate spots. The glass slides were scanned using a GlycoStationReader1200 (Glycotechnica, Sapporo, Japan). MWM: molecular weight markers; MAL: *Mackkia amurensis* lectin; SNA: *Sambucus Nigra* lectin; SSA: *Sambucus sieboldiana* lectin.

2.2. S2,6PSA and S2,3PSA Separation in a Microfluidic Channel Filled with Electrophoresis Leading Buffer Containing Maackia Amurensis Lectin

Simultaneous quantitative measurement of S2,6PSA and S2,3PSA was achieved by performing microchip capillary electrophoresis and liquid-phase binding assay (LBA) on a μTAS Wako i30 auto analyzer with microfluidic chip IO6 (Wako Pure Chemical Industries, Hyogo, Japan) for electrokinetic analyte transport assay (EATA) (Figure 3a–c). Total assay time of μTAS system measuring %S2,3PSA ratio was 9 min, substantially shorter than the previously developed Luminex method (4 h). The reaction time during transport of DNA conjugate and bound free PSA analyte through the chip channels is short (25–50 s), and the binding kinetics are greatly increased by isotachophoresis (ITP) stacking and concentration of the reactants (Figure 3b) [24,25]. Figure 3c shows a typical electropherogram of S2,6PSA and S2,3PSA in a microfluidic channel separated by lectin affinity electrophoresis. Because S2,3PSA is reactive to *Mackkia amurensis* lectin (MAA), electrophoretic migration of the sandwich complex of DNA–labeled anti-total PSA Fab′ (DNA–Fab′), S2,3PSA, and HiLyte Fluor 647–labeled anti-free PSA Fab′ (HiLyte–Fab′) in the separation channel is slower than that of the immunocomplex of DNA–Fab′, S2,6PSA, and HiLyte–Fab′.

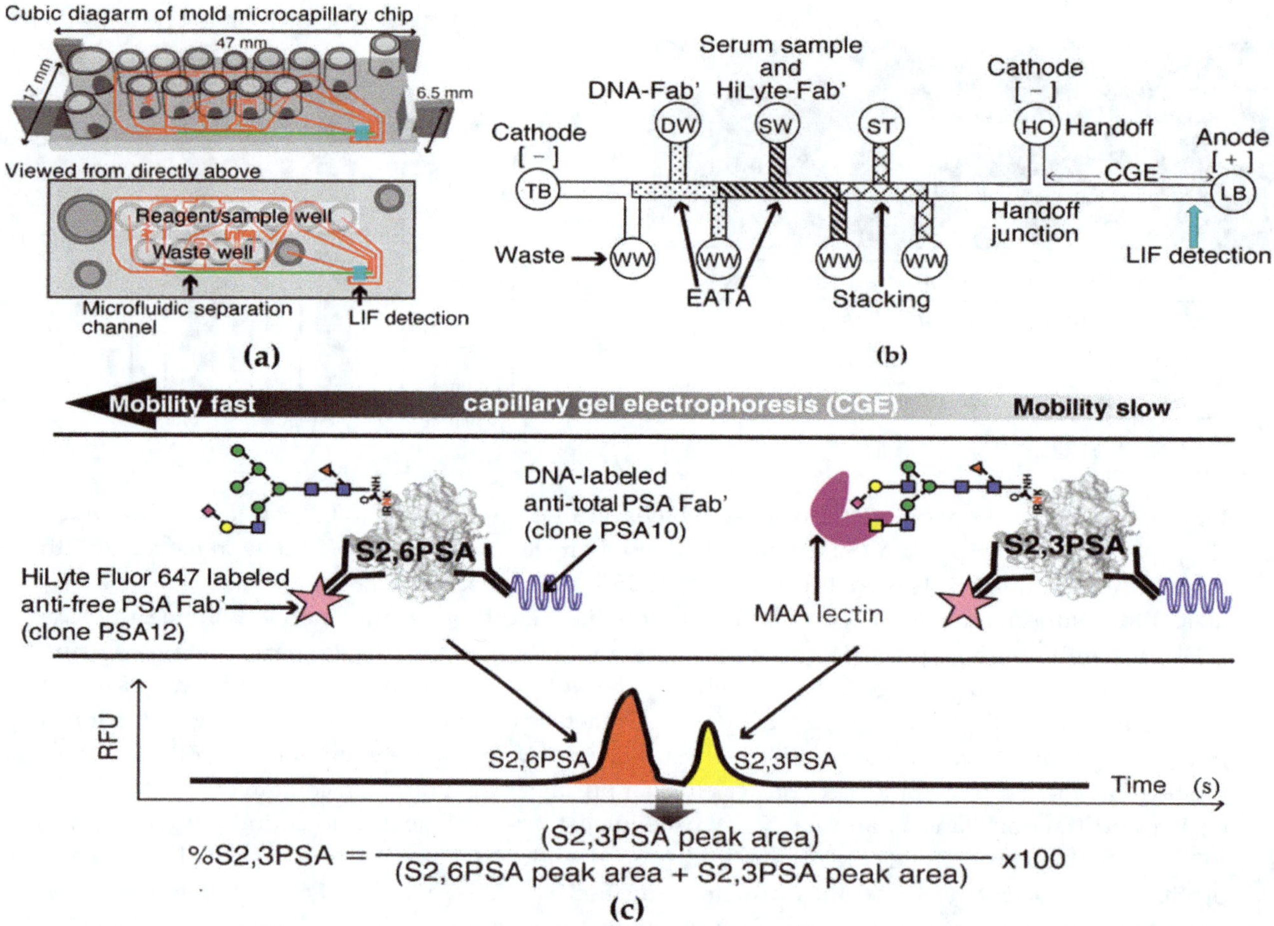

Figure 3. %S2,3PSA test using micro-total immunoassay systems (μTAS)-based microcapillary electrophoresis. (**a**) Molded plastic chip with top wells for reagents and precision microchannels on the bottom. Red line indicates microchannels. Highlight green line indicates microcapillary separation channel. Fluorescence signals are detected through the thin film closing the channels on the bottom of the chip; (**b**) Schematic diagram of a chip showing the electrokinetic analyte transport assay (EATA) method. Waste wells (WWs), trailing buffer (TB) well, leading buffer (LB), handoff (HO), DNA–labeled anti-total PSA Fab′ (DNA–Fab′) (DW), serum sample and HiLyte Fluor 647–labeled anti-free PSA Fab′ (HiLyte–Fab′) mixture (SW), and stacking buffer (ST) wells are shown. Vacuum applied to the WWs loads the reagents and sample-to-chip channel segments and voltage applied between cathode and anode mixes the sample and reagents for the binding reaction. Switching the voltage from the TB well to the HO well switches from isotachophoresis (ITP) stacking mode to capillary gel electrophoresis (CGE) mode. Separation of S2,3PSA from other glyco-isoform of free PSA occurs in the *Mackkia amurensis* lectin (MAA)-filled CGE separation channel prior to laser-induced fluorescence (LIF) detection. (**c**) Typical electropherogram of S2,6PSA and S2,3PSA peak separation. Fluorescent markers have been coelectrophoresed to identify the PSA protein peak positions (data not shown). RFU: relative fluorescence units.

When MAA was eliminated from leading buffer (LB) in the separation channel, both S2,6PSA and S2,3PSA immunocomplex co-migrated to the same position (Figure 4a). Furthermore, using affinity-based separation with MAA lectin against aberrant glycosylation, we also confirmed a capture efficiency of applied S2,3rPSA standard of almost 100% in this assay (Figure 4b,c).

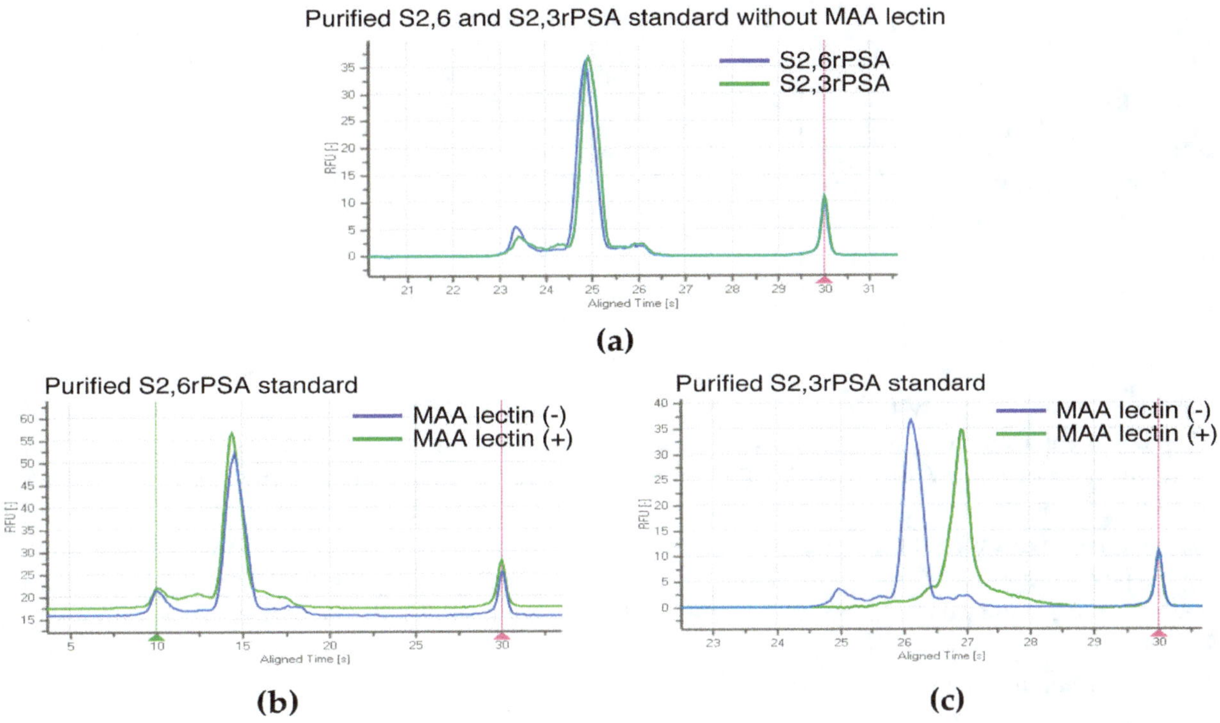

Figure 4. Capture efficiency of applied S2,3PSA standard in µTAS assay. (**a**) Electropherogram of S2,6rPSA and S2,3rPSA without MAA lectin. S2,6rPSA (**b**) and S2,3rPSA (**c**) standard were applied to the detection of peak separation respectively in a microfluidic channel filled with leading buffer (LB) containing MAA lectin (+) or not (−). The capture efficiency was evaluated by the peak mobility shift based on the specific interaction with lectin reactivity.

2.3. Assay Linearity and Sensitivity of %S2,3PSA Test by µTAS System

To demonstrate that our assay is robust for determining %S2,3PSA, recombinant standard samples were serially diluted with control PSA protein and %S2,3PSA determined at a constant concentration of free PSA. As shown in Figure 5a,b, there was a linear relationship between percentage of S2,3PSA and fluorescence intensities in the two prepared samples tested. The assay's sensitivity was determined by testing samples of buffer spiked with serially diluted S2,3PSA with the means ± 2 standard deviations (SD) being calculated for five replicates. As shown in Figure 5c, 0.05 ng/mL S2,3PSA was clearly detectable over the zero sample, there being no overlap of the 2SD range with zero. The reproducibility of the peak area detection for the 0.05 ng/mL level was within 15% coefficient of variation (CV) for %S2,3PSA, indicating that the limits of detection of quantitation of the assay are 0.05 ng/mL.

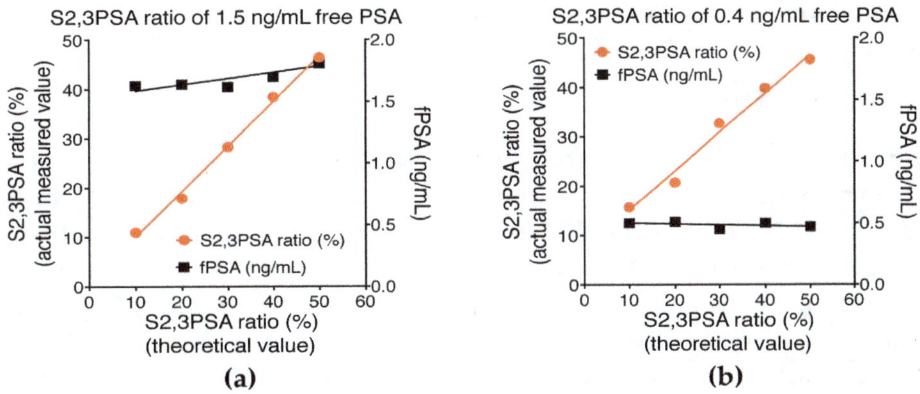

Figure 5. *Cont.*

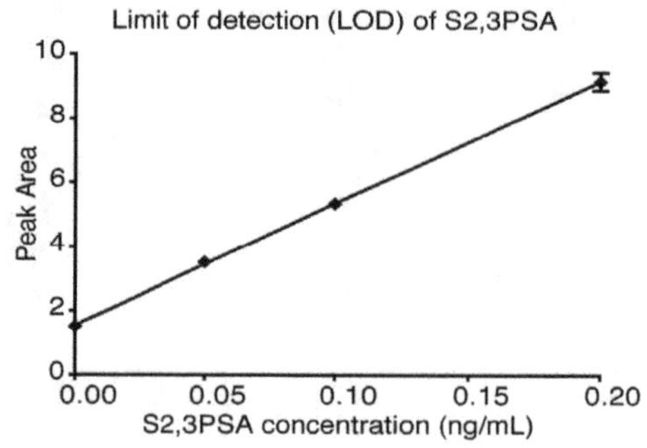

(c)

Figure 5. Assay linearity for measurement of S2,3PSA ratio (%S2,3PSA) and limit of detection of S2,3PSA measurement. (**a**) Sample was a prepared sample, the original sample having an PSA concentration of 1.5 ng/mL and %S2,3PSA of 50.0%; (**b**) Sample was prepared by spiking with PSA (0.4 ng/mL) and %S2,3PSA at 50%. The two samples were serially diluted by control PSA containing S2,6 sialylation or asialo at the same concentration. PSA concentrations and %S2,3PSA were determined by the μTAS system; (**c**) The limit of detection (LOD) was 0.05 ng/mL, this level showing no overlap between the 2 standard deviation (SD) ranges for S2,3PSA concentration and negative control.

2.4. *Assay Reproducibility of %S2,3PSA Test Using the μTAS System*

Assay reproducibility was examined by measuring two samples at each concentration with total of free PSA and %S2,3PSA, using 10 replicate measurements of each sample. We confirmed the assay's very good reproducibility. The CV was calculated to within 3% for free PSA and 4% for %S2,3PSA for all ranges tested (Table 1).

Table 1. Assay reproducibility of S2,3PSA test.

Sample Number	1.0 ng/mL Free PSA		5.0 ng/mL Free PSA	
	Free PSA	%S2,3PSA	Free PSA	%S2,3PSA
1	1.04	50.5	5.06	38.1
2	0.99	50.7	5.08	38.1
3	1.04	49.4	5.00	38.3
4	1.05	50.1	5.07	37.9
5	1.04	47.7	5.05	37.7
6	1.03	50.4	5.24	37.7
7	1.13	50.3	5.13	38.3
8	1.10	46.8	5.01	37.9
9	1.05	47.1	5.04	38.1
10	1.01	48.5	5.21	37.9
Ave. [1]	1.04	49.1	5.09	38.0
SD [2]	0.03	1.51	0.08	0.21
CV [3]	2.8%	3.1%	1.6%	0.6%

[1] Ave.: average; [2] SD, standard deviation; [3] CV: coefficient variation.

2.5. *Validation of %S2,3PSA Test*

Relevant clinical details of patients from whom samples were obtained are shown in Table 2. In this study, age and PSA level of 100 matched serum samples were assessed, comprising 50 from patients with PCa and 50 from BPH cases (Table 2, Figure 6a). Figure 6c shows that %S2,3PSA was significantly higher in patients with PCa than in patients with BPH ($p < 0.0001$). Total PSA level was not significantly different between the groups (Figure 6d). Receiver operating characteristic curve analyses were then used to compare the diagnostic potential of total PSA and %S2,3PSA (Figure 6e). The area under the curve (AUC) showed that results of conventional PSA testing did not differ between patients with BPH and PCa (AUC 0.5062, 95% CI 0.3922–0.6202), whereas there was a good separation for %S2,3PSA (AUC 0.8340, 95% CI 0.7555–0.9125, $p < 0.0001$) without any correlation between each assay (Figure 6b). The optimum cutoff point giving high specificity (72.0%) at 80% sensitivity was determined to be 42.20% of %S2,3PSA, with positive and negative predictive values of 75.5% and 78.7%, respectively, and much superior total PSA specificity (14.0%) at 80% sensitivity was determined to be 4.45 ng/mL of total PSA, with positive and negative predictive values of 48.2% and 41.2%, respectively. In this validation sample set, 54% ($n = 27/50$) of patients with PCa were found to be in the low Grade Group (GG) [26], with GG 1 (Gleason Score, GS 3 + 3) and GG 2 (GS 3 + 4) tumors. In addition, 46% ($n = 23/50$) of patients with PCa were found to have a greater than GG 3 (GS 4 + 3) tumor by prostate biopsy (Pbx) (Table 2). Figure 6g,f shows the total PSA and %S2,3PSA ratio of PCa patients classified by the prostate biopsy grade group (Pbx GG). The %S2,3PSA and total PSA level showed no significant difference between Pbx GG ≤ 2 and Pbx GG ≥ 3. In the case of greater than 50% S2,3PSA ratio, %S2,3PSA of Pbx GG ≥ 3 patients (range 50.7%–71.7%)(47%, $n = 11/23$) was significantly higher than that of Pbx GG ≤ 2 patients (range 50.3%–52.6%) (26%, $n = 7/27$) ($p = 0.0019$).

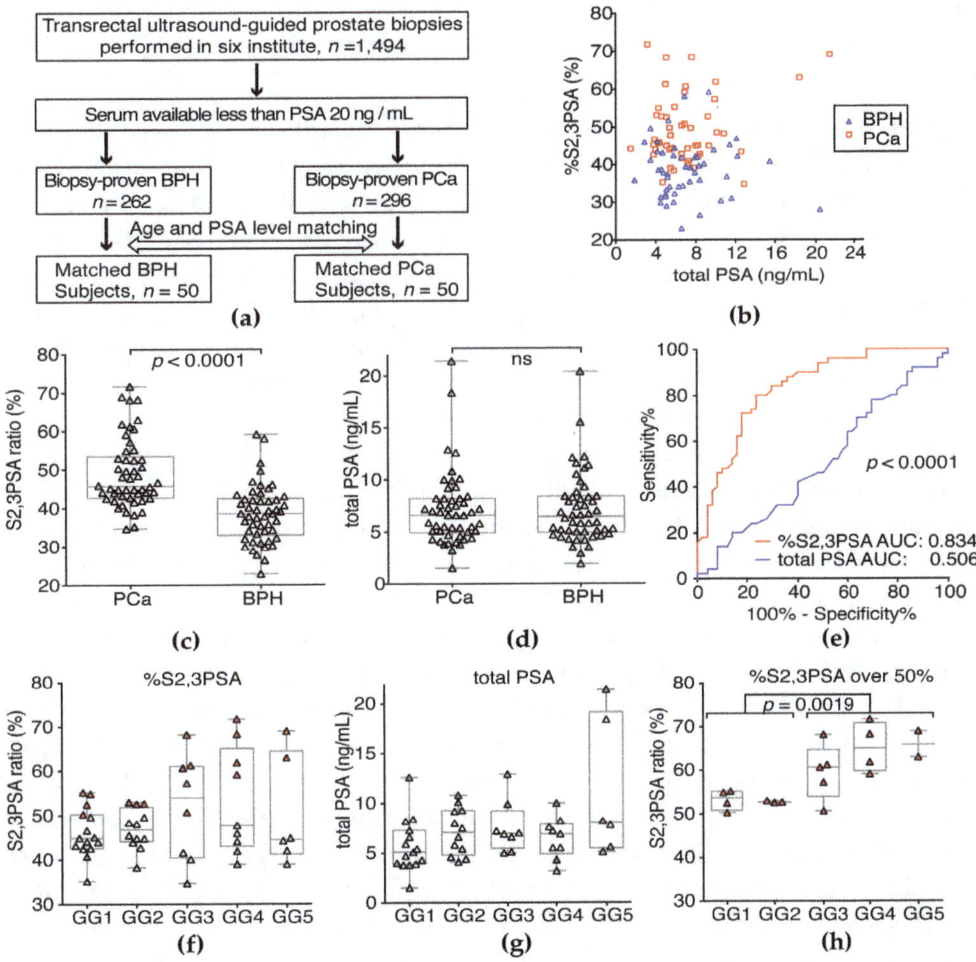

Figure 6. Serum %S2,3PSA and total PSA level in the validation sample set. (**a**) Fifty patients with PCa were pair-matched for age and PSA level with the same number of patients with BPH; (**b**) Correlations between %S2,3PSA and total PSA value in patient serum samples; (**c**) Serum %S2,3PSA was significantly higher in patients with PCa than BPH ($p < 0.0001$). The grand mean represents the overall mean of the Y variable; (**d**) Serum total PSA was not significantly different between PCa and BPH (**e**) Receiver operating characteristics (ROC) curve analysis for detection of PCa showed that the areas under the curve (AUC) for %S2,3PSA and conventional total PSA tests were 0.8340 and 0.5062, respectively; (**f**) %S2,3PSA among PCa patients classified by the Pbx GG; (**g**) total PSA level of PCa patients classified by the Pbx GG. Red triangle indicates %S2,3PSA over 50%; (**h**) Comparison between Pbx GG ≤ 2 and Pbx GG ≥ 3 patients that had an %S2,3PSA ratio over 50% ($p = 0.0019$).

Table 2. Age and total PSA BPH and PCa patients in the validation study.

Characteristics	BPH [a]	PCa [b]	p ([a] vs. [b])
n = 100	50	50	
Age, median (range)	66.5 (51–85)	67 (51–86)	ns [1]
PSA [2], ng/mL, median (range)	6.45 (1.9–20.4)	6.6 (1.5–21.4)	ns [1]
%S2,3PSA, median (range)	38.55 (22.9–59.1)	45.70 (34.7–71.7)	<0.0001
pbx GG [3]		n (%)	
GG 1		15 (30%)	
GG 2		12 (24%)	
GG 3		8 (16%)	
GG 4		9 (18%)	
GG 5		6 (12%)	

[1] no significant difference; [2] total PSA; [3] pbx GG: prostate biopsy grade group; [a] benign prostatic hyperplasia; [b] prostate cancer.

3. Discussion

The use of aberrant PSA glycosylation for early detection of prostate cancer has been reported [27–30]. In particular, we have previously identified that the terminal *N*-glycan structure of PSA from patients with PCa is rich in sialic acid α2,3-linked to the galactose residue, whereas the terminal *N*-glycan structures of PSA from seminal plasma are exclusively α2,6-linked [17]. We have also developed a magnetic bead-based S2,3PSA assay (Luminex method, [19]) that more accurately diagnoses early PCa than conventional PSA testing; however, this method is not sufficiently versatile and does not have enough quantitative capability for clinical application. To overcome these issues, we here developed an automated microcapillary electrophoresis-based immunoassay system (μTAS system) to be able to measure serum %S2,3PSA in clinical settings.

In this study, we developed a μTAS system based on the principles of EATA and LBA, precision-injection molded microfluidic plastic chips, and instrumentation optimized for running microfluidic chips and demonstrated that this EATA method can utilize affinity-based separation involving noncovalent interaction between the immunocomplex of α2,3-linked sialylated PSA glyco-isoform and MAA to simultaneously determine concentrations of total free PSA and its glyco-isoform, S2,3PSA. We have previously demonstrated that the migration speed of an immunocomplex of DNA–Fab in a microfluidic channel can be controlled by changing the length of the DNA fragment [31]; capillary gel electrophoresis (CGE) is also known to be capable of separating molecules on the basis of size and charge.

In this study, we established an assay standard with recombinant S2,3PSA protein expressed by CHO cells and a standard curve for the quantitative measurement of %S2,3PSA according to assay linearity (Figure 5a,b). We also confirmed a capture efficiency of applied S2,3PSA standard of almost 100% in this assay (Figure 4b,c). By using specific lectin MAA to recognize α2,3-linked sialylation directly, the calculating analyte percentage excluded an unspecified factor contributed by different glyco-isoforms like asialo-type glycan as compared to the indirect assay with other lectin-based approaches [32]. These observations suggest that our assay strategy allows the reliable determination of the percentage ratio of S2,3PSA without loss of capturing the specific PSA glyco-isoform.

In terms of assay performance, the sensitivity for detection of S2,3PSA was 0.05 ng/mL using the μTAS immunoassay system. As noted in previous studies of EATA methods [33], up to 140-fold concentrations of sample and reagent mixtures can be achieved by ITP stacking, greatly enhancing assay sensitivity and binding kinetics. The newly developed μTAS system has higher analytical sensitivity than our previous methods [18,19] and %S2,3PSA can be determined at lower free PSA concentrations. This higher analytical sensitivity enables low CVs (<4%) for a precise percentage ratio of S2,3PSA and should improve the clinical utility of %S2,3PSA in patients with small tumors. Clinical studies employing the μTAS system are currently underway; the results will be published separately.

In addition to its high sensitivity, the μTAS in %S2,3PSA assay also shortens time to first result from the 4 h required for our previous assay using the Luminex method, [19] to less than 10 min. We achieved this improvement by combining the LBA principle and microchip capillary electrophoresis. Because LBA does not rely on diffusion of antigen to antibody immobilized on the surfaces of a solid phase, the immunoreaction is quick and stoichiometric. Furthermore, in the on-chip system, electrophoresis can be performed quickly by applying higher voltage under better thermal control; the principle of EATA results in a concentration of reactants that shortens binding and separation times [25,33].

In the present study, a novel assay system for measuring %S2,3PSA with a μTAS system discriminated patients with PCa from patients with BPH with 72.0% specificity at 80.0% sensitivity with a α2,3-sialic acid percentage cut-off of 42.20%, as indicated by an AUC of 0.8340 which was significantly higher than that for conventional PSA testing (0.5062, $p < 0.0001$ Figure 6e). According to some reports [10–12], combination assay containing multiple biomarkers such as the 4K test or Prostate Health Index would be applicable for improving diagnostic accuracy. In contrast, since %S2,3PSA test is a single biomarker assay based on the measurement of aberrant glycosylation, this simple assay strategy would achieve easy-to-use clinical application with a higher accuracy of diagnosis of PCa. Additionally, %S2,3PSA of Pbx GG ≥ 3 patients (range 50.7%–71.7%) was significantly higher than that of Pbx GG ≤ 2 patients (range 50.3%–52.6%) in the case of an over-50% S2,3PSA ratio ($p = 0.0019$) (Figure 6h). Although sample size was small, this result suggests that an over-50% S2,3PSA ratio holds the promise to discriminate between GG 2 and GG 3 tumors and may be used as a predictor for a prostate biopsy to discriminate between non-aggressive and aggressive tumors in the active surveillance program. To address this issue, we would need larger cohort study in the future.

4. Materials and Methods

4.1. Immunoassay Reagents

DNA (245-bp) and HiLyte Fluor 647 dye (AnaSpec, San Jose, CA, USA) were coupled to Fab′ prepared from anti-total PSA and anti-free PSA monoclonal antibodies (clones PSA10 and PSA12, respectively) that had been selected from our panel of mouse immunoglobulin G antibodies. These antibodies were digested with pepsin, followed by reduction of F(ab′)2 using 50 mM 2-aminoethanethiol to form Fab′. Each Fab′ was purified by Diol 200 gel filtration column chromatography (Wako Pure Chemical Industries, Osaka, Japan).

DNA-labeled anti-total PSA Fab′ (clone PSA10) was prepared as follows, a 245-bp DNA fragment was amplified by polymerase chain reaction using lambda DNA as a template and 5′ amine-modified primer as a forward primer to provide the amino group needed to couple the DNA fragment to anti-total PSA (clone PSA10) Fab′ antibody via bifunctional linker. Gene Taq polymerase (Wako Pure Chemical Industries) was used as polymerase. The DNA fragment was purified by using Diol-200 gel filtration and DEAE ion exchange chromatography on a DEAE-P5 W column (Tosoh, Tokyo, Japan). Next, 10 μM of the 245-bp DNA fragment was reacted with 10 mM *N*-(6-maleimidocaproyloxy)succinimide (EMCS) linker (Wako Pure Chemical Industries), a bifunctional linker having both maleimide and succinimide groups, at 37 °C for 30 min in 50 mM phosphate-buffered saline (PBS, pH 7.5). The linker-modified, 245-bp DNA fragment was purified by Diol-200 gel filtration, concentrated to 10 μM, and reacted with 500 μM PSA10 Fab′ at 4 °C for 3 h in 50 mM PBS (pH 6.5). To remove DNA-coupled Fab′ that had more than one DNA fragment, the conjugate was further purified by both Diol-200 gel filtration and DEAE column chromatography.

HiLyte Fluor 647 labeled anti-free PSA Fab′ (clone PSA12) was prepared as follows, anti-free PSA monoclonal antibody (clone PSA12) Fab′ was reacted with 1 mM HiLyte Fluor 647 C2 maleimide (Wako Pure Chemical Industries) at 4 °C for 2 h in 50 mM PBS (pH 7.5), after which 1 mM *N*-ethylmaleimide was added to the reaction mixture to block free thiol groups on the Fab′ molecule after the labeling reaction. Excess unreacted HiLyte Fluor 647 C2 maleimide was removed by Diol-200 gel filtration.

Electrophoresis leading buffer (LB) and trailing buffer (TB) for isotachophoresis (ITP) and capillary electrophoresis (CE) were formulated by adding nonionic surfactants to block the plastic chip surface and facilitate chip filling. The composition of the LB was 4.5% (*w*/*v*) polyethylene glycol (PEG8000), 3% (*w*/*v*) glycerol, 75 mM Tris–HCl (pH 7.5), 10 mM NaCl, 6.0% (*w*/*v*) dextran sulfate, 0.01% bovine serum albumin (BSA), and 4 mg/mL *Maackia amurensis* lectin (MAA). The composition of the sample buffer (SB) was 5.0% (*w*/*v*) PEG20000, 3% (*w*/*v*) glycerol, 75 mM Tris–HCl (pH 7.5), 150 mM NaCl, 0.01% BSA, and 10 mM 2-(*N*-morpholino)ethanesulfonic acid (MES). The TB consisted of 2.0% (*w*/*v*) PEG20000, 3% (*w*/*v*) glycerol, 75 mM Tris, 0.01% BSA, and 125 mM Hepes. The stacking buffer (ST) was composed of 2.0% (*w*/*v*) PEG20000, 3% (*w*/*v*) glycerol, 75 mM Tris–HCl (pH 7.5), and 0.01% BSA.

4.2. Microfluidic Electrophoresis Assay

Simultaneous quantitative measurement of S2,6PSA and S2,3PSA was achieved by performing microchip capillary electrophoresis and liquid-phase binding assay (LBA) on a μTAS Wako i30 auto analyzer with microfluidic chip IO6 (Figure 2a,b; Wako Pure Chemical Industries) for electrokinetic analyte transport assay (EATA). The details of the EATA method have been described by us previously [24] and are shown in Figure 2b. In brief, HyLite–Fab′ was mixed with the serum sample in SB and the resulting mixture loaded into a sample well. DNA–Fab′, the LB containing MAA, and the TB were also loaded into their designated wells, and the ST and focusing dye solutions into the ST well and focusing dye solution well, respectively. After all buffers and sample had been loaded, positive pressure (+20 psi) was applied to all wells to equilibrate all zones. Next, an electrical field was applied from the cathode to the anode to initiate ITP stacking of the DNA–Fab′. The stacked DNA–Fab′ migrated from the DNA–Fab′ zone into the sample + HiLyte–Fab′ zone to initiate formation of the sandwich immunocomplex of DNA–Fab′, PSA, and HiLyte–Fab′. The resulting immunocomplex was then further transported to the separation zone by ITP. During the ITP step, unreacted HiLyte–Fab′ was left behind in the serum sample and HiLyte–Fab′ zone. When the boundary of TB and LB reached the handoff junction, the electrical field was automatically switched from cathode–anode wells to handoff–anode wells and capillary gel electrophoresis (CGE) started to both separate the remaining noise components from the immunocomplex and S2,3PSA from S2,6PSA by affinity electrophoresis in an MAA-containing separation gel. Fluorescence signals from laser-induced fluorescence (LIF) detection were analyzed by software developed to use internal fluorescent markers to align and identify the peaks for S2,6PSA and S2,3PSA. The analyte peaks were integrated for peak area, which was then used to quantitate their ratio, as shown in Figure 2c.

4.3. Prostate Biopsy and Serum Samples

Between June 2007 and June 2016, 1494 transrectal ultrasound-guided prostate biopsies were performed in response to detection in regional PCa screening programs of PSA concentrations of ≥4.0 ng/mL or palpable prostate nodules in Hirosaki University Hospital, Akita University hospital, Tohoku University Hospital and McMaster University (Juravinski Hospital, Hamilton, ON, Canada). Serum samples were obtained from all patients at the time of biopsy and stored at −80 °C until use. The final diagnoses were established by histopathological examination of prostate biopsies. The grade group of prostate biopsy specimens were evaluated according to the International Society of Urological Pathology (ISUP) guidelines [26]. This study was performed in accordance with the ethical standards of the Declaration of Helsinki and was approved by the Ethics Committees of all participating institute including Hirosaki University Graduate School of Medicine ("The Study about Carbohydrate Structure Change in Urological Disease"; approval number: 2014–195). Informed consent was obtained from all patients. Table 2 shows relevant clinical characteristics of the study subjects. To evaluate diagnostic performance of serum S2,3PSA ratio, fifty patients with biopsy-proven PCa were pair-matched for age and PSA level with the same number of BPH patients selected from our serum bank.

4.4. Forced Expression of FLAG-Tag-Fused S2,3 and S2,6PSA in Chinese Hamster Ovary (CHO)-K1 Cells

CHO-K1 cells were obtained from the American Type Culture Collection and grown in Ham's F12 Nutrient Mixture medium supplemented with penicillin, streptomycin, and 10% fetal bovine serum at 37 °C with 5% CO_2. FLAG-tag (N-DYKDDDDK-C)-fused human PSA (kallikrein-3, KLK3) cDNA was amplified from RNA isolated from the prostate of a patient with benign prostatic hyperplasia using the primers hPSA-F1 5′-CCCAAGCTTACCACCTGCAC-3′ and hPSA-FLAG-Xho-R1 5′-TTTCTCGAGCTACTTGTCATCGTCGTCCTTGTAATCAGCGGGGTTGGCCACGATGGT-3′ and subcloned into the PCaG-Neo vector (Wako Pure Chemical Industries). The PSA–FLAG vector was then transiently transfected into CHO-K1 cells. After transfection, recombinant PSA was purified using a FLAG-tag system (Sigma, St. Louis, MO, USA) from serum free media. S2,3PSA and S2,6PSA containing asialo-type standard protein was purified utilizing an ACG lectin column and gel filtration column chromatography.

4.5. Lectin Microarray

One hundred microliters of purified S2,6PSA and S2,3PSA (31.25–2000 ng/mL) were applied to a lectin array (LecChipver1.0; GlycoTechnica, Sapporo, Japan), including triplicate spots of lectins in each of seven divided incubation baths on glass slides [34]. After incubation at 20 °C for 17 h, the reaction solution was discarded and the glass slides scanned using a GlycoStation Reader1200 (GlycoTechnica). Abbreviation of lectins are as follows: MAL, *maackia amurensis* lectin; SNA, *sambucus nigra* lectin; and SSA, *Sambucus sieboldiana* lectin.

4.6. Statistical Analysis

All calculations for clinical data were performed in the SPSS software, ver. 21.0 (SPSS, Inc., Chicago, IL, USA) and in GraphPad Prism 6.03 (GraphPad Software, San Diego, CA, USA). Intergroup differences were statistically analyzed by a Student's t-test for normally distributed variables or by the Mann–Whitney U-test for non-normally distributed models. Data with $p < 0.05$ were considered significant. Receiver operating characteristics (ROC) curves were developed using the library "rms" in R (available on: http://www.r-project.org/) [25] and the statistical difference of AUCs were calculated by the same program.

5. Conclusions

In conclusion, although the present results are preliminary, they suggest that the newly developed serum %S2,3PSA test may have superior diagnostic accuracy to currently available tests. Additionally, we believe that the %S2,3PSA assay with μTAS system has great potential for further application in the clinical laboratory when rapid and quantitative testing is required. Larger-scale studies are warranted to confirm these findings.

Acknowledgments: All of the authors thank Yukie Nishizawa, Kaname Higuchi, and Satomi Sakamoto, technical assistant of Hirosaki University Graduate School of Medicine, for their invaluable help with sample collection and patient data management. This study was supported by the by the Japan Society for the Promotion of Science (JSPS) KAKENHI grant no. 15K15579 and grant no. 15H02563.

Author Contributions: Tohru Yoneyama and Yuki Tobisawa conceived and designed the experiments; Tomokazu Ishikawa performed the experiments; Tohru Yoneyama analyzed the data; Tomokazu Ishikawa, Tatsuo Kurosawa, and Kenji Nakamura developed the automated μTAS-based immunoassay system; Shingo Hatakeyama, Yasuhiro Hashimoto, Takuya Koie, Shintaro Narita, Koji Mitsuzuka, Wilhelmina Duivenvoorden, Jehonathan H. Pinthus, Tomonori Habuchi, Yoichi Arai, and Chikara Ohyama diagnosed BPH and PCa, and performed biopsies; Chikara Ohyama obtained funding. Chikara Ohyama and Tohru Yoneyama supervised. Yuki Tobisawa critically revised the manuscript for intellectual content; Tomokazu Ishikawa and Tohru Yoneyama wrote the paper.

Abbreviations

μTAS	micro-total analysis system
MAA	*maackia amurensis* lectin
EATA	electrokinetic analyte transport assay
LBA	liquid-phase binding assay
C.V.	coefficient of variation
ITP	isotachophoresis
LIF	laser-induced fluorescence
LB	leading buffer
TB	trailing buffer
CE	capillary electrophoresis
SB	sample buffer
ST	stacking buffer
CGE	capillary gel electrophoresis
LOD	limit of detection
PSA	prostate-specific antigen
PCa	prostate cancer
BPH	benign prostatic hyperplasia
Pbx GG	prostate biopsy grade group
LacdiNAc	GalNAcβ1-4GlcNAc-
Gal	galactose
Man	mannose
Fuc	fucose
Sia	sialic acid
GalNAc	*N*-acetylgalactosamine
GlcNAc	*N*-acetylglucosamine

References

1. Schroder, F.H.; Hugosson, J.; Roobol, M.J.; Tammela, T.L.; Ciatto, S.; Nelen, V.; Kwiatkowski, M.; Lujan, M.; Lilja, H.; Zappa, M.; et al. Screening and prostate-cancer mortality in a randomized European study. *N. Engl. J. Med.* **2009**, *360*, 1320–1328. [CrossRef] [PubMed]
2. Hugosson, J.; Carlsson, S.; Aus, G.; Bergdahl, S.; Khatami, A.; Lodding, P.; Pihl, C.G.; Stranne, J.; Holmberg, E.; Lilja, H. Mortality results from the Goteborg randomised population-based prostate-cancer screening trial. *Lancet Oncol.* **2010**, *11*, 725–732. [CrossRef]
3. Loeb, S.; Catalona, W.J. Prostate-specific antigen in clinical practice. *Cancer Lett.* **2007**, *249*, 30–39. [CrossRef] [PubMed]
4. Ito, K.; Ichinose, Y.; Kubota, Y.; Imai, K.; Yamanaka, H. Clinicopathological features of prostate cancer detected by transrectal ultrasonography-guided systematic six-sextant biopsy. *Int. J. Urol.* **1997**, *4*, 474–479. [CrossRef] [PubMed]
5. Ito, K.; Ohi, M.; Yamamoto, T.; Miyamoto, S.; Kurokawa, K.; Fukabori, Y.; Suzuki, K.; Yamanaka, H. The diagnostic accuracy of the age-adjusted and prostate volume-adjusted biopsy method in males with prostate specific antigen levels of 4.1–10.0 ng/mL. *Cancer* **2002**, *95*, 2112–2119. [CrossRef] [PubMed]
6. Balk, S.P.; Ko, Y.J.; Bubley, G.J. Biology of prostate-specific antigen. *J. Clin. Oncol.* **2003**, *21*, 383–391. [CrossRef] [PubMed]
7. Lazzeri, M.; Haese, A.; de la Taille, A.; Palou Redorta, J.; McNicholas, T.; Lughezzani, G.; Scattoni, V.; Bini, V.; Freschi, M.; Sussman, A.; et al. Serum isoform [−2]proPSA derivatives significantly improve prediction of prostate cancer at initial biopsy in a total PSA range of 2–10 ng/mL: A multicentric European study. *Eur. Urol.* **2013**, *63*, 986–994. [CrossRef] [PubMed]
8. Loeb, S.; Sanda, M.G.; Broyles, D.L.; Shin, S.S.; Bangma, C.H.; Wei, J.T.; Partin, A.W.; Klee, G.G.; Slawin, K.M.; Marks, L.S.; et al. The prostate health index selectively identifies clinically significant prostate cancer. *J. Urol.* **2015**, *193*, 1163–1169. [CrossRef] [PubMed]

9. Foley, R.W.; Gorman, L.; Sharifi, N.; Murphy, K.; Moore, H.; Tuzova, A.V.; Perry, A.S.; Murphy, T.B.; Lundon, D.J.; Watson, R.W. Improving multivariable prostate cancer risk assessment using the Prostate Health Index. *BJU Int.* **2016**, *117*, 409–417. [CrossRef] [PubMed]
10. Fossati, N.; Lazzeri, M.; Haese, A.; McNicholas, T.; de la Taille, A.; Buffi, N.M.; Lughezzani, G.; Gadda, G.M.; Lista, G.; Larcher, A.; et al. Clinical performance of serum isoform [−2]proPSA (p2PSA), and its derivatives %p2PSA and the Prostate Health Index, in men aged <60 years: Results from a multicentric European study. *BJU Int.* **2015**, *115*, 913–920. [PubMed]
11. Punnen, S.; Pavan, N.; Parekh, D.J. Finding the Wolf in Sheep's Clothing: The 4Kscore Is a Novel Blood Test That Can Accurately Identify the Risk of Aggressive Prostate Cancer. *Rev. Urol.* **2015**, *17*, 3–13. [PubMed]
12. Vedder, M.M.; de Bekker-Grob, E.W.; Lilja, H.G.; Vickers, A.J.; van Leenders, G.J.; Steyerberg, E.W.; Roobol, M.J. The added value of percentage of free to total prostate-specific antigen, PCA3, and a kallikrein panel to the ERSPC risk calculator for prostate cancer in prescreened men. *Eur. Urol.* **2014**, *66*, 1109–1115. [CrossRef] [PubMed]
13. Fukuda, M. Possible roles of tumor-associated carbohydrate antigens. *Cancer Res.* **1996**, *56*, 2237–2244. [PubMed]
14. Hakomori, S. Glycosylation defining cancer malignancy: New wine in an old bottle. *Proc. Natl. Acad. Sci. USA* **2002**, *99*, 10231–10233. [CrossRef] [PubMed]
15. Yamashita, K.; Taketa, K.; Nishi, S.; Fukushima, K.; Ohkura, T. Sugar chains of human cord serum α-fetoprotein: Characteristics of N-linked sugar chains of glycoproteins produced in human liver and hepatocellular carcinomas. *Cancer Res.* **1993**, *53*, 2970–2975. [PubMed]
16. Amano, J.; Nishimura, R.; Mochizuki, M.; Kobata, A. Comparative study of the mucin-type sugar chains of human chorionic gonadotropin present in the urine of patients with trophoblastic diseases and healthy pregnant women. *J. Biol. Chem.* **1988**, *263*, 1157–1165. [PubMed]
17. Tajiri, M.; Ohyama, C.; Wada, Y. Oligosaccharide profiles of the prostate specific antigen in free and complexed forms from the prostate cancer patient serum and in seminal plasma: A glycopeptide approach. *Glycobiology* **2008**, *18*, 2–8. [CrossRef] [PubMed]
18. Ohyama, C.; Hosono, M.; Nitta, K.; Oh-eda, M.; Yoshikawa, K.; Habuchi, T.; Arai, Y.; Fukuda, M. Carbohydrate structure and differential binding of prostate specific antigen to Maackia amurensis lectin between prostate cancer and benign prostate hypertrophy. *Glycobiology* **2004**, *14*, 671–679. [CrossRef] [PubMed]
19. Yoneyama, T.; Ohyama, C.; Hatakeyama, S.; Narita, S.; Habuchi, T.; Koie, T.; Mori, K.; Hidari, K.I.; Yamaguchi, M.; Suzuki, T.; et al. Measurement of aberrant glycosylation of prostate specific antigen can improve specificity in early detection of prostate cancer. *Biochem. Biophys. Res. Commun.* **2014**, *448*, 390–396. [CrossRef] [PubMed]
20. Jacobson, S.C.; Ramsey, J.M. Microchip electrophoresis with sample stacking. *Electrophoresis* **1995**, *16*, 481–486. [CrossRef] [PubMed]
21. Koutny, L.B.; Schmalzing, D.; Taylor, T.A.; Fuchs, M. Microchip electrophoretic immunoassay for serum cortisol. *Anal. Chem.* **1996**, *68*, 18–22. [CrossRef] [PubMed]
22. Chiem, N.; Harrison, D.J. Microchip-based capillary electrophoresis for immunoassays: Analysis of monoclonal antibodies and theophylline. *Anal. Chem.* **1997**, *69*, 373–378. [CrossRef] [PubMed]
23. Reyes, D.R.; Iossifidis, D.; Auroux, P.A.; Manz, A. Micro total analysis systems. 1. Introduction, theory, and technology. *Anal. Chem.* **2002**, *74*, 2623–2636. [CrossRef] [PubMed]
24. Kawabata, T.; Wada, H.G.; Watanabe, M.; Satomura, S. Electrokinetic analyte transport assay for α-fetoprotein immunoassay integrates mixing, reaction and separation on-chip. *Electrophoresis* **2008**, *29*, 1399–1406. [CrossRef] [PubMed]
25. Park, C.C.; Kazakova, I.; Kawabata, T.; Spaid, M.; Chien, R.L.; Wada, H.G.; Satomura, S. Controlling data quality and reproducibility of a high-sensitivity immunoassay using isotachophoresis in a microchip. *Anal. Chem.* **2008**, *80*, 808–814. [CrossRef] [PubMed]
26. Humphrey, P.A.; Moch, H.; Cubilla, A.L.; Ulbright, T.M.; Reuter, V.E. The 2016 WHO Classification of Tumours of the Urinary System and Male Genital Organs-Part B: Prostate and Bladder Tumours. *Eur. Urol.* **2016**, *70*, 106–119. [CrossRef] [PubMed]
27. Vermassen, T.; Speeckaert, M.M.; Lumen, N.; Rottey, S.; Delanghe, J.R. Glycosylation of prostate specific antigen and its potential diagnostic applications. *Clin. Chim. Acta* **2012**, *413*, 1500–1505. [CrossRef] [PubMed]

28. Drake, R.R.; Jones, E.E.; Powers, T.W.; Nyalwidhe, J.O. Altered glycosylation in prostate cancer. *Adv. Cancer Res.* **2015**, *126*, 345–382. [PubMed]
29. Sarrats, A.; Comet, J.; Tabares, G.; Ramirez, M.; Aleixandre, R.N.; de Llorens, R.; Peracaula, R. Differential percentage of serum prostate-specific antigen subforms suggests a new way to improve prostate cancer diagnosis. *Prostate* **2010**, *70*, 1–9. [CrossRef] [PubMed]
30. Sarrats, A.; Saldova, R.; Comet, J.; O'Donoghue, N.; de Llorens, R.; Rudd, P.M.; Peracaula, R. Glycan characterization of PSA 2-DE subforms from serum and seminal plasma. *Omics* **2010**, *14*, 465–474. [CrossRef] [PubMed]
31. Kawabata, T.; Watanabe, M.; Nakamura, K.; Satomura, S. Liquid-phase binding assay of α-fetoprotein using DNA-coupled antibody and capillary chip electrophoresis. *Anal. Chem.* **2005**, *77*, 5579–5582. [CrossRef] [PubMed]
32. Llop, E.; Ferrer-Batalle, M.; Barrabes, S.; Guerrero, P.E.; Ramirez, M.; Saldova, R.; Rudd, P.M.; Aleixandre, R.N.; Comet, J.; de Llorens, R.; et al. Improvement of Prostate Cancer Diagnosis by Detecting PSA Glycosylation-Specific Changes. *Theranostics* **2016**, *6*, 1190–1204. [CrossRef] [PubMed]
33. Kagebayashi, C.; Yamaguchi, I.; Akinaga, A.; Kitano, H.; Yokoyama, K.; Satomura, M.; Kurosawa, T.; Watanabe, M.; Kawabata, T.; Chang, W.; et al. Automated immunoassay system for AFP-L3% using on-chip electrokinetic reaction and separation by affinity electrophoresis. *Anal. Biochem.* **2009**, *388*, 306–311. [CrossRef] [PubMed]
34. Hirabayashi, J.; Yamada, M.; Kuno, A.; Tateno, H. Lectin microarrays: Concept, principle and applications. *Chem. Soc. Rev.* **2013**, *42*, 4443–4458. [CrossRef] [PubMed]

12

Epigenetic Signature: A New Player as Predictor of Clinically Significant Prostate Cancer (PCa) in Patients on Active Surveillance (AS)

Matteo Ferro [1], Paola Ungaro [2,*], Amelia Cimmino [3,*], Giuseppe Lucarelli [4], Gian Maria Busetto [5], Francesco Cantiello [6], Rocco Damiano [6] and Daniela Terracciano [7,*]

1 Urologic Surgery Unit, European Institute of Oncology, 20141 Milan, Italy; matteo.ferro@ieo.it
2 Institute of Experimental Endocrinology and Oncology (IEOS-CNR) "G. Salvatore", Via Sergio Pansini, 5, 80131 Naples, Italy
3 Institute of Genetics and Biophysics "A. Buzzati Traverso", National Research Council (CNR), Via Pietro Castellino 111, 80131 Naples, Italy
4 Department of Emergency and Organ Transplantation-Urology, Andrology and Kidney Transplantation Unit, University of Bari, 70124 Bari, Italy; giuseppe.lucarelli@inwind.it
5 Department of Gynecological-Obstetrics Sciences and Urological Sciences, Sapienza Rome University Policlinico Umberto I, 00161 Rome, Italy; gianmaria.busetto@uniroma1.it
6 Department of Urology, Magna Graecia University of Catanzaro, 88100 Catanzaro, Italy; cantiello@unicz.it (F.C.); damiano@unicz.it (R.D.)
7 Department of Translational Medical Sciences, University of Naples Federico II, Via Sergio Pansini, 5, 80131 Naples, Italy
* Correspondence: pungaro@ieos.cnr.it (P.U.); amelia.cimmino@igb.cnr.it (A.C.); daniela.terracciano@unina.it (D.T.)

Academic Editor: Carsten Stephan

Abstract: Widespread prostate-specific antigen (PSA) testing notably increased the number of prostate cancer (PCa) diagnoses. However, about 30% of these patients have low-risk tumors that are not lethal and remain asymptomatic during their lifetime. Overtreatment of such patients may reduce quality of life and increase healthcare costs. Active surveillance (AS) has become an accepted alternative to immediate treatment in selected men with low-risk PCa. Despite much progress in recent years toward identifying the best candidates for AS in recent years, the greatest risk remains the possibility of misclassification of the cancer or missing a high-risk cancer. This is particularly worrisome in men with a life expectancy of greater than 10–15 years. The Prostate Cancer Research International Active Surveillance (PRIAS) study showed that, in addition to age and PSA at diagnosis, both PSA density (PSA-D) and the number of positive cores at diagnosis (two compared with one) are the strongest predictors for reclassification biopsy or switching to deferred treatment. However, there is still no consensus upon guidelines for placing patients on AS. Each institution has its own protocol for AS that is based on PRIAS criteria. Many different variables have been proposed as tools to enrol patients in AS: PSA-D, the percentage of freePSA, and the extent of cancer on biopsy (number of positive cores or percentage of core involvement). More recently, the Prostate Health Index (PHI), the 4 Kallikrein (4K) score, and other patient factors, such as age, race, and family history, have been investigated as tools able to predict clinically significant PCa. Recently, some reports suggested that epigenetic mapping differs significantly between cancer patients and healthy subjects. These findings indicated as future prospect the use of epigenetic markers to identify PCa patients with low-grade disease, who are likely candidates for AS. This review explores literature data about the potential of epigenetic markers as predictors of clinically significant disease.

Keywords: active surveillance; prostate cancer; epigenetic biomarkers

1. Introduction

AS has recently become an accepted alternative for patients with low-risk prostate cancer (PCa)-related mortality, allowing for delayed curative intervention if there is reclassification of cancer risk or evidence of disease progression [1]. It has been widely accepted that pre-treatment prostate-specific antigen (PSA) below 10 ng/mL, a biopsy Gleason score of 6 or less, and clinical stage T1c or T2a identify low-risk PCa [2]. Moreover, Klotz et al. [3] recently suggested that patients with a Gleason score of 3 + 4 PCa may be selected for active surveillance (AS), since most of these patients are at a low risk of progression. Risk factors for reclassification and progression have still not been adequately characterized. Low-risk PCa patients were monitored through PSA levels, clinical examination, and repeated prostate biopsies. Changes in biopsy results suggest a need for intervention. Widespread AS use has been prevented because under-sampling prostate biopsies may result in occult high-grade cancer. Moreover, biopsies are invasive tests, not free from side effects such as bleeding and infection risks, suggesting a need to avoid unnecessary repeated prostate biopsies in AS regimens. Several approaches to selecting patients for AS have been proposed. One of these includes the addition of biomarkers to currently used clinical and demographical variables [4]. Biomarker levels can ideally be obtained non-invasively, allowing for controlled follow-up of patients in AS in order to avoid overtreatment and the consequent impairment of quality of life.

In this review, we focused our attention on the potential use of epigenetic mapping as prognostic factors in the clinical management of PCa patients.

1.1. Biomarkers and Active Surveillance: Current Status

PCa patients are classified at diagnostic biopsy as very low-risk when they meet the following criteria: clinical stage T1c disease, PSA-D less than 0.15 ng/mL, a Gleason score $\leq$6, two or fewer biopsy cores with cancer, and a maximum of 50% involvement of any core with cancer [5]. Thaxton et al. showed that the number of patients eligible for AS, who have fatal disease at radical prostatectomy (RP), depends upon the criteria used for AS selection [6]. However, the optimal patient selection and follow-up protocol is still a matter of debate. Prostate biopsy risks, such as bleeding and infections, highlight the need for non-invasive tools for the selection and follow-up of AS patients [7]. The Prostate Health Index (PHI) may play a role in monitoring men under active surveillance (AS) [8,9]. Tosoian et al. [10] found an association between baseline and longitudinal PHI, but not PCA3 [11] values and reclassification during active surveillance. Sottile et al. [12] demonstrated significantly higher p2PSA and PHI levels in men with metastatic disease as compared to those without clinical metastasis. Collectively, PHI and/or PCA3 improve the selection of eligible patients for AS and decision curve analysis demonstrated that PHI outperforms PCA3 [13]. A Canadian report indicated that neutrophil-to-lymphocyte ratio (NLR) is a less expensive and more easily accessible test able to predict Gleason score upgrading and biochemical recurrence in patients with low-risk PCa eligible for AS [14]. Recently, Ferro et al. [15] found a significant association between low serum testosterone levels and upgrading, upstaging, and unfavorable disease, suggesting a new cheap parameter useful to identify low-risk patients eligible for AS. A recently published preliminary study [16] showed that the presence of primary circulating prostate cells is associated with aggressive disease, suggesting that these patients are not eligible for active surveillance. Several authors have shown that, besides the PHI index, the PCA3 score can improve the Epstein and PRIAS protocol's ability to predict insignificant PCa in subjects eligible for AS [17,18]. Lin et al. found that [19] the combination of urine TMPRSS2-ERG and PCA3 were associated with aggressive cancer in men with low-risk PCa on AS. Berg et al. found a significant association between tissue ERG expression and progression during AS [20]. Other authors have recently shown that Ki67 and DLX2, two cancer cell proliferation markers, are predictive of increased metastasis risk and may aid patient selection for AS [21]. It has been repeatedly demonstrated [22–24] that PTEN loss is uncommon in clinically localized PCa, suggesting the potential use of this histopathological biomarker as a predictor of unfavorable prognosis in patients on AS.

Tissue-based prognostic panels as OncotypeDX1 and Prolaris1 have been validated for routine clinical use on men with low-risk PCa. The first is a quantitative RT-PCR assay performed using biopsy samples. This test measures the expression of several genes involved in four different pathways to calculate the Genomic Prostate Score (GPS), which is predictive of aggressive disease in low- and intermediate-risk PCa patients [25]. The Prolaris 1 test provides a proliferative index, called CCP (cell cycle progression) score, on the basis of the expression of 31 cell cycle progression and 15 housekeeping genes [26]. In a multicentric study, the biopsy CCP score from low-risk patients was associated with aggressiveness at radical prostatectomy [27].

1.2. Epigenetic Biomarkers and PCa Prognosis: Future Challenge

The term "epigenetics" defined heritable changes in gene expression that are independent from those occurring in the genome. The epigenetic mechanisms contribute to gene regulation throughout the whole life course of an organism, by changing chromatin architecture and/or access by transcription factors. They include different processes, such as DNA methylation, histone modifications, and post-transcriptional gene regulation by non-coding RNAs. Together, they regulate gene expression by changing chromatin organization and DNA accessibility.

The most well studied epigenetic modification in human diseases is DNA methylation. It involves an enzymatic process mediated by DNA methyltransferases (DNMTs) that catalyze the addition of a methyl group, using S-adenosyl methionine (SAM) as the methyl supplier, to the 5-carbon of the cytosine within CpG dinucleotides to form 5-methylcytosine. CpG are normally methylated when dispersed in the genome or in DNA repetitive region, but remain unmethylated to enable gene expression when they are clustered as a CpG island at the 5′ ends of many genes [28]. The conventional view is that DNMT1 is responsible for the maintenance of tissue-specific methylation patterns during cell replication, while DNMT3A and DNMT3B catalyze the addition of methyl groups de novo during embryogenesis [29,30]. In tumorigenesis, DNA methylation and demethylation are associated with silencing tumor suppressor genes and activating oncogenes, respectively [31].

Histone post-translational modifications (PTMs) include acetylation, biotinylation, methylation, phosphorylation, ubiquitination, SUMOylation, ADP (adenosine diphosphate) ribosylation, proline isomerization, citrulination, butyrylation, propionylation, and glycosylation, which are known as "the histone code" and strongly contribute to the control of gene expression [32].

Such modifications alter the affinity of the histone tails to the DNA and change the conformation of chromatin structure, resulting in transcriptional genes activation or repression. For instance, di- and trimethylation and poor acetylation of lysine 9 residue on histone H3 are associated with the silencing of gene expression. By contrast, the acetylation of histones H3 and H4, together with the methylation of lysine 4 residue on histone H3, results in gene expression. In general, acetylation promotes transcriptional activity and is catalyzed by histone acetyltransferases (HAT). Conversely, histone deacetylases (HDACs) remove acetyl groups leading to a silent chromatin state. Depending on the specific amino acid residues modified and the number of methyl groups added, histone methylation may be associated with the activation or repression of transcription. In general, histone methyltransferases (HMTs) and histone demethylases (HDMs) catalyze the addition or the removal of methyl groups from histone proteins, respectively [33].

There is good evidence that another epigenetic modification, known as noncoding RNAs (ncRNAs), can influence gene expression [34].

The best-characterized class of non-coding RNAs is represented by microRNA (miRNAs), which are single-stranded RNAs, about 19–24 nucleotides in length. They regulate gene expression through the binding to mRNAs, resulting in degradation or translational inhibition [35]. It was estimated that at least 30% of human genes are regulated by miRNA. In metazoans, each mRNA can be combined with multiple miRNAs and each miRNA regulates multiple mRNAs. It is noteworthy that miRNAs regulate a large spectrum of biological processes and play an important role in tumorigenesis, activating oncogenes or restraining tumor suppressor genes [36,37].

Development and progression of PCa are usually associated with global DNA hypomethylation with a lower overall content of 5-methylcytosine (m5C) found in metastatic tissue [38]. The global DNA hypomethylation in PCa causes a loss of IGF2 imprinting (with expression of both parental alleles) both in cancerous and in distant areas within the peripheral zone, indicating that the epigenetic defect in histologically normal tissue might be employed to identify PCa in patients [39] (Figure 1). Conversely, promoter hypermethylation is widespread during neoplastic transformation of prostate cells; indeed, this is one of the first aberrations, seen early in pre-invasive lesions, and appears to be clonally maintained during metastatic progression of PCa [40]. Thus far, several genes, including tumor suppressor genes, have been described as de novo methylated in morphologically normal prostate tissue and in pre-invasive lesions, such as PIN (Prostatic Intraepithelial Neoplasia), and persisting during prostate carcinogenesis [40]. As an example, the relative frequency of methylation of Ras association domain family protein 1, isoform A (*RASSF1A*) promoter was higher in more aggressive tumors compared to less malignant tumors [41,42]. Aberrant promoter methylation was also found in different genes involved in important molecular pathways of carcinogenesis, such as DNA repair/protection, cell cycle regulation, and signal transduction. As an example, the frequency of methylation at the promoter region of Glutathion S-transferase Pi 1 (*GSTP1*), a gene involved in DNA repair, was found elevated not only in more than 90% of PCa cases, but also in over 50% of PCa precursor lesions, confirming that this is an early event in prostate carcinogenesis [42–44]. Further supporting the relevance of DNA methylation in PCa progression, different authors have related CpG methylation patterns to clinical outcomes and revealed that methylation of certain loci (e.g., *AOX1* and *RARB*) predicted disease progression [45,46].

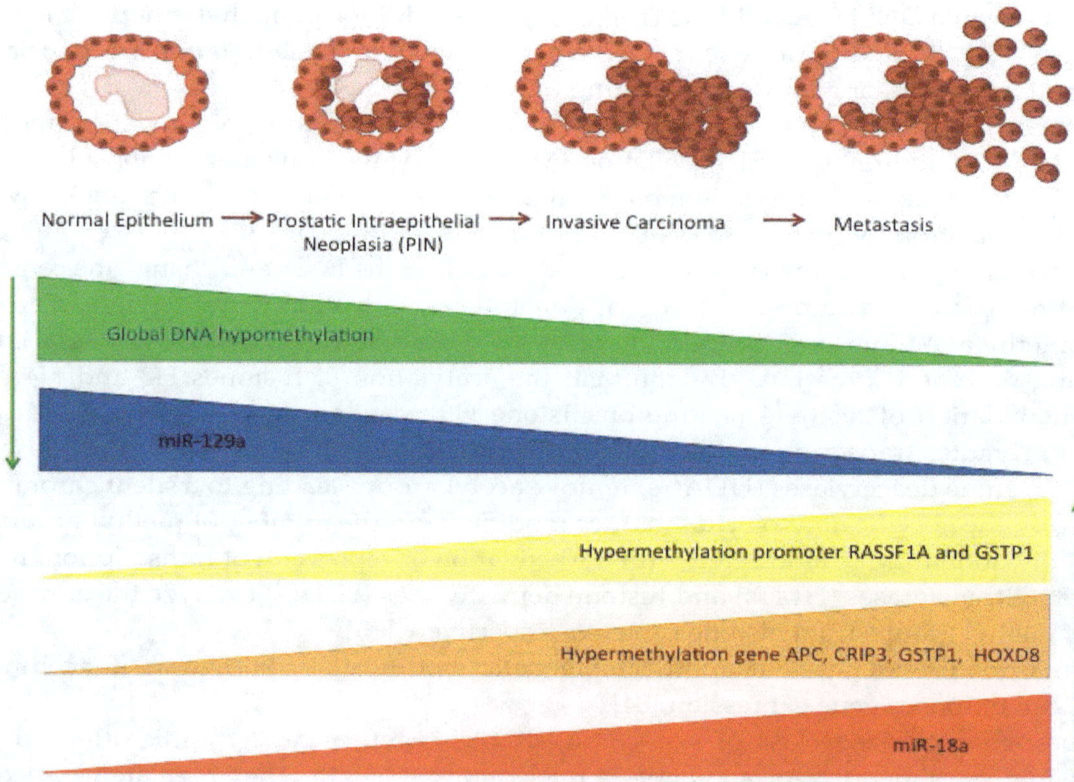

Figure 1. Potential epigenetic biomarkers in patients on AS. The figure shows the epigenetic modifications that have been tested as biomarkers. Green arrows represent down- and up-regulation of epigenetic biomarkers. The aberrant epigenetic changes have been described and cited in the text.

Histone modifications were also found to relate to the pathogenesis of prostate cancer and regulation of cancer cell proliferation. Ellinger and co-authors analyzed H3K4 methylation in patients with advanced PCa and found that this epigenetic modification was a significant predictor of PSA recurrence following radical prostatectomy. Moreover, they also found that H3K4me1, H3K4me2, and H3K4me3 levels were significantly increased in hormone-refractory prostate cancer (HPRC) [47]. One of the most studied epigenetic enzymes in PCa is the histone methyltransferase EZH2 responsible for H3K27 trimethylation. Its overexpression, particularly found in mCRPC [48], correlates with promoter hypermethylation and repression of some tumor suppressor genes [48,49]. Other epigenetic enzymes, such as SET9, SMYD3, JHDM2A, JMJD2C, and LSD1, have been demonstrated to play a role in prostate carcinogenesis [50–54]. LSD1, whose activity is associated to both transcriptional activation or repression, was associated with aggressive CRPC and a high risk of disease relapse [55,56]. Strong expression of all HDACs was accompanied by enhanced tumor cell proliferation. High rates of HDAC1 and HDAC2 expression were significantly associated with tumor dedifferentiation, and HDAC2 expression is associated with shorter PSA relapse time after radical prostatectomy [57,58]. Moreover, AR transcriptional activity is regulated by HAT or HDAC activities, i.e., acetylation facilitates its binding to target DNA sequences, while HDAC1 and HDAC2 abrogate its activity [59]. These data confirm the role of HATs and HDACs in influencing the acetylation status of non-histone proteins. Additionally, the NAD-dependent deacetylase sirtuin-1 (SIRT1) is involved in PCa where its downregulation leads to the upregulation of different oncogenes as a consequence of H2A.Z overexpression [60].

Important biomarkers for PCa have been identified in microRNAs. Recently, Al-Kafaji et al. demonstrated that miR-18a expression increased in peripheral blood of patients with prostate cancer, indicating miR-18a as a potential noninvasive biomarker for prostate cancer tissue [61] (Figure 1). On the contrary, miRNA-129 was found downregulated in prostate cancer. Thus, its overexpression could prevent prostate cancer growth by developing tumor suppressive functions [62].

Zhao et al. [63] recently reported that a 4-gene methylation classifier panel (*APC, CRIP3, GSTP1,* and *HOXD8*) was able to predict patient reclassification on AS.

Epigenetic alterations are commonly found in PCa and play a role in carcinogenesis and tumor spreading. Moreover, new technologies, such as next-generation sequencing (NGS), have been implemented, allowing us both to expand our knowledge on prostate tumorigenesis and to obtain new epigenetic biomarkers useful to PCa patient clinical management.

Collectively, no single epigenetic biomarker has been identified as a marker of aggressive phenotypes.

However, several studies have identified potentially useful epigenetic biomarkers in PCa (Table 1) mainly in tissue samples.

Table 1. Overview of prostate cancer epigenetic biomarkers.

Biomarker	Type of Epigenetic Modification	Sample	References
IGF2	DNA hypo- and hyper-methylation	Tissue	[38–40]
RSSF1A	DNA hypermethylation	Tissue	[41,42]
GSTP1	DNA hypermethylation	Tissue	[42–44]
AOX1	DNA hypermethylation	Tissue	[45,46]
RARB	DNA hypermethylation	Tissue	[45,46]
EZH2	Increased H3K27 trimethylation	Tissue	[48]
SET9, SMYD3, JHDM2A, JMJD2C, LSD1	Histone modifications	Tissue	[50–54]
HAT	Variation in histone acetylation	Tissue	[59]
HDAC1, HDAC2	Histone deacetylation	Tissue	[59]
SIRT1	Downregulation	Tissue	[60]
miR-18a	Overexpression	Peripheral blood	[62]
miRNA-129	Downregulation	Peripheral blood	[62]
APC, CRIP3, GSTP1, HOXD8	DNA hypermethylation	Urinary	[63]

The most studied epigenetic alteration is DNA methylation. Consequently, it is conceivable that methylation markers will be the first that will be translated into clinical practice for the management of PCa patients.

DNA methylation alterations, measured in cell-free circulating and urinary tumor DNA, can potentially be used as PCa biomarkers. A large number of specific DNA methylation alterations are cancer-specific and not detectable in unaffected subjects. Examples of such alterations may be represented by CpG island methylation in the regulatory regions of *GSTP1, APC, PTGS2, RASSF1A*, and *RARB* [64].

GSTP1, RARB, and *RASSF1* DNA promoter methylation has been widely investigated in body fluids as a non-invasive biomarker for the early diagnosis of PCa [65,66]. Other authors [67–69] have suggested that urine cell-free DNA could represent a non-invasive and inexpensive biomarker for assessing specific promoter region methylation.

Chromatin remodeling and non-coding RNA regulation represent an expanding research field.

Collectively, based on literature data and on the improvement of new technologies such as next-generation sequencing (NGS), epigenetic signatures seem to be promising tools for stratifying PCa patients for progression risk. Nevertheless, some obstacles may contribute to the lack of translating such biomarkers for PCa in clinical practice. In particular, an important role was played by the limitation of available methods for analysis, the consistency of experimental design to validate the biomarkers, and the relevance of the epigenetic alteration in prostate carcinogenesis. Moreover, it should be taken into account that epigenetic modifications are affected by aging and prostate cancer is an age-related disease.

Further studies on larger population will define the clinical benefit of epigenetic markers in body fluids.

2. Conclusions

Follow-up of patients on AS can prevent overtreatment and the related impairment of quality of life. Diagnosis of true low-risk PCa is essential to address this therapeutic strategy. As recently reported by Klotz [70], AS is harmless in the medium to long term with a very low cancer-specific mortality of 10–15 years. Many studies have been focused on tools able to provide further improvement of the safety of this conservative therapeutic option.

Several serum and urine biomarkers, including the PHI, the 4K score, and urinary TMPRSS2-ERG or PCA3 mRNA, have been evaluated in men on AS. However, the association with tumor aggressiveness and thus prognostic value remains controversial [71]. Consequently, new players have to be considered to predict cancer progression in an AS regimen.

In this scenario, it could be advantageous to implement epigenetic signature identification of clinically significant PCa in the setting of active surveillance. Such studies represent an urgent need to identify indolent cancer and avoid overtreatment. DNA methylation, histone modifications, and noncoding RNA could potentially provide new tools for prognosis of prostate cancer, affecting clinical management of patients. In particular, since these biomarkers lack specificity, further studies are needed to ascertain if a panel of multiple epigenetic targets may be helpful in planning AS strategies.

Acknowledgments: The authors thank Monica Autiero for critically reading the manuscript. The Italian Association for Cancer Research (MFAG number 11510 to A.C.) supported this work.

Author Contributions: Matteo Ferro and Daniela Terracciano conceived and designed the review; Matteo Ferro, Paola Ungaro, Amelia Cimmino, Daniela Terracciano, Giuseppe Lucarelli, Gian Maria Busetto, Francesco Cantiello and Rocco Damiano performed literature search; Paola Ungaro and Daniela Terracciano wrote the paper.

References

1. Klotz, L. Active surveillance for prostate cancer: Patient selection and management. *Curr. Oncol.* **2010**, *17*, S11–S17. [CrossRef] [PubMed]
2. D'Amico, A.V.; Whittington, R.; Malkowicz, S.B.; Schultz, D.; Blank, K.; Broderick, G.A.; Tomaszewski, J.E.; Renshaw, A.A.; Kaplan, I.; Beard, C.J.; et al. Biochemical outcome after radical prostatectomy, external beam radiation therapy, or interstitial radiation therapy for clinically localized prostate cancer. *JAMA* **1998**, *280*, 969–974. [CrossRef] [PubMed]
3. Klotz, L.; Zhang, L.; Lam, A.; Nam, R.; Mamedov, A.; Loblaw, A. Clinical results of long-term follow-up of a large, active surveillance cohort with localized prostate cancer. *J. Clin. Oncol.* **2010**, *28*, 126–131. [CrossRef] [PubMed]
4. Thomsen, F.B.; Berg, K.D.; Roder, M.A.; Iversen, P.; Brasso, K. Active surveillance for localized prostate cancer: An analysis of patient contacts and utilization of healthcare resources. *Scand. J. Urol.* **2015**, *49*, 43–50. [CrossRef] [PubMed]
5. Weinreb, J.C.; Barentsz, J.O.; Choyke, P.L.; Cornud, F.; Haider, M.A.; Macura, K.J.; Margolis, D.; Schnall, M.D.; Shtern, F.; Tempany, C.M.; et al. Pi-rads prostate imaging—Reporting and data system: 2015, Version 2. *Eur. Urol.* **2016**, *69*, 16–40. [CrossRef] [PubMed]
6. Thaxton, C.S.; Loeb, S.; Roehl, K.A.; Kan, D.; Catalona, W.J. Treatment outcomes of radical prostatectomy in potential candidates for 3 published active surveillance protocols. *Urology* **2010**, *75*, 414–418.
7. Loeb, S.; Carter, H.B.; Berndt, S.I.; Ricker, W.; Schaeffer, E.M. Is repeat prostate biopsy associated with a greater risk of hospitalization? Data from seer-medicare. *J. Urol.* **2013**, *189*, 867–870. [CrossRef] [PubMed]
8. Loeb, S.; Catalona, W.J. The prostate health index: A new test for the detection of prostate cancer. *Ther. Adv. Urol.* **2014**, *6*, 74–77. [CrossRef] [PubMed]
9. Heidegger, I.; Klocker, H.; Pichler, R.; Pircher, A.; Prokop, W.; Steiner, E.; Ladurner, C.; Comploj, E.; Lunacek, A.; Djordjevic, D.; et al. Propsa and the prostate health index as predictive markers for aggressiveness in low-risk prostate cancer-results from an international multicenter study. *Prostate Cancer Prostatic Dis.* **2017**. [CrossRef] [PubMed]
10. Tosoian, J.J.; Loeb, S.; Feng, Z.; Isharwal, S.; Landis, P.; Elliot, D.J.; Veltri, R.; Epstein, J.I.; Partin, A.W.; Carter, H.B.; et al. Association of [−2]proPSA with biopsy reclassification during active surveillance for prostate cancer. *J. Urol.* **2012**, *188*, 1131–1136. [CrossRef] [PubMed]
11. Tosoian, J.J.; Loeb, S.; Kettermann, A.; Landis, P.; Elliot, D.J.; Epstein, J.I.; Partin, A.W.; Carter, H.B.; Sokoll, L.J. Accuracy of PCa3 measurement in predicting short-term biopsy progression in an active surveillance program. *J. Urol.* **2010**, *183*, 534–538. [CrossRef] [PubMed]
12. Sottile, A.; Ortega, C.; Berruti, A.; Mangioni, M.; Saponaro, S.; Polo, A.; Prati, V.; Muto, G.; Aglietta, M.; Montemurro, F. A pilot study evaluating serum pro-prostate-specific antigen in patients with rising PSA following radical prostatectomy. *Oncol. Lett.* **2012**, *3*, 819–824. [PubMed]
13. Hendriks, R.J.; van Oort, I.M.; Schalken, J.A. Blood-based and urinary prostate cancer biomarkers: A review and comparison of novel biomarkers for detection and treatment decisions. *Prostate Cancer Prostatic Dis.* **2017**, *20*, 12–19. [CrossRef] [PubMed]
14. Gokce, M.I.; Tangal, S.; Hamidi, N.; Suer, E.; Ibis, M.A.; Beduk, Y. Role of neutrophil-to-lymphocyte ratio in prediction of gleason score upgrading and disease upstaging in low-risk prostate cancer patients eligible for active surveillance. *Can. Urol. Assoc. J.* **2016**, *10*, E383–E387. [CrossRef] [PubMed]
15. Ferro, M.; Lucarelli, G.; Bruzzese, D.; di Lorenzo, G.; Perdona, S.; Autorino, R.; Cantiello, F.; La Rocca, R.; Busetto, G.M.; Cimmino, A.; et al. Low serum total testosterone level as a predictor of upstaging and upgrading in low-risk prostate cancer patients meeting the inclusion criteria for active surveillance. *Oncotarget* **2016**, *8*, 18424–18434. [CrossRef] [PubMed]
16. Murray, N.P.; Reyes, E.; Fuentealba, C.; Aedo, S.; Jacob, O. The presence of primary circulating prostate cells is associated with upgrading and upstaging in patients eligible for active surveillance. *Ecancermedicalscience* **2017**, *11*, 711. [CrossRef] [PubMed]
17. Cantiello, F.; Russo, G.I.; Ferro, M.; Cicione, A.; Cimino, S.; Favilla, V.; Perdona, S.; Bottero, D.; Terracciano, D.; de Cobelli, O.; et al. Prognostic accuracy of prostate health index and urinary prostate cancer antigen 3 in predicting pathologic features after radical prostatectomy. *Urol. Oncol.* **2015**, *33*, 163.e15–163.e23. [CrossRef] [PubMed]

18. Porpiglia, F.; Cantiello, F.; de Luca, S.; Manfredi, M.; Veltri, A.; Russo, F.; Sottile, A.; Damiano, R. In-parallel comparative evaluation between multiparametric magnetic resonance imaging, prostate cancer antigen 3 and the prostate health index in predicting pathologically confirmed significant prostate cancer in men eligible for active surveillance. *BJU Int.* **2016**, *118*, 527–534. [CrossRef] [PubMed]
19. Lin, D.W.; Newcomb, L.F.; Brown, E.C.; Brooks, J.D.; Carroll, P.R.; Feng, Z.; Gleave, M.E.; Lance, R.S.; Sanda, M.G.; Thompson, I.M.; et al. Urinary tmprss2:ERG and PCa3 in an active surveillance cohort: Results from a baseline analysis in the canary prostate active surveillance study. *Clin. Cancer Res.* **2013**, *19*, 2442–2450. [CrossRef] [PubMed]
20. Berg, K.D.; Vainer, B.; Thomsen, F.B.; Roder, M.A.; Gerds, T.A.; Toft, B.G.; Brasso, K.; Iversen, P. ERG protein expression in diagnostic specimens is associated with increased risk of progression during active surveillance for prostate cancer. *Eur. Urol.* **2014**, *66*, 851–860. [CrossRef] [PubMed]
21. Green, W.J.; Ball, G.; Hulman, G.; Johnson, C.; Van Schalwyk, G.; Ratan, H.L.; Soria, D.; Garibaldi, J.M.; Parkinson, R.; Hulman, J.; et al. KI67 and DLX2 predict increased risk of metastasis formation in prostate cancer—A targeted molecular approach. *Br. J. Cancer* **2016**, *115*, 236–242. [CrossRef] [PubMed]
22. Murphy, S.J.; Karnes, R.J.; Kosari, F.; Castellar, B.E.; Kipp, B.R.; Johnson, S.H.; Terra, S.; Harris, F.R.; Halling, G.C.; Klein, J.L.; et al. Integrated analysis of the genomic instability of pten in clinically insignificant and significant prostate cancer. *Mod. Pathol.* **2016**, *29*, 143–156. [CrossRef] [PubMed]
23. Lotan, T.L.; Carvalho, F.L.; Peskoe, S.B.; Hicks, J.L.; Good, J.; Fedor, H.L.; Humphreys, E.; Han, M.; Platz, E.A.; Squire, J.A.; et al. Pten loss is associated with upgrading of prostate cancer from biopsy to radical prostatectomy. *Mod. Pathol.* **2015**, *28*, 128–137. [CrossRef] [PubMed]
24. Mithal, P.; Allott, E.; Gerber, L.; Reid, J.; Welbourn, W.; Tikishvili, E.; Park, J.; Younus, A.; Sangale, Z.; Lanchbury, J.S.; et al. Pten loss in biopsy tissue predicts poor clinical outcomes in prostate cancer. *Int. J. Urol.* **2014**, *21*, 1209–1214. [CrossRef] [PubMed]
25. Knezevic, D.; Goddard, A.D.; Natraj, N.; Cherbavaz, D.B.; Clark-Langone, K.M.; Snable, J.; Watson, D.; Falzarano, S.M.; Magi-Galluzzi, C.; Klein, E.A.; et al. Analytical validation of the oncotype dx prostate cancer assay—A clinical RT-PCR assay optimized for prostate needle biopsies. *BMC Genom.* **2013**, *14*, 690. [CrossRef] [PubMed]
26. Cuzick, J.; Swanson, G.P.; Fisher, G.; Brothman, A.R.; Berney, D.M.; Reid, J.E.; Mesher, D.; Speights, V.O.; Stankiewicz, E.; Foster, C.S.; et al. Prognostic value of an RNA expression signature derived from cell cycle proliferation genes in patients with prostate cancer: A retrospective study. *Lancet Oncol.* **2011**, *12*, 245–255. [CrossRef]
27. Bishoff, J.T.; Freedland, S.J.; Gerber, L.; Tennstedt, P.; Reid, J.; Welbourn, W.; Graefen, M.; Sangale, Z.; Tikishvili, E.; Park, J.; et al. Prognostic utility of the cell cycle progression score generated from biopsy in men treated with prostatectomy. *J. Urol.* **2014**, *192*, 409–414. [CrossRef] [PubMed]
28. Suzuki, M.; Bird, A. DNA methylation landscapes: Provocative insights from epigenomics. *Nat. Rev. Genet.* **2008**, *9*, 465–476. [CrossRef] [PubMed]
29. Jurkowska, R.Z.; Jukowski, T.P.; Jeltsch, A. Structure and function of mammalian DNA methyltransferases. *ChemBioChem* **2011**, *12*, 206–222. [CrossRef] [PubMed]
30. Okano, M.; Xie, S.; Li, E. Cloning and characterization of a family of novel mammalian DNA (cytosine-5) methyltransferases. *Nat. Genet.* **1998**, *19*, 219–220. [PubMed]
31. Waddington, C.H. "The epigenotype 1942". *Int. J. Epidemiol.* **2012**, *41*, 10–13. [CrossRef] [PubMed]
32. Kouzarides, T. Chromatin modifications and their function. *Cell* **2007**, *128*, 693–705. [CrossRef] [PubMed]
33. Haberland, M.; Montgomery, R.L.; Olson, E.N. The many roles of histone deacetylases in development and physiology: Implications for disease and therapy. *Nat. Rev. Genet.* **2009**, *10*, 32–42. [CrossRef] [PubMed]
34. Rouhi, A.; Mager, D.L.; Humphries, R.K.; Kuchenbauer, F. MiRNAs, epigenetics, and cancer. *Mamm. Genome* **2008**, *19*, 517–525. [CrossRef] [PubMed]
35. He, L.; Hannon, G.J. MicroRNAs: Small RNAs with a big role in gene regulation. *Nat. Rev. Genet.* **2004**, *5*, 522–531. [CrossRef] [PubMed]
36. Farazi, T.A.; Hoell, J.I.; Morozov, P.; Tuschl, T. MicroRNAs in human cancer. *Adv. Exp. Med. Biol.* **2013**, *774*, 1–20.
37. Yoo, C.B.; Jones, P.A. Epigenetic therapy of cancer: Past, present and future. *Nat. Rev. Drug Discov.* **2006**, *5*, 37–50. [CrossRef] [PubMed]

38. Yegnasubramanian, S.; Haffner, M.C.; Zhang, Y.; Gurel, B.; Cornish, T.C.; Wu, Z.; Irizarry, R.A.; Morgan, J.; Hicks, J.; DeWeese, T.L.; et al. DNA hypomethylation arises later in prostate cancer progression than CpG island hypermethylation and contributes to metastatic tumor heterogeneity. *Cancer Res.* **2008**, *68*, 8954–8967. [CrossRef] [PubMed]
39. Jarrad, D.F.; Bussemakers, M.J.; Bova, G.S.; Isaacs, W.B. Regional loss of imprinting of the insulin-like growth factor II gene occurs in human prostate tissues. *Clin. Cancer Res.* **1995**, *12*, 1471–1478.
40. Perry, A.S.; Watson, R.W.; Lawler, M.; Hollywood, D. The epigenome as a therapeutic target in prostate cancer. *Nat. Rev. Urol.* **2010**, *7*, 668–680. [CrossRef] [PubMed]
41. Liu, L.; Yoon, J.H.; Dammann, R.; Pfeifer, G.P. Frequent hypermethylation of the *RASSF1A* gene in prostate cancer. *Oncogene* **2002**, *21*, 6835–6840. [CrossRef] [PubMed]
42. Henrique, R.; Jeronimo, C. Molecular detection of prostate cancer: A role for gstp1 hypermethylation. *Eur. Urol.* **2004**, *46*, 660–669. [CrossRef] [PubMed]
43. Jerónimo, C.; Usadel, H.; Henrique, R.; Oliveira, J.; Lopes, C.; Nelson, W.G.; Sidransky, D. Quantitation of gstp1 methylation in non-neoplastic prostatic tissue and organ-confined prostate adenocarcinoma. *J. Natl. Cancer Inst.* **2001**, *93*, 1747–1752. [CrossRef] [PubMed]
44. Millar, D.S.; Ow, K.K.; Paul, C.L.; Russell, P.J.; Molloy, P.L.; Clark, S.J. Detailed methylation analysis of the glutathione S-transferase-π gene (*GSTP1*) in prostate cancer. *Oncogene* **1999**, *18*, 1313–1324. [CrossRef] [PubMed]
45. Litovkin, K.; van Eynde, A.; Joniau, S.; Lerut, E.; Laenen, A.; Gevaert, T.; Gevaert, O.; Spahn, M.; Kneitz, B.; Gramme, P.; et al. DNA methylation-guided prediction of clinical failure in high-risk prostate cancer. *PLoS ONE* **2015**, *10*, e01300651. [CrossRef] [PubMed]
46. Haldrup, C.; Mundbjerg, K.; Vestergaard, E.M.; Lamy, P.; Wild, P.; Schulz, W.A.; Arsov, C.; Visakorpi, T.; Borre, M.; Høyer, S.; et al. DNA methylation signatures for prediction of biochemical recurrence after radical prostatectomy of clinically localized prostate cancer. *J. Clin. Oncol.* **2013**, *31*, 3250–3258. [CrossRef] [PubMed]
47. Ellinger, J.; Kahl, P.; von der Gathen, J.; Rogenhofer, S.; Heukamp, L.C.; Gutgemann, I.; Walter, B.; Hofstadter, F.; Buttner, R.; Muller, S.C.; et al. Global levels of histone modifications predict prostate cancer recurrence. *Prostate* **2010**, *70*, 61–69. [CrossRef] [PubMed]
48. Varambally, S.; Dhanasekaran, S.M.; Zhou, M.; Barrette, T.R.; Kumar-Sinha, C.; Sanda, M.G.; Ghosh, D.; Pienta, K.J.; Sewalt, R.G.; Otte, A.P.; et al. The polycomb group protein EZH2 is involved in progression of prostate cancer. *Nature* **2002**, *419*, 624–629. [CrossRef] [PubMed]
49. Yu, J.; Rhodes, D.R.; Tomlins, S.A.; Cao, X.; Chen, G.; Mehra, R.; Wang, X.; Ghosh, D.; Shah, R.B.; Varambally, S.; et al. A polycomb repression signature in metastatic prostate cancer predicts cancer outcome. *Cancer Res.* **2007**, *67*, 10657–10663. [CrossRef] [PubMed]
50. Wissmann, M.; Yin, N.; Müller, J.M.; Greschik, H.; Fodor, B.D.; Jenuwein, T.; Vogler, C.; Schneider, R.; Günther, T.; Buettner, R.; et al. Cooperative demethylation by *JMJD2C* and *LSD1* promotes androgen receptor-dependent gene expression. *Nat. Cell Biol.* **2007**, *9*, 347–353. [CrossRef] [PubMed]
51. Gaughan, L.; Stockley, J.; Wang, N.; McCracken, S.R.; Treumann, A.; Armstrong, K.; Shaheen, F.; Watt, K.; McEwan, I.J.; Wang, C.; et al. Regulation of the androgen receptor by set9-mediated methylation. *Nucleic Acids Res.* **2011**, *39*, 1266–1279. [CrossRef] [PubMed]
52. Suikki, H.E.; Kujala, P.M.; Tammela, T.L.; van Weerden, W.M.; Vessella, R.L.; Visakorpi, T. Genetic alterations and changes in expression of histone demethylases in prostate cancer. *Prostate* **2010**, *70*, 889–898. [CrossRef] [PubMed]
53. Vieira, F.Q.; Costa-Pinheiro, P.; Almeida-Rios, D.; Graça, I.; Monteiro-Reis, S.; Simões-Sousa, S.; Carneiro, I.; Sousa, E.J.; Godinho, M.I.; Baltazar, F.; et al. Smyd3 contributes to a more aggressive phenotype of prostate cancer and targets cyclin D2 through H4K20ME3. *Oncotarget* **2015**, *6*, 13644–13657. [CrossRef] [PubMed]
54. Vieira, F.Q.; Costa-Pinheiro, P.; Ramalho-Carvalho, J.; Pereira, A.; Menezes, F.D.; Antunes, L.; Carneiro, I.; Oliveira, J.; Henrique, R.; Jerónimo, C. Deregulated expression of selected histone methylases and demethylases in prostate carcinoma. *Endocr. Relat. Cancer* **2013**, *21*, 51–61. [CrossRef] [PubMed]
55. Kahl, P.; Gullotti, L.; Heukamp, L.C.; Wolf, S.; Friedrichs, N.; Vorreuther, R.; Solleder, G.; Bastian, P.J.; Ellinger, J.; Metzger, E.; et al. Androgen receptor coactivators lysine-specific histone demethylase 1 and four and a half lim domain protein 2 predict risk of prostate cancer recurrence. *Cancer Res.* **2006**, *66*, 11341–11347. [CrossRef] [PubMed]

56. Metzger, E.W.; Wissmann, M.; Yin, N.; Müller, J.M.; Schneider, R.; Peters, A.H.; Günther, T.; Buettner, R.; Schüle, R. LSD1 demethylates repressive histone marks to promote androgen-receptor-dependent transcription. *Nature* **2005**, *437*, 436–439. [CrossRef] [PubMed]
57. Haikidou, K.; Gaughan, L.; Cook, S.; Leung, H.Y.; Neal, D.E.; Robson, C.N. Upregulation and nuclear recruitment of HDAC1 in hormone refractory prostate cancer. *Prostate* **2004**, *59*, 177–189. [CrossRef] [PubMed]
58. Weichert, W.; Röske, A.; Gekeler, V.; Beckers, T.; Stephan, C.; Jung, K.F.; Fritzsche, F.R.N.; Niesporek, S.; Denkert, C.; Dietel, M.; et al. Histone deacetylases 1, 2 and 3 are highly expressed in prostate cancer and hdac2 expression is associated with shorter PSA relapse time after radical prostatectomy. *Br. J. Cancer* **2008**, *98*, 604–610. [CrossRef] [PubMed]
59. Korkmaz, C.G.; Frønsdal, K.; Zhang, Y.; Lorenzo, P.I.; Saatcioglu, F. Potentiation of androgen receptor transcriptional activity by inhibition of histone deacetylation—Rescue of transcriptionally compromised mutants. *J. Endocrinol.* **2004**, *182*, 377–389. [CrossRef] [PubMed]
60. Baptista, T.; Graça, I.; Sousa, E.J.; Oliveira, A.I.; Costa, N.R.; Costa-Pinheiro, P.; Amado, F.; Henrique, R.; Jerónimo, C. Regulation of histone H2A.Z expression is mediated by sirtuin 1 in prostate cancer. *Oncotarget* **2013**, *4*, 1673–1685. [CrossRef] [PubMed]
61. Al-Kafaji, G.; Al-Naieb, Z.T.; Bakhiet, M. Increased oncogenic microRNA-18a expression in the peripheral blood of patients with prostate cancer: A potential novel non-invasive biomarker. *Oncol. Lett.* **2016**, *11*, 1201–1206. [CrossRef] [PubMed]
62. Xu, S.; Yi, X.M.; Zhou, W.Q.; Cheng, W.; Ge, J.P.; Zhang, Z.Y. Downregulation of miR-129 in peripheral blood mononuclear cells is a diagnostic and prognostic biomarker in prostate cancer. *Int. J. Clin. Exp. Pathol.* **2015**, *8*, 14335–14344. [PubMed]
63. Zhao, F.; Olkhov-Mitsel, E.; van der Kwast, T.; Sykes, J.; Zdravic, D.; Venkateswaran, V.; Zlotta, A.R.; Loblaw, A.; Fleshner, N.E.; Klotz, L.; et al. Urinary DNA methylation biomarkers for noninvasive prediction of aggressive disease in patients with prostate cancer on active surveillance. *J. Urol.* **2017**, *197*, 335–341. [CrossRef] [PubMed]
64. Yegnasubramanian, S. Prostate cancer epigenetics and its clinical implications. *Asian J. Androl.* **2016**, *18*, 549–558. [CrossRef] [PubMed]
65. Sunami, E.; Shinozaki, M.; Higano, C.S.; Wollman, R.; Dorff, T.B.; Tucker, S.J.; Martinez, S.R.; Mizuno, R.; Singer, F.R.; Hoon, D.S. Multimarker circulating DNA assay for assessing blood of prostate cancer patients. *Clin. Chem.* **2009**, *55*, 559–567. [CrossRef] [PubMed]
66. Ahmed, H. Promoter methylation in prostate cancer and its application for the early detection of prostate cancer using serum and urine samples. *Biomark. Cancer* **2010**, *2*, 17–33. [CrossRef] [PubMed]
67. Partin, A.W.; Van Neste, L.; Klein, E.A.; Marks, L.S.; Gee, J.R.; Troyer, D.A.; Rieger-Christ, K.; Jones, J.S.; Magi-Galluzzi, C.; Mangold, L.A.; et al. Clinical validation of an epigenetic assay to predict negative histopathological results in repeat prostate biopsies. *J. Urol.* **2014**, *192*, 1081–1087. [CrossRef] [PubMed]
68. Ellinger, J.; Muller, S.C.; Stadler, T.C.; Jung, A.; von Ruecker, A.; Bastian, P.J. The role of cell-free circulating DNA in the diagnosis and prognosis of prostate cancer. *Urol. Oncol.* **2011**, *29*, 124–129. [CrossRef] [PubMed]
69. Roupret, M.; Hupertan, V.; Yates, D.R.; Catto, J.W.; Rehman, I.; Meuth, M.; Ricci, S.; Lacave, R.; Cancel-Tassin, G.; de la Taille, A.; et al. Molecular detection of localized prostate cancer using quantitative methylation-specific PCR on urinary cells obtained following prostate massage. *Clin. Cancer Res.* **2007**, *13*, 1720–1725. [CrossRef] [PubMed]
70. Klotz, L. Active surveillance for low-risk prostate cancer. *Curr. Opin. Urol.* **2017**, *27*, 225–230. [CrossRef] [PubMed]
71. Loeb, S.; Bruinsma, S.M.; Nicholson, J.; Briganti, A.; Pickles, T.; Kakehi, Y.; Carlsson, S.V.; Roobol, M.J. Active surveillance for prostate cancer: A systematic review of clinicopathologic variables and biomarkers for risk stratification. *Eur. Urol.* **2015**, *67*, 619–626. [CrossRef] [PubMed]

13

The Effect of Metformin and GANT61 Combinations on the Radiosensitivity of Prostate Cancer Cells

Annelies Gonnissen [1,2], Sofie Isebaert [1,2,*], Chad M. McKee [3], Ruth J. Muschel [3] and Karin Haustermans [1,2]

1 Laboratory of Experimental Radiotherapy, Department of Oncology, KU Leuven—University of Leuven, 3000 Leuven, Belgium; annelies.gonnissen@kuleuven.be (A.G.); karin.haustermans@uzleuven.be (K.H.)
2 Department of Radiation Oncology, University Hospitals Leuven, 3000 Leuven, Belgium
3 Department of Oncology, CRUK/MRC Oxford Institute for Radiation Oncology, University of Oxford, Oxford OX3 7DQ, UK; chad.mckee@oncology.ox.ac.uk (C.M.M.); ruth.muschel@oncology.ox.ac.uk (R.J.M.)
* Correspondence: sofie.isebaert@uzleuven.be

Academic Editor: Carsten Stephan

Abstract: The anti-diabetes drug metformin has been shown to have anti-neoplastic effects in several tumor models through its effects on energy metabolism and protein synthesis. Recent studies show that metformin also targets Hedgehog (Hh) signaling, a developmental pathway re-activated in several tumor types, including prostate cancer (PCa). Furthermore, we and others have shown that Hh signaling is an important target for radiosensitization. Here, we evaluated the combination of metformin and the Hh inhibitor GANT61 (GLI-ANTagonist 61) with or without ionizing radiation in three PCa cell lines (PC3, DU145, 22Rv1). The effect on proliferation, radiosensitivity, apoptosis, cell cycle distribution, reactive oxygen species production, DNA repair, gene and protein expression was investigated. Furthermore, this treatment combination was also assessed in vivo. Metformin was shown to interact with Hh signaling by inhibiting the effector protein glioma-associated oncogene homolog 1 (GLI1) in PCa cells both in vitro and in vivo. The combination of metformin and GANT61 significantly inhibited PCa cell growth in vitro and enhanced the radiation response of 22Rv1 cells compared to either single agent. Nevertheless, neither the growth inhibitory effect nor the radiosensitization effect of the combination treatment observed in vitro was seen in vivo. Although the interaction between metformin and Hh signaling seems to be promising from a therapeutic point of view in vitro, more research is needed when implementing this combination strategy in vivo.

Keywords: prostate cancer; metformin; hedgehog pathway; radiosensitization; xenograft mouse model

1. Introduction

The biguanide metformin, commonly used for the treatment of patients with type 2 diabetes, has been associated with a decreased incidence and mortality in several tumor types, including prostate cancer (PCa) [1–3]. Metformin has also been shown to have anti-neoplastic effects [4], potentially due to its effects on energy metabolism and protein synthesis by activation of adenosine monophosphate (AMP)-activated protein kinase (AMPK) signaling and inhibition of the mammalian target of rapamycin (mTOR) [5–7]. Additionally, several preclinical studies have shown that metformin can increase the effect of radiotherapy [8–12]. The mechanism of these radiosensitizing effects are not completely understood but include reoxygenation of hypoxic regions [9], impairment of DNA damage response [11] and induction of reactive oxygen species (ROS) [12]. The radiosensitizing effect of metformin has been shown to be highly context-dependent and more research is needed to identify the appropriate treatment conditions and cell populations to induce radiosensitization by metformin.

Some recent studies have identified the Hedgehog (Hh) signaling pathway as a novel target of metformin [13,14]. This pathway is a potential candidate for anti-cancer treatment, since several tumor types are known to have deregulated Hh signaling, including PCa [15–18]. Of note, metformin has been shown to inhibit Hh signaling in breast [13] and pancreatic [14] cancer cells.

We have previously shown that inhibition of Hh signaling at the level of the transcription factors using the small molecule inhibitor GANT61 (GLI-ANTagonist 61) is highly effective in PCa cells and increased radiosensitivity both in vitro and in vivo [19].

In this study, the link between AMPK and Hh signaling was explored in several PCa cell lines. Additionally, we investigated whether simultaneous targeting of both pathways with metformin and GANT61, respectively, could enhance PCa cytotoxicity and/or radiosensitivity both in vitro and in vivo.

2. Results

2.1. Metformin Decreases Cell Growth and Survival of Prostate Cancer (PCa) Cells

Metformin significantly decreased PCa cell growth in a time- and dose-dependent manner (Figure 1A). A high dose of metformin (5 mM) was able to induce a significant decrease in cell survival in all cell lines (Figure 1B). The PC3 cells were the most sensitive with a half maximal inhibitory concentration (IC_{50}) value around 5 mM, whereas the IC_{50} in 22Rv1 and DU145 was between 10–20 mM metformin (Figure S1).

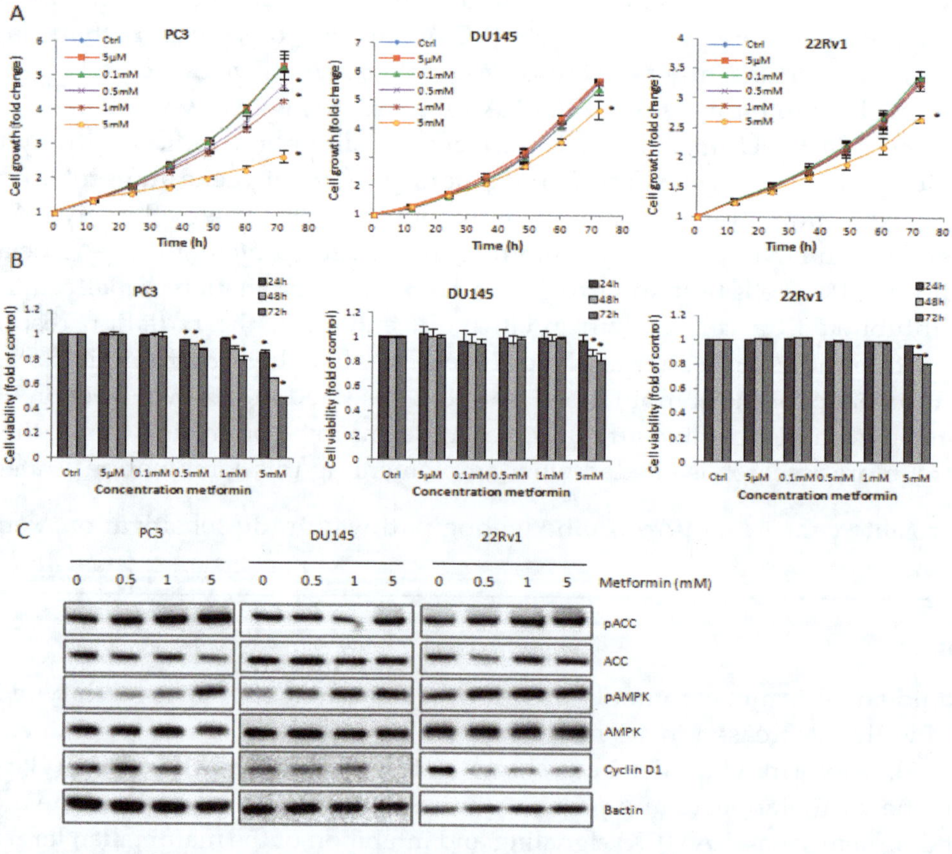

Figure 1. Effect of metformin on prostate cancer (PCa) cells. (**A**) Cell growth and (**B**) cell viability after metformin treatment. Means ± standard error of means (SEM) of three independent experiments. * $p < 0.05$ vs. control; (**C**) Protein expression of the downstream signaling molecules after 72-h metformin treatment. ACC, Acetyl-CoA carboxylase; AMPK, adenosine monophosphate (AMP)-activated protein kinase; pACC, phospho-Acetyl-CoA carboxylase; pAMPK, phospho-Adenosine monophosphate (AMP)-activated protein kinase.

In line with this, cyclin D1 protein expression was drastically decreased after treatment with 5 mM metformin, especially in the rapidly proliferating PC3 and DU145 cell lines (Figure 1C). Additionally, metformin activated its downstream signaling components AMPK and Acetyl-CoA carboxylase (ACC) in a dose-dependent manner in all PCa cell lines (Figure 1C).

2.2. Metformin Increases Radiosensitivity of PCa Cells Independent of Adenosine Monophosphate (AMP)-Activated Protein Kinase (AMPK) Activation

Metformin (5 mM) increased radiosensitivity of DU145 and 22Rv1 cells with a dose-enhancement factor (DEF) of 1.6 ± 0.15 ($p < 0.05$) and 1.36 ± 0.08 ($p < 0.05$) respectively. In contrast, the radiosensitivity of PC3 cells was not affected by metformin (Figure 2A). To evaluate the role of AMPK in the metformin-induced radiosensitization effect in the DU145 and 22Rv1 cells, AMPK was silenced by means of silencing RNA (siRNA). Downregulation of (phospho)AMPK did not affect the intrinsic radiosensitivity of either cell line nor did it change the metformin-induced radiosensitization (Figure 2B).

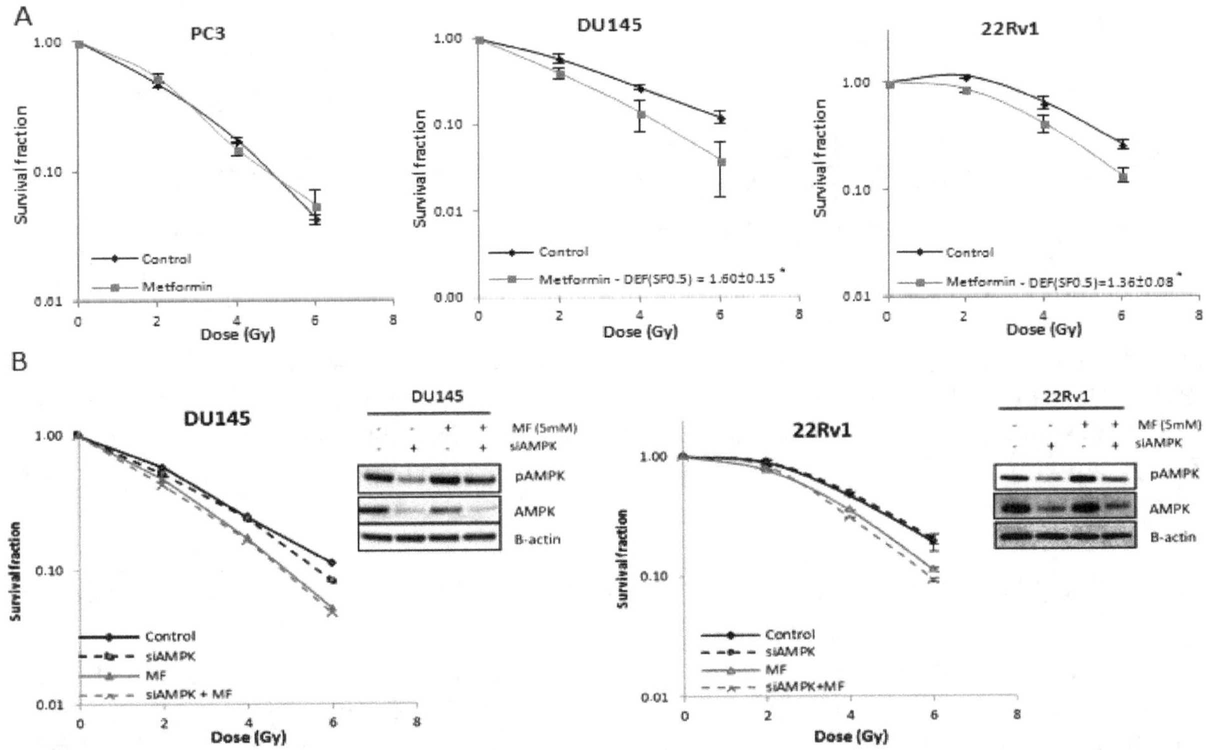

Figure 2. Effect of metformin (MF) on radiosensitivity of PCa cells. (**A**) Clonogenic survival after 72-h treatment with metformin (5 mM) prior to/during ionizing radiation (IR); (**B**) Clonogenic survival of DU145 and 22Rv1 cells transfected with AMPK silencing RNA (siRNA) and 72-h treatment with metformin (5 mM) prior to/during IR. Knockdown was verified with western blotting. Means ± SEM of three independent experiments. * $p < 0.05$ vs. control. DEF: dose-enhancement factor.

2.3. Metformin Regulates Hedgehog Signaling in an AMPK-Dependent Manner

Next, we investigated if there was a link between metformin and Hh signaling in PCa cells. Indeed, metformin (5 mM) significantly decreased glioma-associated oncogene homolog 1 (*GLI1*) and patched 1 (*PTCH1*) gene and protein expression in all cell lines (Figure 3A,B). Although metformin only significantly decreased glioma-associated oncogene homolog 2 (*GLI2*) gene expression in the DU145 cells, we did observe decreased GLI2 protein expression after metformin treatment in all PCa cell lines (Figure 3A,B). In addition, AMPK activation was shown to be inversely correlated with GLI1 protein expression. Silencing AMPK expression with siRNA increased GLI1 expression, whereas activation of AMPK by metformin decreased GLI1 expression in 22Rv1 cells (Figure 3C). This indicates that metformin regulates Hh signaling, probably through AMPK signaling.

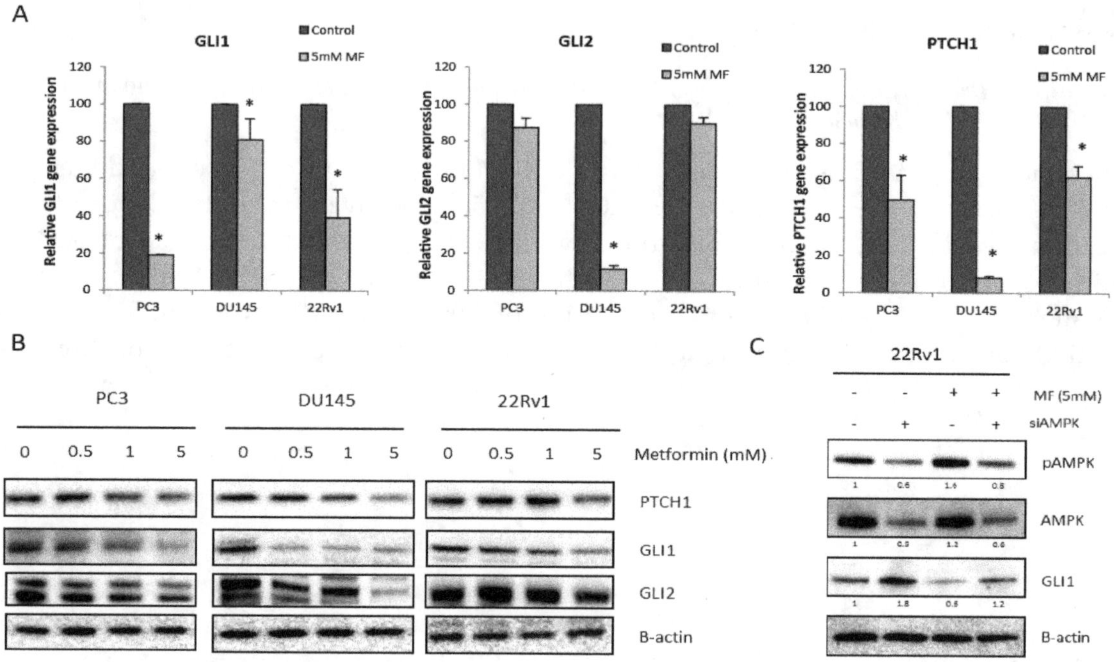

Figure 3. Link between metformin and Hedgehog signaling. (**A**) *GLI1*, *GLI2* and *PTCH1* gene expression after 72-h metformin treatment. Means + SEM of two independent experiments. * $p < 0.05$ vs. control; (**B**) PTCH1, GLI1 and GLI2 protein expression after 72-h metformin treatment; (**C**) (p)AMPK protein and GLI1 expression in 22Rv1 cells transfected with AMPK siRNA and treated with metformin (5 mM) 72-h prior to protein lysis. GLI1, glioma-associated oncogene homolog 1; GLI2, glioma-associated oncogene homolog 2; PTCH1, patched 1.

2.4. Combination of Metformin and GANT61 (GLI-ANTagonist 61) Synergistically Decreases PCa Cell Growth

The link between AMPK and GLI1 led to the question as to whether the combination of metformin with Hh inhibitors could enhance the cytotoxic effect of the individual drugs. We have previously shown that the GLI1/2 inhibitor GANT61 significantly decreased cell survival of PC3 and 22Rv1 cells [19]. Indeed, combining metformin and GANT61 significantly decreased cell growth of all PCa cell lines, resulting in an almost complete blockage of cell growth in PC3 and 22Rv1 cells (Figure 4A). Additionally, we confirmed decreased *GLI1* gene expression in all cells treated with the drug combination (Figure S2). Cell cycle analyses revealed that the drug combination in the PC3 cells led to a G2/M-arrest after only 24 h, which persisted until 72 h of treatment (Figure 4B). This corresponds to the dramatic decrease in cell growth already observed after 24 h of treatment. The drug combination also significantly increased the sub-G1 population which peaked at 48 h (Figure 4C). In the DU145 cells, no significant cell cycle effects were observed after 24–72 h of either treatment (Figure 4B), whereas the combination treatment did significantly increase apoptosis after 72 h compared to either single agent (Figure 4C). In the 22Rv1 cells, GANT61 induced a G1-arrest after only 24 h. Metformin alone did not have a significant effect on cell cycle, however, the combination of both drugs resulted in a much more pronounced G1-arrest after 72 h of treatment compared to GANT61 alone (Figure 4B). Apoptosis was also significantly induced by both individual drugs and even more by the drug combination (Figure 4C). Moreover, we observed that both drugs and their combination induced DNA damage in all cell lines after 72 h of treatment assessed by means of γH2AX staining (Figure S3).

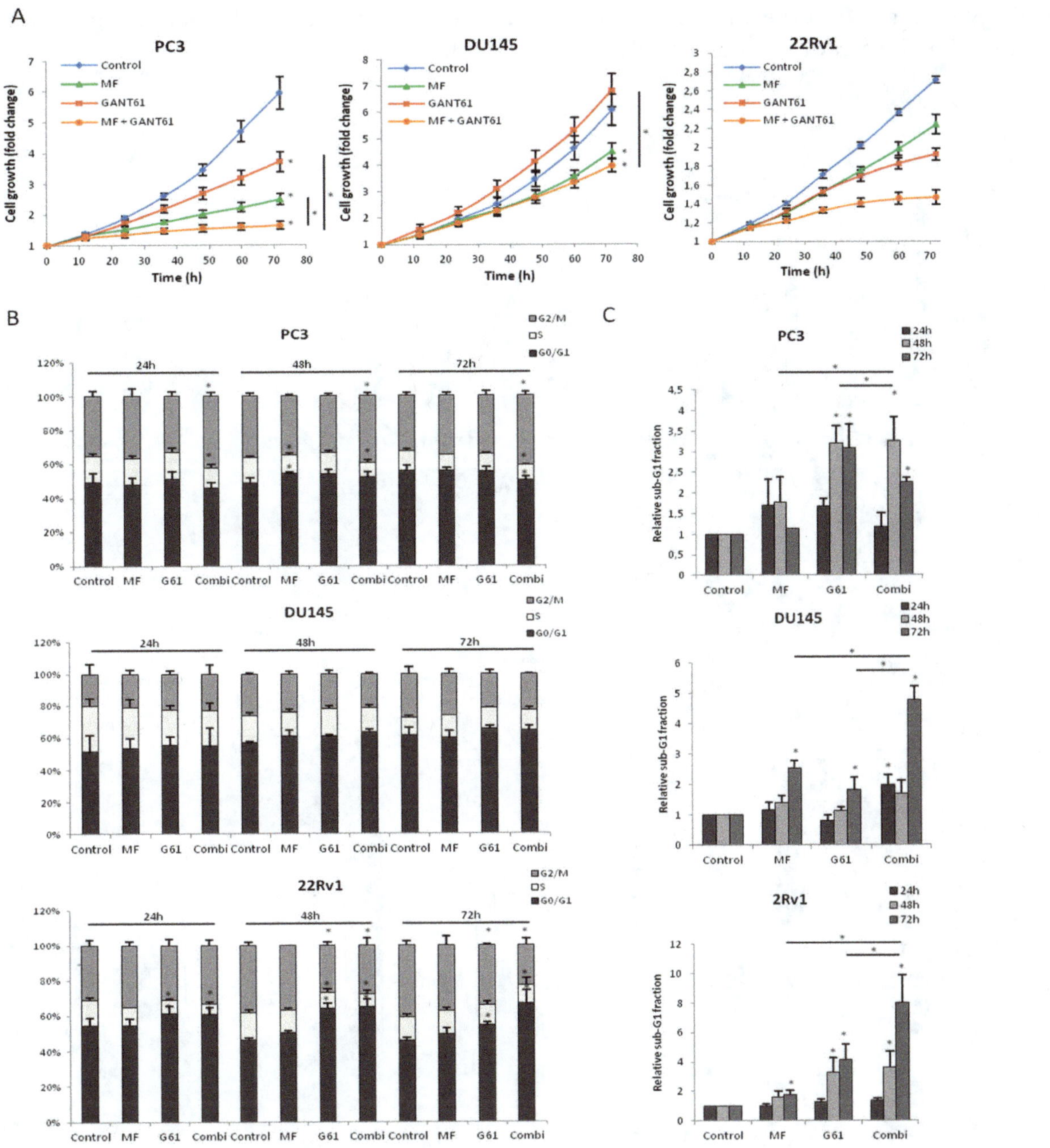

Figure 4. Combination of metformin and GANT61 (GLI-ANTagonist 61) in PCa cells (**A**) Cell growth; (**B**) cell cycle distribution and (**C**) sub-G1 population after treatment with metformin (5 mM), GANT61 (10 μM) or combination; (**B**,**C**) Cells were fixed at 24, 48 and 72 h of treatment. Means ± SEM of three independent experiments. * $p < 0.05$ vs. control.G61, GANT61.

2.5. Combining Metformin and GANT61 Enhances the Effect of Ionizing Radiation In Vitro

Short-term survival analyses illustrated that the combination of metformin and GANT61 with ionizing radiation (IR) significantly decreased cell survival in all cell lines (Figure 5A). In the PC3 and DU145 cells, the response to IR in the combination treatment is most likely due to metformin since addition of GANT61 did not significantly decrease cell survival any further. In contrast, in the 22Rv1 cells, a significant decrease in cell survival in the combination group compared to metformin alone was observed. To assess the effect on the intrinsic radiosensitivity, clonogenic survival assays were performed. Consistent with previous results, the combination of metformin and GANT61 significantly enhanced radiosensitivity of 22Rv1 cells compared to either single agent (Figure 6B). In the PC3 cells, we did not observe an effect of the combination treatment or either single agent, whereas only metformin had a radiosensitizing effect in the DU145 cells (Figure 5B).

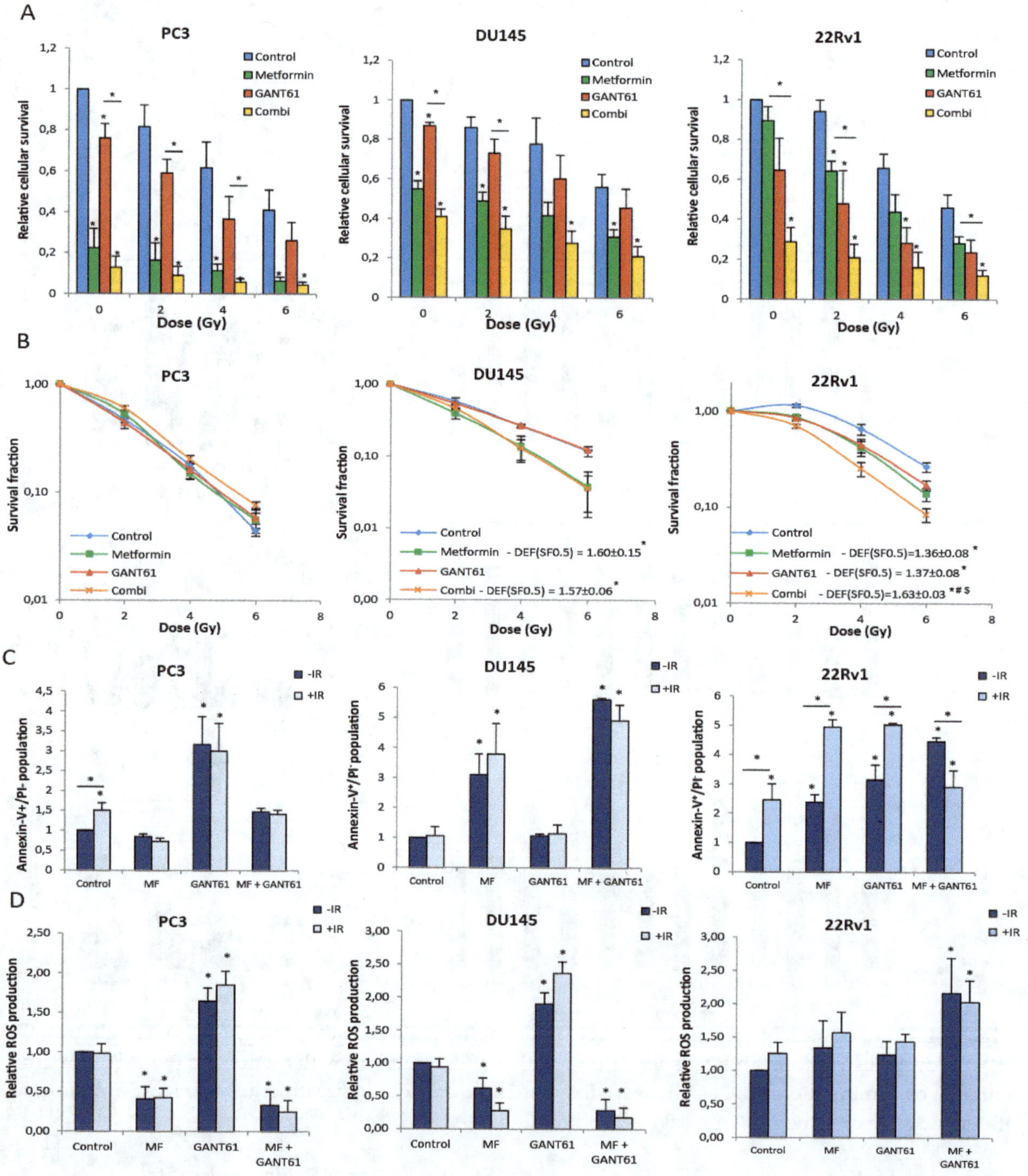

Figure 5. Effect of the combination of metformin and GANT61 on radiosensitivity of PCa cells. (**A**) Relative short-term cell survival 7 days after treatment with increasing doses of ionizing radiation after 72-h pretreatment with metformin, GANT61 or combination; (**B**) Clonogenic survival after 72-h treatment with metformin, GANT61 or combination prior to/during IR; (**C**) AnnexinV$^+$/propidium iodide (PI)$^-$ cells and (**D**) Reactive oxygen species (ROS) production at 24-h post-IR after 72-h pretreatment with metformin (5 mM), GANT61 (10 µM) or combination. Means ± SEM of three independent experiments. * $p < 0.05$ vs. control.

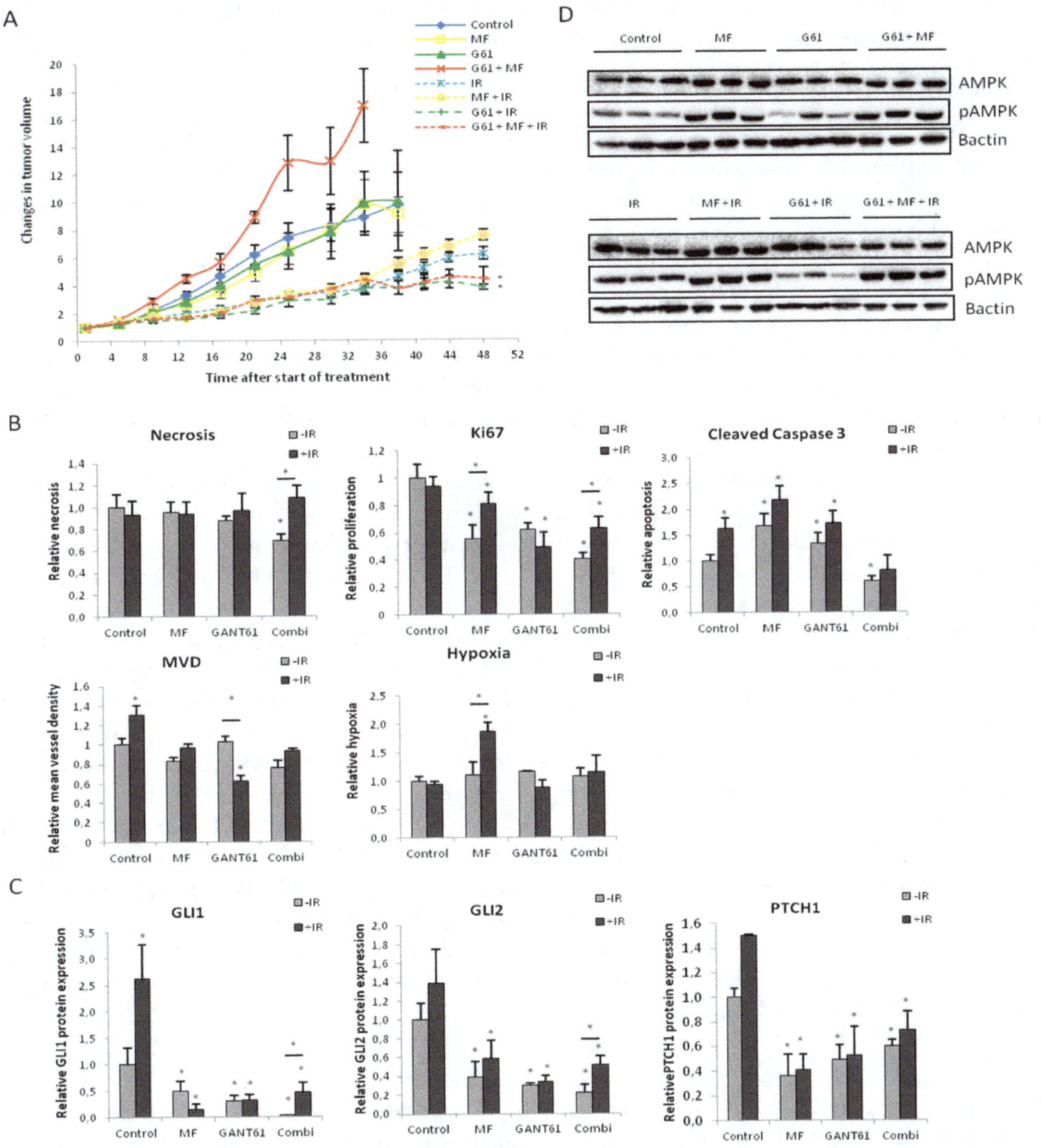

Figure 6. Effect of the combination of metformin and GANT61 on radiosensitivity in a 22Rv1 xenograft model. (**A**) Relative tumor growth of 22Rv1 xenograft mice treated with metformin (250 mg/kg), GANT61 (50 mg/kg) or combination. At treatment day 5, tumors were irradiated with a single dose of 6Gy (six mice/group); (**B**) Immunohistochemical analyses of necrosis, Ki67, cleaved caspase 3, mean vessel density (MVD), hypoxia and (**C**) Hedgehog (Hh) target proteins GLI1, GLI2 and PTCH1 (six mice/group, $n \leq 12$ tumors). * $p < 0.05$ vs. control; (**D**) Protein expression of pAMPK and AMPK in 22Rv1 xenograft tumors ($n = 3$ tumors/treatment group).

The combination of IR with either single agent increased apoptosis in the 22Rv1 cells. However, in the drug combination treatment, addition of IR did not further increase apoptosis; on the contrary, apoptosis was decreased in this condition indicating that other mechanisms might be important here (Figure 5C). In the PC3 and DU145 cells, apoptosis was not (further) increased upon addition of IR

(Figure 5C). Furthermore, we observed that ROS were increased in the 22Rv1 cells when using the drug combination; an effect which could attribute to the increased radiosensitivity (Figure 5D).

2.6. Combination of Metformin and GANT61 Stimulates Tumor Growth In Vivo

Since the drug combination enhanced the radiosensitivity of 22Rv1 cells in vitro, we used a 22Rv1 xenograft model to assess the effect of the drug combination in vivo. Surprisingly, although we observed a robust decrease of cell proliferation in vitro, the combination of GANT61 and metformin appeared to be pro-proliferative in vivo. Metformin and GANT61 alone did not have any effect on tumor growth (Figure 6A). To investigate why the combination of both drugs resulted in a paradoxical effect, we looked deeper into the molecular changes that occurred in these tumors. Tumors treated with the drug combination were less necrotic and had fewer apoptotic cells compared to control tumors or those treated with either single agent (Figure 6B). In addition, these tumors contained fewer blood vessels compared to controls or the GANT61-treated tumors. No changes in hypoxia were observed. Although the drug combination increased tumor growth, this was not reflected by Ki67 expression, which was significantly lower in these tumors compared to controls and either single agent (Figure 6B). This implies that the growth stimulatory effect of the drug combination is more likely due to pro-survival effects rather than effects on proliferation.

As for the combination with IR, metformin did not increase radiosensitivity of 22Rv1 tumors, while GANT61 did result in enhanced radiosensitivity. The combination of metformin and GANT61 with IR also significantly decreased tumor growth, however this was most likely attributed to the effect of GANT61 (Figure 6A). As previously shown [19], the GANT61-induced radiosensitization is attributed to decreased proliferation and increased apoptosis. In the tumors treated with the drug combination, the radiosensitizing effect can also, at least partially, be ascribed to effects on proliferation. In contrast, the amount of apoptosis is lower in these tumors compared to controls or tumors treated with a single agent, but we observed more necrosis in the tumors treated with the combined modality, which could also attribute to the decreased tumor growth (Figure 6B).

Finally, we verified whether both drugs reached their target in the tumors to verify their specificity in vivo. Immunohistochemical analyses of GLI1, GLI2 and PTCH1 demonstrated that GANT61 was able to specifically inhibit Hh signaling in the tumor (Figure 6C). We also provide evidence that metformin targets AMPK signaling as phospho-AMPK (pAMPK) was significantly increased in all tumor of metformin-treated mice (Figure 6D). Additionally, we showed that the link between metformin and Hh signaling also exists in vivo. Both metformin also significantly decreased protein expression of GLI1, GLI2 and PTCH1 (Figure 6C).

3. Discussion

Contradicting findings have been reported in PCa patients regarding an association between metformin use in diabetic PCa patients and biochemical recurrence (BCR) and metastasis. Several studies have shown that metformin had no effect on BCR-free survival of PCa patients after radical prostatectomy [20–23]. In contrast, a retrospective study by He et al. [24] did find a beneficial effect of metformin on overall survival (OS) of PCa patients treated with radical prostatectomy [24]. In a study by Spratt et al. [25] the authors specifically looked at PCa patients treated with external-beam radiotherapy (EBRT) and found a significant positive correlation between metformin use and BCR-free survival and OS [25]. These studies demonstrate that metformin might be an important treatment option for PCa patients, especially in the combination setting with EBRT.

In this study, we first evaluated the effect of metformin on cell growth and radiosensitivity of PCa cells. In line with a previous study by Sahra et al. [4], we found that metformin (5 mM) decreased cell growth of all cell lines, which coincided with reduced protein levels of cyclin D1. The fact that we could only observe a significant inhibition of cell growth at high doses of metformin is in accordance with multiple studies using different tumor cell types [4,8,26–28]. Several preclinical studies have already investigated the effect of metformin on the radiosensitivity of different tumor types and multiple mechanisms have been associated with the enhanced radiation sensitivity after metformin treatment [8–12]. Here, a radiosensitizing effect of metformin was observed in the DU145 and 22Rv1 cells, but not in the PC3 cells. This lack of radiosensitization in the PC3 cells could be a result of the higher sensitivity of PC3 cells to metformin leading to the absence of any additional effect upon IR. Data also suggest that metformin may enhance radiation response specifically in certain genetic backgrounds (p53, liver kinase B1 (LKB1)), but more research is needed to gain better insight in the specific interactions between metformin and important oncogenic and tumor suppressor genes [28].

We show that metformin also interacts with the Hh signaling pathway, specifically by decreasing gene and protein expression of the Hh target genes *GLI1* and *PTCH1*. Similar interactions were described recently in breast [13] and pancreatic [14] cancer cells. Our data demonstrate that this interaction is mediated by the activation of AMPK signaling, which is in line with the data of Nakamura et al. [14]. Accordingly, two recent studies have shown the AMPK phosphorylates GLI1, which results in the proteasomal degradation of GLI1 [29,30]. On top of that, we demonstrate that metformin also decreased Hh signaling in vivo. Interestingly, we observed a differential inhibition of Hh signaling in the three PCa cell lines at the gene level. In the PC3 and 22Rv1 cells, metformin significantly inhibited *GLI1* and *PTCH1* gene expression, whereas in the DU145 cells, metformin strongly inhibited *GLI2* gene expression in addition to inhibiting *GLI1* and *PTCH1*. Nevertheless, we did not observe a different phenotype in these cell lines in response to metformin treatment.

In a previous study by our group, we demonstrated that Hh inhibition increased the intrinsic radiosensitivity of 22Rv1 cells and not of PC3 and DU145 cells, which appeared to be dependent on functional p53 signaling [19]. Furthermore, it seems unlikely that the effect of metformin on radiosensitivity is through its effects on Hh signaling, as we have shown that metformin regulates Hh signaling in an AMPK-dependent manner, whereas it increases radiosensitivity of PCa cells independent of AMPK activation. Therefore, Hh inhibition and metformin both increase radiosensitivity of PCa cells but in a different manner.

This interesting interaction between metformin and Hh signaling suggests that the combination of metformin with Hh inhibition has the potential to further enhance the cytotoxic and/or radiosensitizing effect of either single agent. To our best knowledge, this combination has never been tested before. Our results show that this combination treatment is highly effective against PCa proliferation in vitro. This was associated with an increase of apoptosis and the induction of DNA damage in all cell lines. Additionally, we observed G2/M-arrest after just 24 h in the PC3 cells, these being the most sensitive to this drug combination. In the 22Rv1 cells, the cells treated with the drug combination experienced G1-arrest, which was at least partially ascribed to GANT61. In contrast with the high cytotoxicity of the drug combination observed in vitro, combining metformin and GANT61 appeared to be pro-proliferative in a 22Rv1 xenograft mouse model. Strangely, the amount of proliferation in these tumors was significantly decreased compared to control or either single agent, suggesting that the increased tumor growth was more likely attributed to decreased apoptosis and necrosis.

Our data also suggest that the combination of metformin and GANT61 only increases radiosensitivity of cells that are sensitized by both individual drugs, as was the case with the 22Rv1 cells. The PC3 cells were not radiosensitized by either drug or the combination, whereas the DU145 cells were only sensitized by metformin and not by GANT61 due to its p53 mutation [19], resulting in no extra benefit upon drug combination. In the 22Rv1 cells we observed a radiosensitizing effect of both metformin and GANT61 which was further enhanced by the drug combination. This was not the case in the in vivo situation, where we only observed a radiosensitizing effect of GANT61 and no additive effect on radiosensitivity by metformin. In line with our previously published data, the GANT61-induced radiosensitization was associated with decreased proliferation and increased cell death [19]. In tumors treated with the drug combination and IR, the amount of necrosis was significantly increased. One potential reason for the lack of radiosensitization of metformin in vivo might be the dosage of metformin used. In vitro, high-doses of metformin (5 mM) are needed to induce cytotoxic and radiosensitizing effects. These high levels of metformin are typically not achieved in an in vivo situation. We used 250 mg/kg intraperitoneally, which is also considered quite high compared to the typical metformin dosing in diabetic patients which lies around 30 mg/kg orally. However, considering the interspecies differences between mice and humans, the Food and Drug Administration (FDA) applies a standard scaling factor of 12.3 [31] which makes our in vivo dosage used definitely acceptable.

Several Smoothened (SMO) inhibitors are currently in the early stages of clinical investigation in PCa patients. Despite the high efficacy of SMO inhibition in patients with basal cell carcinoma and medulloblastoma, which are characterized by the presence of Hh mutations, the efficacy of these inhibitors in ligand-dependent Hh-activated cancer types such as PCa has not yet been established. Early phase clinical trials demonstrated little or no responsiveness to Hh inhibition in these tumor types so far. Multiple clinical trials are currently ongoing to investigate the potential of Hh inhibition as monotherapy or in combination with hormonal therapy in PCa [32]. The use of Hh inhibitors more downstream the signaling cascade has not yet been investigated in patients. Based on our results, the combination of GANT61 with radiotherapy might also be a promising strategy to test in the clinic [19].

Although the combination of metformin and GANT61 therapy appeared very effective in an in vitro situation, the interaction of metformin and GANT61 in the in vivo setting resulted in a paradoxical (pro-survival) effect. This suggests that the tumor microenvironment could play an important role in the anti-tumor activity of drug combinations in vivo. We have previously shown that Hh inhibition indeed also targets the stromal compartment of the tumor and that this results in an increased efficacy of radiotherapy and Hh inhibition in two PCa xenograft models [19]. This was in line with other reports indicating that the tumor-associated stroma is also influenced by Hh inhibition and this might have an impact on the tumor cells [33,34]. Additionally, metformin has also been shown to influence the tumor microenvironment. A study by Martin et al. [35] has found that metformin induced vascular endothelial growth factor A (VEGF-A) expression in a BRAF-driven melanoma tumor model. This resulted in increased angiogenesis and accelerated tumor growth [35]. Although we also observed an enhanced tumor growth in the combination group, we did not observe any changes in microvessel density in our study.

This observation highlights the importance of testing drug interactions in an in vivo setting. The effect of drug interactions is often overlooked in preclinical studies, resulting in the failure of many novel medications in clinical trials. Therefore, more research into the interaction between Hh inhibition and metformin should be performed in multiple tumor models to guarantee the safety of Hh inhibition in diabetic patients using metformin.

4. Materials and Methods

4.1. Cell Culture and Drug Exposure

The androgen-unresponsive PCa cell lines PC3 and DU145 were obtained from the American Type Culture Collection (ATCC; Manassas, VA, USA). The PC3 cells were grown in minimal essential medium (MEM, Life Technologies, Carlsbad, CA, USA) supplemented with 10% fetal bovine serum (FBS; Life Technologies). The DU145 cells were cultured in MEM (Life Technologies) supplemented with 10% FBS, 1% sodium pyruvate (Life Technologies) and 1% non-essential amino acids (Life Technologies). The androgen-responsive 22Rv1 cells (European Collection of Cell Cultures, ECACC, Salisbury, UK) were cultured in RPMI 1640 medium without phenol red (Sigma-Aldrich, St. Louis, MA, USA), supplemented with 10% FBS, 1% L-glutamine and 1% 4-(2-hydroxyethyl)-1-piperazineethanesulfonic acid (HEPES) buffer (Life Technologies). All cells were maintained at 37 °C in a humidified incubator with 5% CO_2/95% O_2 atmosphere.

Stock solutions of metformin (Sigma-Aldrich) were prepared in sterile water or saline for in vitro and in vivo experiments, respectively. For in vitro experiments, stock solutions of GANT61 were prepared in dimethyl sulfoxide (DMSO; Adipogen, San Diego, CA, USA). For the in vivo experiment,

GANT61 (Tocris, Bristol, UK) was dissolved in 100% EtOH and was further dissolved in saline (9:1 saline:EtOH). Control conditions were treated with the corresponding drug solvent.

4.2. Cell Growth and Survival

Cells were seeded in a 96-well plate at a density of 2.5–45 × 10^4 cells per well and treated for 72 h with different concentrations of the inhibitors. Cell growth was assessed using the Incucyte Zoom system (Essen BioScience, Ann Arbor, MI, USA). Short-term survival assays were performed by pretreating the cells with GANT61 (10 μM) and metformin (5 mM) for 72 h followed by IR (2, 4, or 6 Gy). After 24 h, fresh medium was added and cell survival was assessed 7 days thereafter by means of sulforhodamine B (SRB) assay [36].

4.3. Quantitative Real-Time Polymerase Chain Reaction (qPCR)

RNA isolation and quantitative Polymerase Chain Reaction (qPCR) reactions were performed as previously described [19]. Primer sequences for glyceraldehyde 3-phosphate dehydrogenase (GAPDH), PTCH1, GLI1 and GLI2 are enlisted in Supplemental Table S1. Gene expression was calculated as expression per 100,000 copies of the household gene *GAPDH*.

4.4. Immunoblot Analysis

Immunoblotting was performed as done before [19]. Primary antibodies against ACC (#3662, 1:1000), phospho-acetyl-CoA carboxylase (pACC) (#3661, 1:500), AMPK (#2532, 1:1000), pAMPK (#2535, 1:500), GLI1 (#2534, 1:500) from Cell Signaling Technologies (Beverly, MA, USA), cyclin D1 (CCND1) (sc-8396, 1:200) and PTCH1 (sc-6149, 1:200) from Santa Cruz (Dallas, TX, USA) and GLI2 (600-401-845, 1:1000) from Rockland Immunochemicals (Limerick, PA, USA) were used. Β-actin (Cell Signaling Technologies, #4967, 1:1000) was used as loading control. An enhanced chemiluminescence detection system (Perkin Elmer, Waltham, MA, USA) was used to visualize immune-reactive proteins using Fujifilm LAS-3000 mini camera (Fujifilm, Germany). Protein expression was quantified using ImageJ 1.50.

4.5. Flow Cytometry

Apoptotic cell populations (AnnexinV$^+$/PI$^-$),DNA damage and cell cycle distribution were measured as previously described [19]. Reactive oxygen species (ROS) were detected using 2′,7′-dichlorodihydrofluorescein diacetate [37]. FACSVerse Flow cytometer (BD Biosciences, Franklin Lakes, NJ, USA) was used for flow cytometric analysis.

4.6. Colony Formation

Clonogenic formation assays were performed as previously described [19]. After 72-h drug treatment, cells were seeded at low density and irradiated with 2, 4 and 6 Gy using a Baltograph (Balteau NDT, Hermalle-sous-argenteau, Belgium) or mock irradiated. Fresh medium was added 16 h post-irradiation. After 11–21 days post-irradiation, cells were fixed with 2.5% glutaraldehyde in phosphate buffered saline (PBS) and stained with 0.4% crystal violet. The colonies containing ≥50 cells were counted with ColCount (Oxford Optronix, Oxford, UK). Survival fractions normalized for drug-induced toxicity. Dose-enhancement factor (DEF) was calculated as the ratio of the dose needed for the control cells to the dose needed for the treated cells to reach a survival fraction of 0.5 (DEF0.5).

4.7. Animal Experiments

Animal experiments were approved by the ethics committee of KU Leuven (P131/2014). Male NMRI Nu/Nu mice (Janvier, France) were inoculated in both flanks with 2 × 10^6 22Rv1 cells in 100:100 μL medium/Matrigel (VWR, Radnor, PA, USA). Once tumors reached a volume of 150 mm^3, mice were treated by intraperitoneal injection with solvent (9:1 saline/EtOH), metformin (250 mg/kg, every day), GANT61 (50 mg/kg every other day) or the combination of both drugs for 7 weeks. At day 5 of drug treatment, tumors were irradiated with a single dose of 6 Gy. During the entire treatment period, tumor growth was followed by 2-weekly caliper measurements and tumor volumes were calculated ($V = (\text{length} \times \text{width} \times \text{height}) \times \pi/6$). In addition, the body weight of the mice was monitored to assess potential treatment toxicity. Mice were euthanized at the end of drug treatment or when tumors reached the maximum ethically permitted volume of 2×10^3 mm^3. Thirty min before euthanasia, pimonidazole was intraperitoneally injected. Afterwards, tumors were excised and half of the tumor was fixed in formalin and embedded in paraffin for immunohistochemical analysis and the other half was snap-frozen for protein analysis.

4.8. Immunohistochemistry

Immunohistochemistry for Ki67, cleaved caspase3, pimonidazole, cluster of differentiation 31 (CD31), GLI1, GLI2 and PTCH1 was performed as previously described [19]. Protein expression was quantified using ImageJ.

4.9. Statistical Analysis

One-way ANOVA with Tukey's multiple comparison test or a two-tailed student's *t*-test were used for the in vitro experiments. For the in vivo experiment, a Kolmogorov–Smirnov method was used to test for normality. Thereafter, either a two-tailed student's *t*-test was used when the data were normally distributed with equal variance or nonparametric analysis using the Mann–Whitney rank-sum test in other conditions. All statistical tests were performed using the software package Statistica 12 (StatSoft Inc., Tulsa, OK, USA). A *p*-value of <0.05 was considered statistically significant.

Acknowledgments: Annelies Gonnissen and Sofie Isebaert were sponsored by a grant from the National Cancer Plan Action 29 Belgium (KPC_29_023). Karin Haustermans is a clinical research fellow of the Research Foundation Flanders.

Author Contributions: Annelies Gonnissen, Sofie Isebaert, Chad M. McKee, Ruth J. Muschel and Karin Haustermans conceived and designed the experiments; Annelies Gonnissen performed the experiments; Annelies Gonnissen and Sofie Isebaert analyzed the data; Karin Haustermans contributed reagents/materials/analysis tools; Annelies Gonnissen, Sofie Isebaert, Chad M. McKee, Ruth J. Muschel and Karin Haustermans wrote the paper.

Abbreviations

ACC	Acetyl-CoA carboxylase
AMP	Adenosine monophosphate
AMPK	AMP-activated protein kinase
CCND1	Cyclin D1
CD31	Cluster of differentiation 31
qPCR	Quantitative Polymerase Chain Reaction
DEF	Dose-enhancement factor
DMSO	Dimethyl sulfoxide
EBRT	External-beam radiotherapy
ECACC	European Collection of Cell Cultures
FBS	Fetal bovine serum
GANT61	GLI-ANTagonist 61
GAPDH	Glyceraldehyde 3-phosphate dehydrogenase
GLI	Glioma-associated oncogene homolog
HEPES	4-(2-hydroxyethyl)-1-piperazineethanesulfonic acid
Hh	Hedgehog

IC_{50}	Half maximal inhibitory concentration
IR	Ionizing radiation
LKB1	Liver kinase B1
MEM	Minimal essential medium
MF	Metformin
mTOR	Mammalian target of rapamycin
MVD	Microvessel density
OS	Overall survival
pACC	Phospho Acetyl-CoA carboxylase
pAMPK	Phospho AMP-activated protein kinase
PBS	Phosphate buffered saline
PI	Propidium iodide
PTCH1	Patched 1
PCa	Prostate cancer
ROS	Reactive oxygen species
SEM	Standard error of means
siRNA	Silencing RNA
SMO	Smoothened
VEGF-A	Vascular endothelial growth factor A

References

1. Noto, H.; Goto, A.; Tsujimoto, T.; Noda, M. Cancer risk in diabetic patients treated with metformin: A systematic review and meta-analysis. *PLoS ONE* **2012**, *7*, e33411. [CrossRef] [PubMed]
2. Pollak, M.N. Investigating metformin for cancer prevention and treatment: The end of the beginning. *Cancer Discov.* **2012**, *2*, 778–790. [CrossRef] [PubMed]
3. Del, B.S.; Vazquez-Martin, A.; Cufi, S.; Oliveras-Ferraros, C.; Bosch-Barrera, J.; Joven, J.; Martin-Castillo, B.; Menendez, J.A. Metformin: Multi-faceted protection against cancer. *Oncotarget* **2011**, *2*, 896–917.
4. Ben, S.I.; Laurent, K.; Loubat, A.; Giorgetti-Peraldi, S.; Colosetti, P.; Auberger, P.; Tanti, J.F.; Le Marchand-Brustel, Y.; Bost, F. The antidiabetic drug metformin exerts an antitumoral effect in vitro and in vivo through a decrease of cyclin D1 level. *Oncogene* **2008**, *27*, 3576–3586.
5. Kourelis, T.V.; Siegel, R.D. Metformin and cancer: New applications for an old drug. *Med. Oncol.* **2012**, *29*, 1314–1327. [CrossRef] [PubMed]
6. Dowling, R.J.; Zakikhani, M.; Fantus, I.G.; Pollak, M.; Sonenberg, N. Metformin inhibits mammalian target of rapamycin-dependent translation initiation in breast cancer cells. *Cancer Res.* **2007**, *67*, 10804–10812. [CrossRef] [PubMed]
7. Zakikhani, M.; Dowling, R.; Fantus, I.G.; Sonenberg, N.; Pollak, M. Metformin is an AMP kinase-dependent growth inhibitor for breast cancer cells. *Cancer Res.* **2006**, *66*, 10269–10273. [CrossRef] [PubMed]
8. Song, C.W.; Lee, H.; Dings, R.P.; Williams, B.; Powers, J.; Santos, T.D.; Choi, B.H.; Park, H.J. Metformin kills and radiosensitizes cancer cells and preferentially kills cancer stem cells. *Sci. Rep.* **2012**, *2*, 362. [CrossRef] [PubMed]
9. Zannella, V.E.; Dal, P.A.; Muaddi, H.; McKee, T.D.; Stapleton, S.; Sykes, J.; Glicksman, R.; Chaib, S.; Zamiara, P.; Milosevic, M.; et al. Reprogramming metabolism with metformin improves tumor oxygenation and radiotherapy response. *Clin. Cancer Res.* **2013**, *19*, 6741–6750. [CrossRef] [PubMed]
10. Storozhuk, Y.; Hopmans, S.N.; Sanli, T.; Barron, C.; Tsiani, E.; Cutz, J.C.; Pond, G.; Wright, J.; Singh, G.; Tsakiridis, T. Metformin inhibits growth and enhances radiation response of non-small cell lung cancer (NSCLC) through ATM and AMPK. *Br. J. Cancer* **2013**, *108*, 2021–2032. [CrossRef] [PubMed]
11. Zhang, T.; Zhang, L.; Zhang, T.; Fan, J.; Wu, K.; Guan, Z.; Wang, X.; Li, L.; Hsieh, J.T.; He, D.; et al. Metformin sensitizes prostate cancer cells to radiation through EGFR/p-DNA-PKCS in vitro and in vivo. *Radiat. Res.* **2014**, *181*, 641–649. [CrossRef] [PubMed]
12. Kim, E.H.; Kim, M.S.; Cho, C.K.; Jung, W.G.; Jeong, Y.K.; Jeong, J.H. Low and high linear energy transfer radiation sensitization of HCC cells by metformin. *J. Radiat. Res.* **2014**, *55*, 432–442. [CrossRef] [PubMed]

13. Fan, C.; Wang, Y.; Liu, Z.; Sun, Y.; Wang, X.; Wei, G.; Wei, J. Metformin exerts anticancer effects through the inhibition of the Sonic hedgehog signaling pathway in breast cancer. *Int. J. Mol. Med.* **2015**, *36*, 204–214. [CrossRef] [PubMed]
14. Nakamura, M.; Ogo, A.; Yamura, M.; Yamaguchi, Y.; Nakashima, H. Metformin suppresses sonic Hedgehog expression in pancreatic cancer cells. *Anticancer Res.* **2014**, *34*, 1765–1769. [PubMed]
15. Karhadkar, S.S.; Bova, G.S.; Abdallah, N.; Dhara, S.; Gardner, D.; Maitra, A.; Isaacs, J.T.; Berman, D.M.; Beachy, P.A. Hedgehog signalling in prostate regeneration, neoplasia and metastasis. *Nature* **2004**, *431*, 707–712. [CrossRef] [PubMed]
16. Gonnissen, A.; Isebaert, S.; Haustermans, K. Hedgehog signaling in prostate cancer and its therapeutic implication. *Int. J. Mol. Sci.* **2013**, *14*, 13979–14007. [CrossRef] [PubMed]
17. Teglund, S.; Toftgard, R. Hedgehog beyond medulloblastoma and basal cell carcinoma. *Biochim. Biophys. Acta* **2010**, *1805*, 181–208. [CrossRef] [PubMed]
18. Onishi, H.; Katano, M. Hedgehog signaling pathway as a therapeutic target in various types of cancer. *Cancer Sci.* **2011**, *102*, 1756–1760. [CrossRef] [PubMed]
19. Gonnissen, A.; Isebaert, S.; McKee, C.M.; Dok, R.; Haustermans, K.; Muschel, R.J. The hedgehog inhibitor GANT61 sensitizes prostate cancer cells to ionizing radiation both in vitro and in vivo. *Oncotarget* **2016**, *7*, 84286–84298. [CrossRef] [PubMed]
20. Kaushik, D.; Karnes, R.J.; Eisenberg, M.S.; Rangel, L.J.; Carlson, R.E.; Bergstralh, E.J. Effect of metformin on prostate cancer outcomes after radical prostatectomy. *Urol. Oncol.* **2014**, *32*, 43–47. [CrossRef] [PubMed]
21. Patel, T.; Hruby, G.; Badani, K.; Abate-Shen, C.; McKiernan, J.M. Clinical outcomes after radical prostatectomy in diabetic patients treated with metformin. *Urology* **2010**, *76*, 1240–1244. [CrossRef] [PubMed]
22. Rieken, M.; Kluth, L.A.; Xylinas, E.; Fajkovic, H.; Becker, A.; Karakiewicz, P.I.; Herman, M.; Lotan, Y.; Seitz, C.; Schramek, P.; et al. Association of diabetes mellitus and metformin use with biochemical recurrence in patients treated with radical prostatectomy for prostate cancer. *World J. Urol.* **2014**, *32*, 999–1005. [CrossRef] [PubMed]
23. Allott, E.H.; Abern, M.R.; Gerber, L.; Keto, C.J.; Aronson, W.J.; Terris, M.K.; Kane, C.J.; Amling, C.L.; Cooperberg, M.R.; Moorman, P.G.; et al. Metformin does not affect risk of biochemical recurrence following radical prostatectomy: Results from the SEARCH database. *Prostate Cancer Prostatic Dis.* **2013**, *16*, 391–397. [CrossRef] [PubMed]
24. He, X.X.; Tu, S.M.; Lee, M.H.; Yeung, S.C. Thiazolidinediones and metformin associated with improved survival of diabetic prostate cancer patients. *Ann. Oncol.* **2011**, *22*, 2640–2645. [CrossRef] [PubMed]
25. Spratt, D.E.; Zhang, C.; Zumsteg, Z.S.; Pei, X.; Zhang, Z.; Zelefsky, M.J. Metformin and prostate cancer: Reduced development of castration-resistant disease and prostate cancer mortality. *Eur. Urol.* **2013**, *63*, 709–716. [CrossRef] [PubMed]
26. Liu, J.; Li, M.; Song, B.; Jia, C.; Zhang, L.; Bai, X.; Hu, W. Metformin inhibits renal cell carcinoma in vitro and in vivo xenograft. *Urol. Oncol.* **2013**, *31*, 264–270. [CrossRef] [PubMed]
27. Zhang, T.; Guo, P.; Zhang, Y.; Xiong, H.; Yu, X.; Xu, S.; Wang, X.; He, D.; Jin, X. The antidiabetic drug metformin inhibits the proliferation of bladder cancer cells in vitro and in vivo. *Int. J. Mol. Sci.* **2013**, *14*, 24603–24618. [CrossRef] [PubMed]
28. Koritzinsky, M. Metformin: A Novel Biological Modifier of Tumor Response to Radiation Therapy. *Int. J. Radiat. Oncol. Biol. Phys.* **2015**, *93*, 454–464. [CrossRef] [PubMed]
29. Li, Y.H.; Luo, J.; Mosley, Y.Y.; Hedrick, V.E.; Paul, L.N.; Chang, J.; Zhang, G.; Wang, Y.K.; Banko, M.R.; Brunet, A.; et al. AMP-Activated Protein Kinase Directly Phosphorylates and Destabilizes Hedgehog Pathway Transcription Factor GLI1 in Medulloblastoma. *Cell Rep.* **2015**, *12*, 599–609. [CrossRef] [PubMed]
30. Di, M.L.; Basile, A.; Coni, S.; Manni, S.; Sdruscia, G.; D'Amico, D.; Antonucci, L.; Infante, P.; De, S.E.; Cucchi, D.; et al. The energy sensor AMPK regulates Hedgehog signaling in human cells through a unique Gli1 metabolic checkpoint. *Oncotarget* **2016**, *7*, 9538–9549.
31. Sharma, V.; McNeill, J.H. To scale or not to scale: The principles of dose extrapolation. *Br. J. Pharmacol.* **2009**, *157*, 907–921. [CrossRef] [PubMed]
32. Suzman, D.L.; Antonarakis, E.S. Clinical Implications of Hedgehog Pathway Signaling in Prostate Cancer. *Cancers* **2015**, *7*, 1983–1993. [CrossRef] [PubMed]

33. Zeng, J.; Aziz, K.; Chettiar, S.T.; Aftab, B.T.; Armour, M.; Gajula, R.; Gandhi, N.; Salih, T.; Herman, J.M.; Wong, J.; et al. Hedgehog Pathway Inhibition Radiosensitizes Non-Small Cell Lung Cancers. *Int. J. Radiat. Oncol. Biol. Phys.* **2013**, *86*, 143–149. [CrossRef] [PubMed]
34. Karlou, M.; Lu, J.F.; Wu, G.; Maity, S.; Tzelepi, V.; Navone, N.M.; Hoang, A.; Logothetis, C.J.; Efstathiou, E. Hedgehog signaling inhibition by the small molecule smoothened inhibitor GDC-0449 in the bone forming prostate cancer xenograft MDA PCa 118b. *Prostate* **2012**, *72*, 1638–1647. [CrossRef] [PubMed]
35. Martin, M.J.; Hayward, R.; Viros, A.; Marais, R. Metformin accelerates the growth of BRAF V600E-driven melanoma by upregulating VEGF-A. *Cancer Discov.* **2012**, *2*, 344–355. [CrossRef] [PubMed]
36. De, S.H.; Kimpe, M.; Isebaert, S.; Nuyts, S. A systematic assessment of radiation dose enhancement by 5-Aza-2′-deoxycytidine and histone deacetylase inhibitors in head-and-neck squamous cell carcinoma. *Int. J. Radiat. Oncol. Biol. Phys.* **2009**, *73*, 904–912.
37. Isebaert, S.F.; Swinnen, J.V.; McBride, W.H.; Begg, A.C.; Haustermans, K.M. 5-aminoimidazole-4-carboxamide riboside enhances effect of ionizing radiation in PC3 prostate cancer cells. *Int. J. Radiat. Oncol. Biol. Phys.* **2011**, *81*, 1515–1523. [CrossRef] [PubMed]

14

Does the Prostate Health Index Depend on Tumor Volume?—A Study on 196 Patients after Radical Prostatectomy

Frank Friedersdorff [1,*], Britt Groß [1], Andreas Maxeiner [1], Klaus Jung [1,2], Kurt Miller [1], Carsten Stephan [1,2], Jonas Busch [1,†] and Ergin Kilic [3,†]

1 Department of Urology, Charité University Hospital, 10098 Berlin, Germany; grossbritt@yahoo.de (B.G.); andres.maxeiner@charite.de (A.M.); klaus.jung@charite.de (K.J.); kurt.miller@charite.de (K.M.); carsten.stephan@charite.de (C.S.); Jonas.busch@charite.de (J.B.)

2 Berlin Institute for Urologic Research, 10115 Berlin, Germany

3 Department of Pathology, Charité University Hospital, 10098 Berlin, Germany; ergin.kilic@charite.de

* Correspondence: frank.friedersdorff@charite.de

† These authors contributed equally to this work.

Academic Editors: Jack A. Schalken and William Chi-shing Cho

Abstract: The Prostate Health Index (PHI) has been used increasingly in the context of prostate cancer (PCa) diagnostics since 2010. Previous studies have shown an association between PHI and a tumor volume of >0.5 cm^3. The aim of this study was to investigate the correlation between PHI and tumor volume as well as the Gleason score. A total of 196 selected patients with prostate cancer treated with radical prostatectomy at our institution were included in our study. The tumor volume was calculated and preoperative serum parameters total prostate-specific antigen (tPSA), free PSA (fPSA), [−2]proPSA, and PHI were evaluated. The association between the pathological findings such as Gleason score, pathological T-stage (pT stage), and tumor volume were evaluated. We further used logistic regression and Cox proportional hazard regression analyses for assessing the association between tumor volume and PHI and for predicting biochemical recurrence. With an area under the curve (AUC) of 0.79, PHI is the most accurate predictor of a tumor volumes >0.5 cm^3. Moreover, PHI correlates significantly with the tumor volume (r = 0.588), which is significantly different (p = 0.008) from the correlation of the Gleason score with tumor volume (r = 0.385). PHI correlates more strongly with the tumor volume than does the Gleason score. Using PHI improves the prediction of larger tumor volume and subsequently clinically significant cancer.

Keywords: prostate cancer; Prostate Health Index; tumor volume

---

1. Introduction

Prostate cancer (PCa) is still one of the most frequent illnesses in men. Since the introduction of screening with prostate-specific antigen (PSA) in the early 1990s, the incidence of PCa has risen sharply, though the age at first diagnosis has been shifting toward younger patients with less advanced stages of PCa [1]. The number of deaths from PCa has been reduced in recent years, though not proportionally with the rise in incidence.

The degree of tumor expansion is the most important factor for both PCa prognosis and therapy [2]. The PCa tumor volume has a substantial influence on the course of the illness. Growth exceeding the capsule and lymph node metastases occurs mainly with larger tumors [3–5]. There is an approximately proportional relationship between the tumor volume and the stage of differentiation. Tumors that are smaller than 0.5 cm^3 are classified as "insignificant", since the tumor grows so slowly that there is a high probability that it will never reach a significant size before the death of the patient [6]. The probability of the existence of a tumor larger than 0.5 cm^3 can be calculated, for example, with a nomogram [7].

The Prostate Health Index (PHI) is currently one of the most promising new markers of PCa. Initial studies have shown that PHI preferentially detects aggressive carcinomas and, due to its high specificity, can reduce the number of unnecessarily performed biopsies [8,9]. Furthermore, tumors larger than 0.5 cm^3 have significantly higher PHI values than tumors with smaller volumes [10–12]. However, it is still not known whether PHI correlates continuously with tumor volume. A marker that is able to reliably predict the tumor volume would be advantageous for therapeutic decision-making. PHI and [−2]proPSA are currently the best available serum parameters for PCa detection [9]. At 90% sensitivity, the specificity of PHI for PCa detection is on average 31.6% [9]. The use of PHI in the framework of PCa screening reduces the use of biopsies by 15%–41%, in comparison to classic screening with only total prostate-specific antigen (tPSA) measurement [8,13]. Moreover, there is an association between PHI and carcinomas with unfavorable prognostic characteristics [12,14].

The use of PHI appears quite promising in patients with diagnosed PCa who are following an active surveillance strategy. Approximately 30%–37% of these tumors advance to stages requiring intervention [15,16]. With a PHI score >43, there is a 3.6 times higher risk for disease progression, according to a study by Hirama et al. [15]. Carcinomas with an elevated tendency for deterioration can be identified earlier this way and subjected to a definitive therapy. Overall, the integration of PHI into active surveillance appears to be also economically useful. The increased expenditures from this additional blood test would be outweighed since the reduction of unnecessary biopsies, doctor visits, and laboratory tests would reduce the costs in comparison to examinations based only on tPSA [17,18].

The aim of the present study was to determine if there is a continuous correlation between PHI and tumor volume over the entire range of values commonly seen.

2. Results

2.1. Clinicopathological Characteristics of the Study Cohort

All clinicopathological characteristics are summarized in Table 1. One-third of the patients ($n = 65$) had a well-differentiated tumor (Gleason < 7). A total of 131 patients had a poorly differentiated tumor (Gleason ≥ 7). Within this group, a Gleason 7 tumor was found in 57.6% of the patients and 9.7% of the patients had a Gleason 8 or 9, Table 1). About 80% of the patients had a locally confined tumor (pT $\leq$ 2c). An "insignificant" carcinoma ($\leq$0.5 cm^3, range 0.03 to 0.48 cm^3) was found in 39 specimens (20%) and a "significant" tumor (>0.5 cm^3, range 0.57 to 22.8 cm^3) in 157 cases (80%).

Table 1. Clinicopathological data (median and range) of the study cohort.

Variable	Median (Range)	Mean ± S.D.
Age (years)	71 (49–85)	70 ± 7
Prostate volume (cm^3)	36.7 (9.2–264)	42.9 ± 27.1
Tumor volume (cm^3)	1.57 (0.03–22.8)	2.76 ± 3.47
Percentage of tumor volume	4.3 (0.02–80.4)	7.8 ± 10.6
	Number (Percent)	
Pathological tumor stage		
≤2c	154 (78.6)	
3a	29 (14.8)	
3b	11 (5.6)	
4	2 (1.0)	
Gleason Score		
<7	65 (33.2)	
7a (3 + 4)	77 (39.2)	
7b (4 + 3)	36 (18.4)	
≥8	18 (9.2)	
Resection margin status		
R0	143 (73.0)	
R1	50 (25.5)	
Rx	3 (1.5)	

2.2. PSA Parameters in Relation to Clinicopathololological Factors and Tumor Volume

In Table 2, the data of all four PSA derivatives and the prostate and tumor volumes are compiled in relation to the pathological Gleason score (well and poorly differentiated tumors) and the pathological stage (locally limited and advanced tumors). While percent free PSA (%fPSA) did not differ between the two tumor staging groups nor prostate volume both between the Gleason and staging groups, all other parameters were significantly different. The highest significance levela of $p < 0.0001$ were reached for the tumor volume and the percentage of tumor as well as for [−2]proPSA and PHI. In addition, Table 3 shows that all four serum parameters had significantly higher (tPSA, [−2]proPSA, PHI) or lower (%fPSA) values in patients with tumor volumes larger than 0.5 cm^3, the so-called significant tumors. Additional details are summarized in the Supplementary Table S1.

Table 2. Prostate volume, tumor volume, and prostate-specific antigen (PSA) analytes (median and range) in dependence on Gleason score and pathological tumor stage.

Variable	All Patients	Gleason Score <7 ≥7		*p*-Value	pT Stage ≤2c ≥3		*p*-Value
	(*n* = 196)	(*n* = 65)	(*n* = 131)		(*n* = 154)	(*n* = 42)	
Prostate volume (cm^3)	36.7 (9.2–264)	36.8 (17.6–167)	36.1 (9.2–264)	0.568	35.3 (14.7–167)	39.8 (9.2–264)	0.295
Tumor volume (cm^3)	1.58 (0.03–22.8)	0.66 (0.03–10.9)	2.26 (0.04–22.8)	<0.0001	1.21 (0.03–18.6)	4.36 (0.87–22.8)	<0.0001
Percentage of tumor (%)	4.3 (0.02–80.4)	1.4 (0.02–40.3)	6.6 (0.1–80.4)	<0.0001	3.1 (0.02–50.0)	10.0 (3.1–80.4)	<0.0001
tPSA (ng/mL)	5.0 (0.7–61.6)	4.2 (0.7–17.7)	5.4 (0.7–61.6)	<0.001	4.6 (0.7–61.6)	5.6 (1.8–32.6)	0.005
%fPSA (%)	12.3 (4.0–76.6)	14.4 (4.9–36.9)	11.3 (4.0–76.6)	<0.001	12.7 (4.0–76.6)	11.5 (4.9–28.2)	0.154
[−2]proPSA (pg/mL)	12.3 (2.3–117)	10.0 (2.3–46.7)	14.2 (3.2–117)	<0.0001	11.7 (2.3–117)	17.4 (3.7–58.2)	0.0005
Prostate Health Index (PHI)	47.6 (9.3–228)	37.5 (10.5–102)	55.3 (9.3–228)	<0.0001	43.4 (9.3–211)	67.1 (22.3–228)	<0.0001

Statistical significances were calculated using the Mann–Whitney *U*-test.

Table 3. PSA parameters (medians and ranges) in dependence on the tumor volume.

Variable	Tumor Volume		*p*-Value
	≤0.5 cm^3 (*n* = 39)	>0.5 cm^3 (*n* = 157)	
tPSA (ng/mL)	2.8 (0.7–10.8)	5.4 (0.7–61.6)	<0.0001
%fPSA	15.8 (6.0–35.0)	11.7 (4.0–76.6)	0.0006
[−2]proPSA (pg/mL)	9.4 (2.3–32.0)	13.6 (3.2–117)	<0.0001
PHI	32.9 (16.1–66.4)	53.7 (9.3–228)	<0.0001

Statistical significance calculated using the Mann–Whitney *U*-test.

The further associations between the clinicopathological variables and the PSA analytes were examined using correlation calculations and receiver-operating characteristi (ROC) curve analyses. Table 4 shows the correlations between the serum PSA parameters and the clinicopathological variables. PHI showed a significantly higher correlation to tumor volume than Gleason score (0.588 vs. 0.385; $p = 0.008$). Moreover, [−2]proPSA showed a significantly higher correlation with tumor volume than Gleason score (0.659 vs. 0.385, $p = 0.0002$). Interestingly, [−2]proPSA correlated significantly more with tumor volume than pT stage (0.659 vs. 0.522; $p = 0.037$). The correlation comparison between PHI and [−2]proPSA showed no difference ($p = 0.25$). PHI correlated significantly better with tumor volume than PSA (0.588 vs. 0.363; $p = 0.004$). The scatter plots of the PHI values in relation to the tumor volume as well as to the Gleason score categories and pT classifications are displayed in Figure 1A–C.

The areas under the ROC curves (AUCs) of the individual serum parameters are presented in Table 5. At 0.79, PHI reaches the greatest AUC value in differentiating tumor volumes ≤0.5 cm^3 from those >0.5 cm^3. In general, PHI is the best parameter to predict aggressive PCa with Gleason score (GS) ≥ 7 and locally advanced stages with ≥pT3a. Furthermore, PHI reached a significantly higher AUC than that of the pT stage in predicting a tumor volume of >0.5 cm^3 (0.79 vs. 0.69; $p = 0.04$). Thus, to show the mutual influence and interdependence between all these variables, we performed a logistic regression analysis as a multivariable approach. For that purpose, the categorized Gleason score and pT stage in combination with PHI were analyzed to differentiate between the two tumor volume categories. All three variables showed a significant odds ratio (Gleason score: 6.61 with a 95% confidence interval of 2.72 to 16.1), *p*-value < 0.001; pT stage: (1.60 (1.01–2.55), *p* = 0.047; PHI: 1.04 (1.02–1.07, *p* = 0.002)). This combination distinctly increased the AUC value to 0.87 (0.82–0.91) indicating the improved prediction between the insignificant and significant tumor volume.

Table 4. Pearson correlation of the serum parameters and the pathology findings.

Parameter	Tumor Volume (cm^3)	Tumor (%)	Gleason Score (≤6, 7a, 7b, ≥8)	pT Stage (≤2c, 3a, 3b, 4)
tPSA	0.363 (<0.0001)	0.287 (<0.0001)	0.153 (0.032)	0.237 (0.0008)
%fPSA	−0.101 (0.158)	−0.145 (0.043)	−0.157 (0.028)	−0.071 (0.324)
[−2]proPSA	0.659 (<0.0001)	0.389 (<0.0001)	0.246 (0.0005)	0.344 (<0.0001)
PHI	0.588 (<0.0001)	0.478 (<0.0001)	0.309 (<0.0001)	0.317 (<0.0001)
Gleason Score	0.385 (<0.0001)	0.373 (<0.0001)	-	0.397 (<0.0001)
pT Stage	0.522 (<0.0001)	0.486 (<0.0001)	0.397 (<0.0001)	-

The table presents the *r* values, with the *p*-values in parentheses.

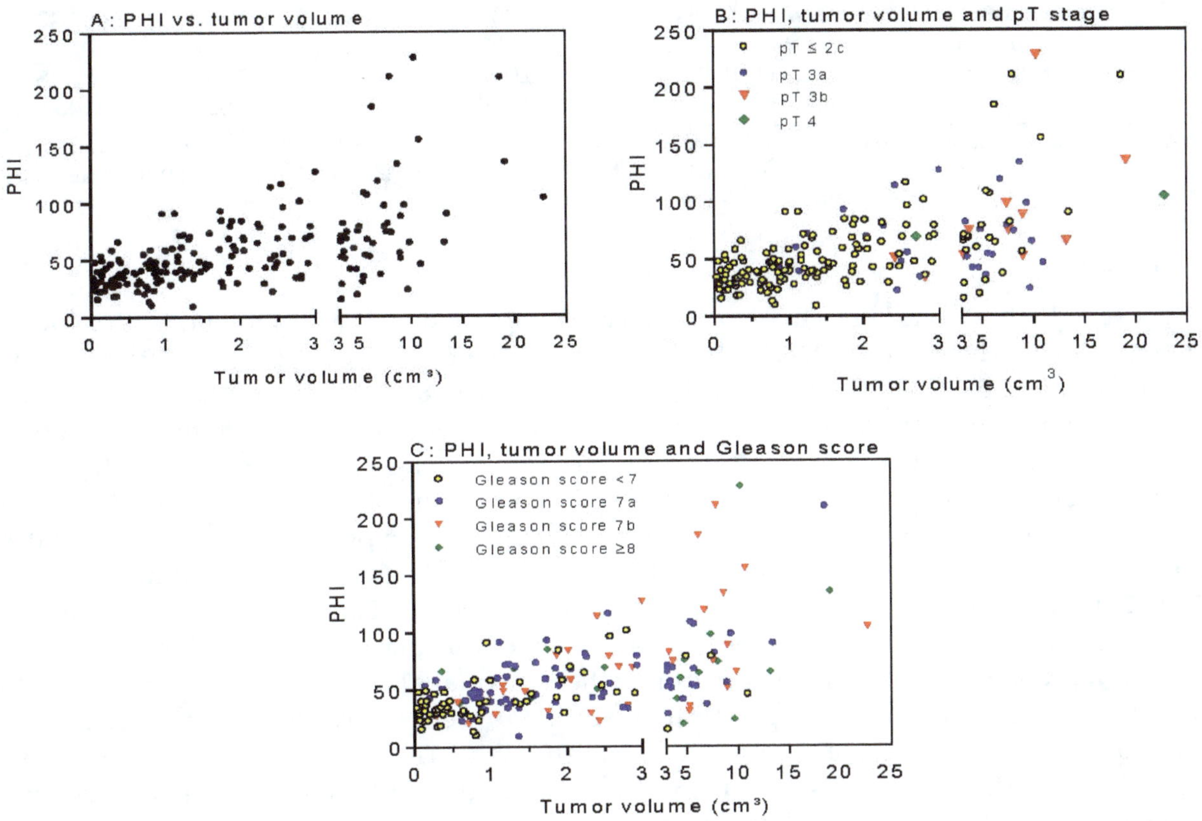

Figure 1. PHI values in relation to tumor volume, pT stage and Gleason score as indicated in (**A**–**C**).

Table 5. Calculated areas under the receiver operating characteristic (ROC) curves of the serum parameters (left column) to predict tumors with particular characteristics (top row). The 95% confidence intervals of the area under the curves (AUCs) are given in parentheses.

Parameter	Gleason Score ≥ 7 vs. <7	pT Stage ≥3a vs. ≤2c	Tumor Volume >0.5 vs. ≤0.5 cm^3
tPSA	0.64 (0.56–0.73)	0.64 (0.55–0.73)	0.74 (0.65–0.83)
%fPSA	0.64 (0.56–0.72)	0.57 (0.48–0.67)	0.68 (0.58–0.77)
[−2]proPSA	0.66 (0.59–0.74)	0.68 (0.58–0.77)	0.72 (0.64–0.81)
PHI	0.72 (0.65–0.80)	0.70 (0.62–80.0)	0.79 (0.72–0.86)

2.3. PHI and Tumor Volume as Independent Predictors of Biochemical Relapse

To evaluate the relationships between the conventional clinicopathological variables (Gleason score, pathological tumor stage, resection status) and age, tumor value, and PHI as predictors of the biochemical recurrence, we performed Cox regression analyses (Table 6). Both tumor volume and PHI were statistically significant predictors of a biochemical recurrence (follow-up time: 37 months (95% confidence interval 31 to 44)) in the univariate Cox regression model but also remained, despite the limited number of patients and events ($n = 25$) and the independent factors in the multivariable model ($p = 0.048$ and 0.0009).

Table 6. Cox proportional hazard regression analyses of tumor volume and PHI in relation to conventional clinicopathological variables for predicting biochemical recurrence after radical prostatectomy.

Variable [a]	Univariable Analysis		Multivariable Analysis [b]	
	Hazard Ratio (95% CI [c])	*p*-Value	Hazard Ratio (95% CI)	*p*-Value
Age (continuous)	1.05 (0.98–1.12)	0.159	not included	
pT stage	4.27 (1.91–9.56)	0.0004	3.92 (1.60–9.56)	0.003
Gleason Score	1.97 (1.22–3.18)	0.006	1.91 (1.01–3.57)	0.042
Margin resection status	3.34 (1.52–7.35)	0.003	1.65 (0.67–4.01)	0.273
Tumor volume	1.12 (1.01–1.24)	0.047	0.83 (0.68–0.99)	0.048
PHI	1.02 (1.01–1.03)	<0.0001	1.02 (1.01–1.03)	0.0009

[a] Age and tumor volume were used with their continuous values, the pathological factors as categorized data as indicated in the previous tables; [b] The multivariable analysis included all variables with *p*-values < 0.10 obtained in the univariable analysis; [c] CI = confidence interval.

3. Discussion

The use of PHI as a marker with high specificity for aggressive PCa and tumors with a low grade of differentiation has been proven [10,11,19]. In the present study, PHI correlates significantly with the tumor volume ($r = 0.588$). This is significantly stronger ($p = 0.008$) than the correlation of the Gleason score with tumor volume ($r = 0.385$). The hypothesis was supported by the significantly higher PHI value for tumor volumes >0.5 cm^3 [10–12,14]. Furthermore, it seems plausible that the PHI values rise with increasing carcinoma volumes, since there is a proven relationship between tumor size and tumor differentiation [4,5,12,20]. Previous studies have shown that PHI can predict a tumor volume >0.5 cm^3 even more precisely (AUC: 0.72–0.94) than Gleason score $\geq$7 (AUC: 0.64–0.74) or a pT-stage $\geq$ 3a (AUC: 0.72–0.85) [10,11,14,21,22]. The strong correlation between PHI and tumor volume found in this study describes a further partial aspect of the association of this marker with aggressive carcinomas.

PHI as a preoperative parameter shows significant explanatory power to predict a significant tumor volume in the prostatectomy preparation. In the present study, PHI reached a test strength (AUC) of 0.79 in the detection of clinical significant tumors. The portion of substantial tumors in our analysis was 80%. Comparable results for the test strength of PHI were reported in the work by Guazzoni et al. [11]. In 350 preparations, PHI detected tumors >0.5 cm^3 with an AUC of 0.8. In that study, the portion of substantial tumors was 93%. Somewhat lower AUC values were found in the work from Tallon et al. [21]. In the framework of that study, 154 prostate preparations were examined. A volume >0.5 cm^3 was found in 88% of the study participants. The calculated AUC value of PHI for the detection of substantial tumors was 0.72. In that study and in the present study, T3 tumors were included. In a study by Ferro et al., the AUC of PHI for the detection of substantial tumors was 0.94 [10]. The more advantageous results of that study might be explainable by the different composition of their study sample. On the one hand, that study limited itself to locally limited tumors (T1–T2); on the other hand, a comparatively smaller portion of the carcinomas (17%) had a substantial size ($\geq$0.5 cm^3). In the most recent study on 135 Asian patients by Chiu et al. [12], PHI reached a comparable high AUC of 0.82 to predict a tumor volume of >0.5 cm^3, but only about half (52.3%) of all patients had a tumor volume >0.5 cm^3. Since the portion of significant tumor volumes was

80% in our present study, comparability seems to be given more with the studies by Guazzoni et al. and Tallon et al. [11,21]. Furthermore, there is an association between the serum marker PHI and the pathological Gleason score. In our present study, PHI was the best parameter to detect tumors with a Gleason score $\geq$7 (AUC: 0.72) while the other parameters tPSA, %fPSA, and [−2]proPSA showed comparatively smaller AUCs of 0.64, 0.64, and 0.66, respectively. In other studies, the calculated AUC of PHI for the detection of tumors with a Gleason score $\geq$7 was between 0.67 and 0.74 [11,19,22]. In the work by Ferro et al. [10], an exceptionally high-test strength (AUC: 0.83) of PHI was found for the detection of tumors with a Gleason score $\geq$7. In addition, in this case, the clearly advantageous results from the research group of Ferro et al. [10] might be due to a different composition of the study group. Chiu et al. [12] provided only data for prediction of pathological Gleason score $\geq$7 or pathological pT3 stage and reached an AUC of exactly 0.8.

The relationship between PHI and biopsy Gleason score has already been investigated in numerous studies. According to a meta-analysis from 2014, PHI detects carcinomas with a Gleason $\geq$7 with an AUC of 0.90 [19]. That value is clearly above the calculated test strength of the present study for the detection of low differentiated tumors (AUC: 0.72). One possible source of such a large difference in results is that the biopsy Gleason score and the pathological Gleason score differ in many cases. The tissue samples of the core needle biopsy harbor a comparatively higher risk to incorrectly evaluate the Gleason grade more favorably than it actually is, since this technique of examination is inherently not capable of imaging the entire PCa. Since the Gleason score can differ according to the methods chosen, that meta-analysis is only conditionally comparable with the present study. Moreover, the processing of a prostatectomy preparation is the more precise method to characterize a PCa and, thus, to estimate the relation of Gleason score and PHI.

There is an association between PHI and the extensiveness of the local tumor. In the present study, PHI detected tumors with growth exceeding the capsule with an AUC of 0.70. The AUCs of other parameters were lower (tPSA: 0.64, %fPSA: 0.57, [−2]proPSA: 0.68). In other studies, the AUC for the detection of T3 tumors was reported as 0.69–0.72 [11,20], which is comparable to our study. In the study by Ferro et al. [10], PHI detected tumors exceeding the capsule with an AUC of 0.85.

In the present study, it is apparent that PHI shows the highest AUCs for the prediction of the tumor characteristics (0.79 for tumor volume, 0.72 for Gleason score $\geq$7, 0.70 for pT $\leq$ 3a). In other studies, it has been shown that PHI predicts the tumor volume more precisely than the Gleason score of the T-stage does [10–12,14,21]. Consequently, it can be assumed that the levels of PSA, fPSA, and [−2]proPSA (the components of the PHI) are influenced not only by the cell differentiation but likewise by the amount of carcinoma cells (tumor volume). According to the results of this study, it is conceivable that the tumor volume is the strongest determining factor. This is also supported by the high Pearson's correlation factors of 0.588 and 0.478 for PHI with the tumor volume and the percentage of tumor, respectively. The correlation of PHI with the Gleason score (r = 0.309) and pT stage (r = 0.317) is weaker in our cohort. All these correlation data were unfortunately not provided by all previous studies. Furthermore, tumor volume (borderline significance with p = 0.048) and PHI (p = 0.0009) remained as independent factors in multivariable analysis to predict a biochemical recurrence (Table 6) beside the known pathological data pT stage and Gleason score. For example, the resection margin status could not reach significance (p = 0.27) in this Cox proportional hazard regression model, which emphasizes the importance of tumor volume and PHI.

The tumor volume is an important predictor of the further disease course and, correspondingly, should be kept in mind in planning therapy including focal therapy. Our method very precisely estimates tumor volume and has not been described before. Other earlier studies do not focus on methodological aspects. In the present work, the median tumor volume was 1.58 cm^3, and the median PHI was 47.6. The results of this work show that a high PHI value is most likely connected with a large tumor volume, which could be a contraindication for a therapy approach of active surveillance. The integration of PHI into active surveillance could reduce the frequency of biopsies. Larger intervals between follow-up biopsies would be a clear advantage for the patient. Nevertheless, large-scale studies about this are needed in order to rule out the possibility that a lower frequency of biopsies in combination with regular PHI determinations leads to a worse outcome for the patient. The use of PHI in the preparation of a prostatectomy is likewise conceivable. High PHI values indicate a large tumor volume, which in turn makes the possibility of performing a nerve-sparing operation more improbable. Correspondingly, it could be advantageous to advise the patient of this aspect before operating. Future studies might be able to answer the question of whether there is a PHI limit value, above which a nerve-sparing operation becomes very improbable. This could lead to a more transparent risk prognosis before surgery.

The serum markers PHI and [−2]proPSA are accurate predictors of the tumor volume in prostatectomy preparations. Further, it was shown in the AUC analysis that PHI shows a stronger association to tumor volume than the established predictive parameters of the Gleason score and T-stage. It is important to integrate PHI into active surveillance of PCa patients, since an estimate of the tumor volume, as an important predictor of the illness progression, could support an adequate therapy decision.

4. Materials and Methods

4.1. Study Population

The study was approved by the Charité Ethics Committee. All patients provided written informed consent for this research study. Preoperative serum samples (tPSA, free PSA (fPSA), [−2]proPSA) were collected from 460 men who underwent radical prostatectomy between 2001 and 2014. The surgical approach was retroperitoneal, laparoscopic, or da Vinci based. The exclusion criteria were incomplete (n = 233) or missing pathological sections (n = 24), lack of appropriate serum samples (n = 2), or use of neoadjuvant therapies (n = 5) so that finally 196 patients were included in the analysis.

The study groups (Table 1) were defined as follows: carcinomas with a pathological GS of 4–6 were assembled into the GS < 7 group (well differentiated, n = 65) and carcinomas with a GS of 7–10 (n = 131) were assembled into the GS ≥ 7 group (poorly differentiated). The stage "locally limited" (n = 154) included tumors with pathological T-stage (pT stage) 2a, 2b, and 2c. The stage "locally advanced" included tumors in the pT-stages 3a, 3b, and 4 (n = 42). The volume of the tumors was divided into two categories: "insignificant" (≤0.5 cm^3, n = 39) and "significant" (>0.5 cm^3, n = 157) according to the Epstein criteria [23].

The prognostic potential of the tumor volume in relation to the other clinicopathological parameters including PHI was assessed to predict tumor recurrence after radical prostatectomy. The conventional criterion of biochemical recurrence of increased PSA after surgery was used. Biochemical recurrence was defined as the first postoperative PSA value of >0.1 ng/mL following a nadir PSA level after surgery and confirmed by persistent increased PSA values >0.1 ng/mL. The interval between radical prostatectomy and biochemical recurrence was calculated in months as time to the development of this event, while patients without biochemical recurrence were censored at the last follow-up visit.

4.2. Pathology Assessment

After the macroscopic assessment, the preparations were weighed and measured in three planes (apico-basal, horizontal, ventro-dorsal). The prostates were sliced first medially along the urethra and then the apex and base were cut off. Both mid-pieces, the apex, and the base were each divided into approximately 5 mm thick tissue blocks and then embedded in paraffin. The entire paraffin blocks were sliced by machine into 2–4 μm thin sections and then mounted onto specimen slides. They were then stained with hematoxyline and eosin (H&E). The prostatectomy preparations of this study had a mean (range) of 28 (10–63) sections; in total, over 5500 H&E sections were examined microscopically.

4.3. Serological Diagnosis and Volumetric Analysis

The preoperative determination of serum tPSA, fPSA, and [−2]proPSA was performed on the fully automated immunoassay device Access® (Beckman Coulter, Brea, CA, USA) as described before [24]. PHI was calculated according to the equation $[-2]\text{proPSA}/\text{fPSA} \times \sqrt{\text{PSA}}$.

All tissue sections were examined under a microscope, and carcinomas were outlined in color. The appraisal of the preparation was performed together with an experienced pathologist (EK).

As Figure 2 illustrates, carcinomas were surrounded with a hand-drawn line. The surfaces of the prostate and the surface of the tumor on the H&E sections were identified by means of a gridwork screen (3 mm × 3 mm). The gridwork screen was placed on the slides, and the surfaces were enumerated. The boxes were evaluated as "1", "0.5", and "0" when they were covered with clearly more than 50%, approximately with 50%, or clearly less than 50% by tumor, respectively. For each H&E section, the number of boxes for prostate and for cancer were recorded separately. Periprostatic soft tissue and intraprostatic parts of the seminal vesicle were excluded from the evaluation. The volume of the prostate was calculated with the aid of the ellipsis formula ($\pi/6 \times$ height $\times$ width $\times$ depth). The percentage portion of the carcinoma was calculated as follows: %tumor = (total number of tumor boxes/total number of prostate boxes) × 100. The tumor volume was then calculated with the following formula: tumor volume = (%tumor × prostate volume)/100.

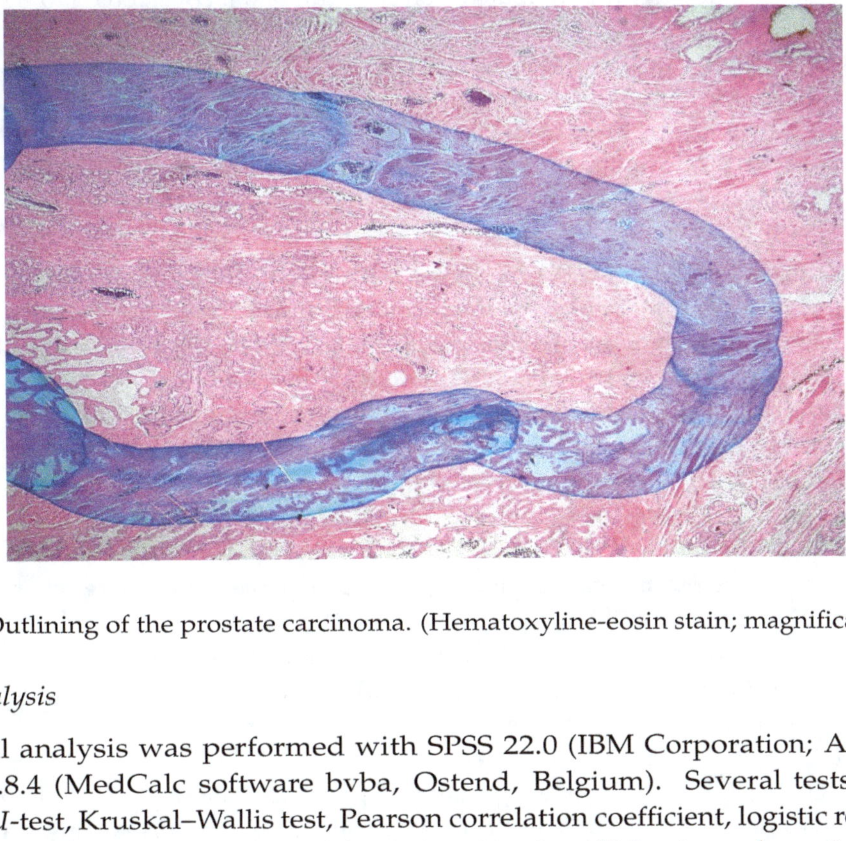

Figure 2. Outlining of the prostate carcinoma. (Hematoxyline-eosin stain; magnification: 20×).

4.4. Statistical Analysis

All statistical analysis was performed with SPSS 22.0 (IBM Corporation; Armonk, NY, USA) and MedCalc 16.8.4 (MedCalc software bvba, Ostend, Belgium). Several tests were performed (Mann–Whitney *U*-test, Kruskal–Wallis test, Pearson correlation coefficient, logistic regression, and Cox hazard regression). ROC analysis was used for estimating the AUCs. A p-value < 0.05 was considered statistically significant.

Acknowledgments: We thank Silke Rabenhorst and Sabine Becker for their valuable technical assistance.

Author Contributions: This manuscript is part of the doctoral thesis of Britt Groß. Frank Friedersdorff and Britt Groß designed the study and drafted the manuscript; Andreas Maxeiner, Carsten Stephan, and Jonas Busch provided the clinical specimens for this study; Klaus Jung, Carsten Stephan, and Kurt Miller supervised the research, analyzed the data, and edited the paper; Britt Groß and Klaus Jung performed the statistical analysis and the data processing; Ergin Kilic and Britt Groß performed the pathological analysis. All authors read and approved the final manuscript.

References

1. The American Cancer Society. Cancer Facts & Figures 2015. Available online: Http://www.Cancer.Org/research/cancerfactsstatistics (accessed on 15 May 2015).
2. European Association of Urology. Guidelines on Prostate-Cancer 2015. Available online: Http://uroweb.Org/guideline/prostate-cancer/ (accessed on 4 June 2015).
3. Epstein, J.I.; Amin, M.; Boccon-Gibod, L.; Egevad, L.; Humphrey, P.A.; Mikuz, G.; Newling, D.; Nilsson, S.; Sakr, W.; Srigley, J.R.; et al. Prognostic factors and reporting of prostate carcinoma in radical prostatectomy and pelvic lymphadenectomy specimens. *Scand. J. Urol. Nephrol. Suppl.* **2005**, *216*, 34–63. [CrossRef] [PubMed]
4. McNeal, J.E.; Villers, A.A.; Redwine, E.A.; Freiha, F.S.; Stamey, T.A. Capsular penetration in prostate cancer. Significance for natural history and treatment. *Am. J. Surg. Pathol.* **1990**, *14*, 240–247. [CrossRef] [PubMed]
5. McNeal, J.E.; Villers, A.A.; Redwine, E.A.; Freiha, F.S.; Stamey, T.A. Histologic differentiation, cancer volume, and pelvic lymph node metastasis in adenocarcinoma of the prostate. *Cancer* **1990**, *66*, 1225–1233. [PubMed]
6. Stamey, T.A.; Freiha, F.S.; McNeal, J.E.; Redwine, E.A.; Whittemore, A.S.; Schmid, H.P. Localized prostate cancer. Relationship of tumor volume to clinical significance for treatment of prostate cancer. *Cancer* **1993**, *71*, 933–938. [CrossRef]
7. Kattan, M.W.; Eastham, J.A.; Wheeler, T.M.; Maru, N.; Scardino, P.T.; Erbersdobler, A.; Graefen, M.; Huland, H.; Koh, H.; Shariat, S.; et al. Counseling men with prostate cancer: A nomogram for predicting the presence of small, moderately differentiated, confined tumors. *J. Urol.* **2003**, *170*, 1792–1797. [CrossRef] [PubMed]
8. De la Calle, C.; Patil, D.; Wei, J.T.; Scherr, D.S.; Sokoll, L.; Chan, D.W.; Siddiqui, J.; Mosquera, J.M.; Rubin, M.A.; Sanda, M.G. Multicenter evaluation of the prostate health index to detect aggressive prostate cancer in biopsy naive men. *J. Urol.* **2015**, *194*, 65–72. [CrossRef] [PubMed]
9. Filella, X.; Gimenez, N. Evaluation of [−2]proPSA and prostate health index (PHI) for the detection of prostate cancer: A systematic review and meta-analysis. *Clin. Chem. Lab. Med.* **2013**, *51*, 729–739. [CrossRef] [PubMed]
10. Ferro, M.; Lucarelli, G.; Bruzzese, D.; Perdona, S.; Mazzarella, C.; Perruolo, G.; Marino, A.; Cosimato, V.; Giorgio, E.; Tagliamonte, V.; et al. Improving the prediction of pathologic outcomes in patients undergoing radical prostatectomy: The value of prostate cancer antigen 3 (PCa3), prostate health index (PHI) and sarcosine. *Anticancer Res.* **2015**, *35*, 1017–1023. [PubMed]
11. Guazzoni, G.; Lazzeri, M.; Nava, L.; Lughezzani, G.; Larcher, A.; Scattoni, V.; Gadda, G.M.; Bini, V.; Cestari, A.; Buffi, N.M.; et al. Preoperative prostate-specific antigen isoform p2PSA and its derivatives, %p2PSA and prostate health index, predict pathologic outcomes in patients undergoing radical prostatectomy for prostate cancer. *Eur. Urol.* **2012**, *61*, 455–466. [CrossRef] [PubMed]
12. Chiu, P.K.; Lai, F.M.; Teoh, J.Y.; Lee, W.M.; Yee, C.H.; Chan, E.S.; Hou, S.M.; Ng, C.F. Prostate health index and %p2PSA predict aggressive prostate cancer pathology in Chinese patients undergoing radical prostatectomy. *Ann. Surg. Oncol.* **2016**, *23*, 2707–2714. [CrossRef] [PubMed]
13. Lazzeri, M.; Haese, A.; de la Taille, A.; Palou Redorta, J.; McNicholas, T.; Lughezzani, G.; Scattoni, V.; Bini, V.; Freschi, M.; Sussman, A.; et al. Serum isoform [−2]proPSA derivatives significantly improve prediction of prostate cancer at initial biopsy in a total PSA range of 2–10 ng/mL: A multicentric European study. *Eur. Urol.* **2013**, *63*, 986–994. [CrossRef] [PubMed]
14. Cantiello, F.; Russo, G.I.; Ferro, M.; Cicione, A.; Cimino, S.; Favilla, V.; Perdona, S.; Bottero, D.; Terracciano, D.; de Cobelli, O.; et al. Prognostic accuracy of prostate health index and urinary prostate cancer antigen 3 in predicting pathologic features after radical prostatectomy. *Urol. Oncol.* **2015**, *33*, 163.e115–163.e123. [CrossRef] [PubMed]
15. Hirama, H.; Sugimoto, M.; Ito, K.; Shiraishi, T.; Kakehi, Y. The impact of baseline [−2]proPSA-related indices on the prediction of pathological reclassification at 1 year during active surveillance for low-risk prostate cancer: The Japanese multicenter study cohort. *J. Cancer Res. Clin. Oncol.* **2014**, *140*, 257–263. [CrossRef] [PubMed]
16. Klotz, L.; Zhang, L.; Lam, A.; Nam, R.; Mamedov, A.; Loblaw, A. Clinical results of long-term follow-up of a large, active surveillance cohort with localized prostate cancer. *J. Clin. Oncol.* **2010**, *28*, 126–131. [CrossRef] [PubMed]

17. Nichol, M.B.; Wu, J.; An, J.J.; Huang, J.; Denham, D.; Frencher, S.; Jacobsen, S.J. Budget impact analysis of a new prostate cancer risk index for prostate cancer detection. *Prostate Cancer Prostatic Dis.* **2011**, *14*, 253–261. [CrossRef] [PubMed]
18. Nichol, M.B.; Wu, J.; Huang, J.; Denham, D.; Frencher, S.K.; Jacobsen, S.J. Cost-effectiveness of prostate health index for prostate cancer detection. *BJU Int.* **2012**, *110*, 353–362. [CrossRef] [PubMed]
19. Wang, W.; Wang, M.; Wang, L.; Adams, T.S.; Tian, Y.; Xu, J. Diagnostic ability of %p2PSA and prostate health index for aggressive prostate cancer: A meta-analysis. *Sci. Rep.* **2014**, *4*, 5012. [CrossRef] [PubMed]
20. Stamey, T.A.; Yemoto, C.M.; McNeal, J.E.; Sigal, B.M.; Johnstone, I.M. Prostate cancer is highly predictable: A prognostic equation based on all morphological variables in radical prostatectomy specimens. *J. Urol.* **2000**, *163*, 1155–1160. [CrossRef]
21. Tallon, L.; Luangphakdy, D.; Ruffion, A.; Colombel, M.; Devonec, M.; Champetier, D.; Paparel, P.; Decaussin-Petrucci, M.; Perrin, P.; Vlaeminck-Guillem, V. Comparative evaluation of urinary PCa3 and tmprss2: ERG scores and serum PHI in predicting prostate cancer aggressiveness. *Int. J. Mol. Sci.* **2014**, *15*, 13299–13316. [CrossRef] [PubMed]
22. Fossati, N.; Buffi, N.M.; Haese, A.; Stephan, C.; Larcher, A.; McNicholas, T.; de la Taille, A.; Freschi, M.; Lughezzani, G.; Abrate, A.; et al. Preoperative prostate-specific antigen isoform p2PSA and its derivatives, %p2PSA and prostate health index, predict pathologic outcomes in patients undergoing radical prostatectomy for prostate cancer: Results from a multicentric European prospective study. *Eur. Urol.* **2015**, *68*, 132–138. [CrossRef] [PubMed]
23. Kryvenko, O.N.; Epstein, J.I. Definition of insignificant tumor volume of Gleason score 3 + 3 = 6 (grade group 1) prostate cancer at radical prostatectomy: Is it time to increase the threshold? *J. Urol.* **2016**, *196*, 1664–1669. [CrossRef] [PubMed]
24. Stephan, C.; Vincendeau, S.; Houlgatte, A.; Cammann, H.; Jung, K.; Semjonow, A. Multicenter evaluation of [-2]proprostate-specific antigen and the prostate health index for detecting prostate cancer. *Clin. Chem.* **2013**, *59*, 306–314. [CrossRef] [PubMed]

Permissions

All chapters in this book were first published by MDPI; hereby published with permission under the Creative Commons Attribution License or equivalent. Every chapter published in this book has been scrutinized by our experts. Their significance has been extensively debated. The topics covered herein carry significant findings which will fuel the growth of the discipline. They may even be implemented as practical applications or may be referred to as a beginning point for another development.

The contributors of this book come from diverse backgrounds, making this book a truly international effort. This book will bring forth new frontiers with its revolutionizing research information and detailed analysis of the nascent developments around the world.

We would like to thank all the contributing authors for lending their expertise to make the book truly unique. They have played a crucial role in the development of this book. Without their invaluable contributions this book wouldn't have been possible. They have made vital efforts to compile up to date information on the varied aspects of this subject to make this book a valuable addition to the collection of many professionals and students.

This book was conceptualized with the vision of imparting up-to-date information and advanced data in this field. To ensure the same, a matchless editorial board was set up. Every individual on the board went through rigorous rounds of assessment to prove their worth. After which they invested a large part of their time researching and compiling the most relevant data for our readers.

The editorial board has been involved in producing this book since its inception. They have spent rigorous hours researching and exploring the diverse topics which have resulted in the successful publishing of this book. They have passed on their knowledge of decades through this book. To expedite this challenging task, the publisher supported the team at every step. A small team of assistant editors was also appointed to further simplify the editing procedure and attain best results for the readers.

Apart from the editorial board, the designing team has also invested a significant amount of their time in understanding the subject and creating the most relevant covers. They scrutinized every image to scout for the most suitable representation of the subject and create an appropriate cover for the book.

The publishing team has been an ardent support to the editorial, designing and production team. Their endless efforts to recruit the best for this project, has resulted in the accomplishment of this book. They are a veteran in the field of academics and their pool of knowledge is as vast as their experience in printing. Their expertise and guidance has proved useful at every step. Their uncompromising quality standards have made this book an exceptional effort. Their encouragement from time to time has been an inspiration for everyone.

The publisher and the editorial board hope that this book will prove to be a valuable piece of knowledge for researchers, students, practitioners and scholars across the globe.

List of Contributors

Ragheed Saoud
Department of Surgery (Section of Urology), University of Chicago, Chicago, IL 60637, USA

Nassib Abou Heidar
Department of Surgery (Division of Urology), American University of Beirut Medical Center, Beirut 11-0236, Lebanon

Alessia Cimadamore
Section of Pathological Anatomy, Polytechnic University of the Marche Region, School of Medicine, 60126 Ancona, Italy

Gladell P. Paner
Department of Surgery (Section of Urology), University of Chicago, Chicago, IL 60637, USA
Department of Pathology, University of Chicago, Chicago, IL 60637, USA

Dilys Lam
Epigenetics Research Laboratory, Genomics and Epigenetics Division, Garvan Institute of Medical Research, Sydney, New South Wales 2010, Australia

Susan Clark, Clare Stirzaker and Ruth Pidsley
Epigenetics Research Laboratory, Genomics and Epigenetics Division, Garvan Institute of Medical Research, Sydney, New South Wales 2010, Australia
St. Vincent's Clinical School, University of New South Wales, Sydney, New South Wales 2010, Australia

Prakash Kulkarni
Institute for Bioscience and Biotechnology Research, University of Maryland, Rockville, MD 20850, USA

Vladimir N. Uversky
Department of Molecular Medicine, Morsani College of Medicine, University of South Florida, Tampa, FL 33612, USA
Laboratory of New methods in Biology, Institute for Biological Instrumentation, Russian Academy of Sciences, Pushchino 142290, Moscow Region, Russia

Kazuhisa Hagiwara, Yuki Tobisawa, Shingo Hatakeyama, Kazuyuki Mori and Takuya Koie
Department of Urology, Hirosaki University Graduate School of Medicine, Hirosaki 036-8562, Japan

Takatoshi Kaya, Tomonori Kaneko and Yoshihiko Suda
Corporate R&D Headquarters, Konica Minolta, Inc., Hino-shi, Tokyo 191-8511, Japan

Yasuhiro Hashimoto
Department of Advanced Transplant and Regenerative Medicine, Hirosaki University Graduate School of Medicine, Hirosaki 036-8562, Japan

Chikara Ohyama and Tohru Yoneyama
Department of Urology, Hirosaki University Graduate School of Medicine, Hirosaki 036-8562, Japan
Department of Advanced Transplant and Regenerative Medicine, Hirosaki University Graduate School of Medicine, Hirosaki 036-8562, Japan

Katrin Schlack, Andres Jan Schrader, Axel Semjonow, Stefan Thomes, Julie Steinestel and Martin Boegemann
Department of Urology, Prostate Center, University Hospital Muenster, Albert-Schweitzer-Campus 1, GB A1, Muenster D-48149, Germany

Laura-Maria Krabbe
Department of Urology, Prostate Center, University Hospital Muenster, Albert-Schweitzer-Campus 1, GB A1, D-48149 Muenster, Germany
Department of Urology, University of Texas Southwestern Medical Center, Dallas, TX 75390-9110, USA

Manfred Fobker
Center for Laboratory Medicine, University Hospital Muenster, Albert-Schweitzer-Campus 1, GB A1, Muenster D-48149, Germany

Xavier Filella and Laura Foj
Department of Biochemistry and Molecular Genetics (CDB), Hospital Clínic, IDIBAPS, C/Villarroel, 170, 08036 Barcelona, Catalonia, Spain

Jiun-Hung Geng
Department of Urology, Kaohsiung Medical University Hospital, Kaohsiung 807, Taiwan
Department of Urology, Kaohsiung Municipal Hsiao-Kang Hospital, Kaohsiung 812, Taiwan

Victor C. Lin
Department of Urology, E-Da Hospital, Kaohsiung 824, Taiwan
School of Medicine for International Students, I-Shou University, Kaohsiung 840, Taiwan

Chia-Cheng Yu
Division of Urology, Department of Surgery, Kaohsiung Veterans General Hospital, Kaohsiung 813, Taiwan
Department of Urology, School of Medicine, National Yang-Ming University, Taipei 112, Taiwan
Department of Pharmacy, Tajen University, Pingtung 907, Taiwan

Chao-Yuan Huang
Department of Urology, National Taiwan University Hospital, College of Medicine, National Taiwan University, Taipei 100, Taiwan
Department of Urology, National Taiwan University Hospital Hsin-Chu Branch, Hsinchu 300, Taiwan

Hsin-Ling Yin
Department of Pathology, Kaohsiung Medical University Hospital, Kaohsiung 807, Taiwan
Department of Pathology, Faculty of Medicine, College of Medicine, Kaohsiung Medical University, Kaohsiung 807, Taiwan

Ta-Yuan Chang
Department of Occupational Safety and Health, China Medical University, Taichung 404, Taiwan

Te-Ling Lu
Department of Pharmacy, China Medical University, Taichung 404, Taiwan

Shu-Pin Huang
Department of Urology, Kaohsiung Medical University Hospital, Kaohsiung 807, Taiwan
Department of Urology, Faculty of Medicine, College of Medicine, Kaohsiung Medical University, Kaohsiung 807, Taiwan
Graduate Institute of Medicine, College of Medicine, Kaohsiung Medical University, Kaohsiung 807, Taiwan

Bo-Ying Bao
Department of Pharmacy, China Medical University, Taichung 404, Taiwan
Sex Hormone Research Center, China Medical University Hospital, Taichung 404, Taiwan
Department of Nursing, Asia University, Taichung 413, Taiwan

Lorenzo Bascetta, Arianna Oliviero, Monica Evangelista and Alberto Mercatanti
Non-Coding RNA Laboratory, Institute of Clinical Physiology (IFC), National Research Council (CNR), via G. Moruzzi 1, 56124 Pisa, Italy

Romina D'Aurizio and Marco Pellegrini
Laboratory for Integrative System Medicine (LISM), Institute of Informatics and Telematics (IIT), National Research Council (CNR), via G. Moruzzi 1, 56124 Pisa, Italy

Francesca Marrocolo
Department of Oncology, San Donato Hospital, Azienda USL Toscana Sud-Est, via P. Nenni 20, 52100 Arezzo, Italy

Sergio Bracarda
Department of Oncology, San Donato Hospital, Azienda USL Toscana Sud-Est, via P. Nenni 20, 52100 Arezzo, Italy
Istituto Toscano Tumori (ITT), via T. Alderotti 26/N, 50139 Firenze, Italy

Milena Rizzo
Non-Coding RNA Laboratory, Institute of Clinical Physiology (IFC), National Research Council (CNR), via G. Moruzzi 1, 56124 Pisa, Italy
Istituto Toscano Tumori (ITT), via T. Alderotti 26/N, 50139 Firenze, Italy

Kambiz Rahbar
Department of Nuclear Medicine, Muenster University Medical Center, Albert-Schweitzer-Campus 1, GB A1, D-48149 Muenster, Germany

Martin Aringer
Department of Rheumatology, Dresden University Medical Center, Fetscherstraße 74, D-01307 Dresden, Germany

Shubham Dayal, Jun Zhou, Praveen Manivannan, Mohammad Adnan Siddiqui, Omaima Farid Ahmad, Matthew Clark, Sahezeel Awadia, Rafael Garcia-Mata, Lirim Shemshedini and Krishnamurthy Malathi
Department of Biological Sciences, 2801 W. Bancroft St., University of Toledo, Toledo, OH 43606, USA

Tomokazu Ishikawa
Department of Urology, Hirosaki University Graduate School of Medicine, Hirosaki 036-8562, Japan
Diagnostics Research Laboratories, Wako Pure Chemical Industries, Hyogo 661-0963, Japan

Tatsuo Kurosawa and Kenji Nakamura
Diagnostics Research Laboratories, Wako Pure Chemical Industries, Hyogo 661-0963, Japan

Shintaro Narita and Tomonori Habuchi
Department of Urology, Akita University Graduate School of Medicine, Akita 010-8543, Japan

Koji Mitsuzuka and Yoichi Arai
Department of Urology, Tohoku University Graduate School of Medicine, Sendai 980-8574, Japan

Wilhelmina Duivenvoorden and Jehonathan H. Pinthus
Department of Surgery, McMaster University, Hamilton, ON L8S4L8, Canada

Matteo Ferro
Urologic Surgery Unit, European Institute of Oncology, 20141 Milan, Italy

Paola Ungaro
Institute of Experimental Endocrinology and Oncology (IEOS-CNR) "G. Salvatore", Via Sergio Pansini, 5, 80131 Naples, Italy

Amelia Cimmino
Institute of Genetics and Biophysics "A. Buzzati Traverso", National Research Council (CNR), Via Pietro Castellino 111, 80131 Naples, Italy

Giuseppe Lucarelli
Department of Emergency and Organ Transplantation-Urology, Andrology and Kidney Transplantation Unit, University of Bari, 70124 Bari, Italy

Gian Maria Busetto
Department of Gynecological-Obstetrics Sciences and Urological Sciences, Sapienza Rome University Policlinico Umberto I, 00161 Rome, Italy

Francesco Cantiello and Rocco Damiano
Department of Urology, Magna Graecia University of Catanzaro, 88100 Catanzaro, Italy

Daniela Terracciano
Department of Translational Medical Sciences, University of Naples Federico II, Via Sergio Pansini, 5, 80131 Naples, Italy

Annelies Gonnissen, Sofie Isebaert and Karin Haustermans
Laboratory of Experimental Radiotherapy, Department of Oncology, KU Leuven—University of Leuven, 3000 Leuven, Belgium
Department of Radiation Oncology, University Hospitals Leuven, 3000 Leuven, Belgium

Chad M. McKee and Ruth J. Muschel
Department of Oncology, CRUK/MRC Oxford Institute for Radiation Oncology, University of Oxford, Oxford OX3 7DQ, UK

Frank Friedersdorff, Britt Groß, Andreas Maxeiner, Kurt Miller and Jonas Busch
Department of Urology, Charité University Hospital, 10098 Berlin, Germany

Klaus Jung and Carsten Stephan
Department of Urology, Charité University Hospital, 10098 Berlin, Germany
Berlin Institute for Urologic Research, 10115 Berlin, Germany

Ergin Kilic
Department of Pathology, Charité University Hospital, 10098 Berlin, Germany

Index